nutrition

for the eye

The Top 50 Nutrients to Know
from the Basics to the Details
the Myths, the Realities, & the Scientific Evidence

N. A. Adams, MD

Chairman of Department
Department of Ophthalmology
Paul L. Foster School of Medicine
Texas Tech University Health Sciences Center
El Paso, Texas

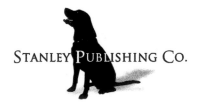

STANLEY PUBLISHING CO.

www.stanleypublishing.com

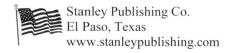

Stanley Publishing Co.
El Paso, Texas
www.stanleypublishing.com

ISBN 987-0-9790350-5-0

Notice

Ophthalmology and the eye sciences are ever changing fields.
Standard safety precautions must be followed. There are numerous
side effects of dietary supplements as well as interactions with over-
the-counter and prescribed medications. Dietary supplements should
be taken only under the advice and supervision of a knowledgeable
healthcare provider. Furthermore, controlled safety studies of many of
these nutrients during pregnancy and breast-feeding are not available,
so the use of these nutrients during pregnancy and breast-feeding
should only be taken under the supervision of a knowledgeable
healthcare provider after understanding and addressing the risks and
benefits of supplementation. In addition, children's bodies often
behave differently than that of adults, and it is often improper to
simply adjust doses according to weight. A pediatrician should be
consulted regarding the use of nutritional supplements for children.

**Dr. Adams recommends that you speak with your physician to
ensure that the diet and supplement choices are right for you.**

For More Information Regarding
The Collaborative Vision Research Foundation

please visit: www.collaborativevision.org
or email to: cvrf@collaborativevision.org

Dedicated
To
My Wife and Children

Table of Contents

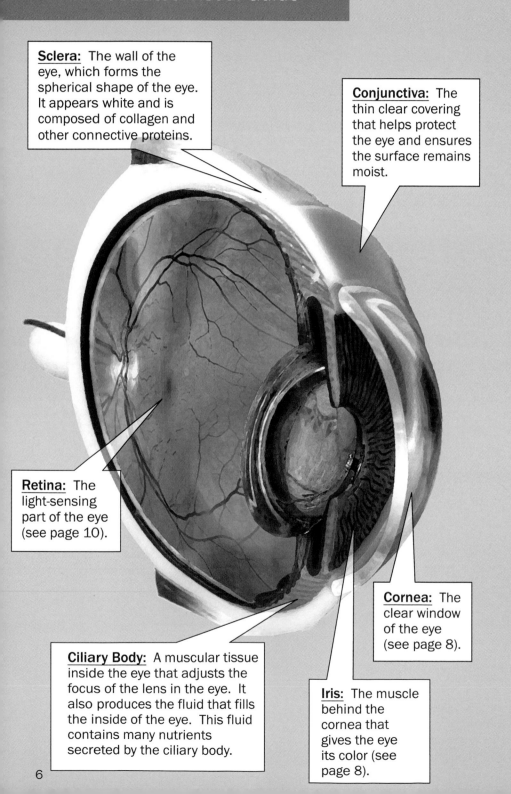

Sclera: The wall of the eye, which forms the spherical shape of the eye. It appears white and is composed of collagen and other connective proteins.

Conjunctiva: The thin clear covering that helps protect the eye and ensures the surface remains moist.

Retina: The light-sensing part of the eye (see page 10).

Ciliary Body: A muscular tissue inside the eye that adjusts the focus of the lens in the eye. It also produces the fluid that fills the inside of the eye. This fluid contains many nutrients secreted by the ciliary body.

Cornea: The clear window of the eye (see page 8).

Iris: The muscle behind the cornea that gives the eye its color (see page 8).

Diseases of the Conjunctiva

- Pink eye is also called conjunctivitis and is an infection of the conjunctiva. It is often caused by a virus but can be caused by bacteria.

- Allergies of the eye can occur in the conjunctiva. Symptoms include intense itching and burning and it may mimic pink eye.

E

F P

T O Z

Diseases of the Ciliary Body

- Fluid build-up in the eye is a risk factor for the disease glaucoma (see page 15).

- Uveitis and iritis are inflammations inside the eye caused by disease or injury to the iris or ciliary body. They can be painful and can be caused by infections or systemic diseases (or disorders that occur throughout different organs in the body).

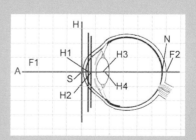

Iris: Also known as the "diaphragm" of the eye. The iris can adjust the size of the opening in the center of the iris (known as the pupil) in order to adjust the amount of light entering the eye.

Cornea: Light enters the eye through the cornea. In fact, the cornea is remarkable in its clarity. It also serves as a powerful filter of UV light. There are stem cells around the cornea that replace the surface of the cornea every 7 to 10 days. For protection, the cornea is incredible in its sensitivity to touch or injury. There are more sensory nerve endings in the cornea per square-millimeter than anywhere else in the body.

Lens: The light that enters the eye is focused by the lens to the back of the eye and onto the light-sensing retina.

The lens acts like a magnifying glass. It's the most transparent cellular tissue in the human body! It sits in a thin sack.

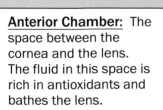

Anterior Chamber: The space between the cornea and the lens. The fluid in this space is rich in antioxidants and bathes the lens.

Diseases of the Cornea

- When the eye does not produce enough tears to keep the entire cornea moist and lubricated, dry eye occurs. Dry eye can cause irritation, redness, and blurred vision.

- Infections of the cornea are often serious and can result in ulcers, or erosions of the surface of the cornea.

- Injury or trauma to the cornea can result in corneal scars. Often, the scar is opaque, and if it is in the center of the cornea, severe loss of vision can occur.

- Astigmatism is when the curvature of the cornea is too steep in one direction. Astigmatism is often easily corrected with glasses or contact lenses. On the other hand, keratoconus occurs when the curvature of the cornea is severely abnormal, with thinning of the cornea.

- In Fuchs' disease, the pump cells of the cornea fail and the cornea swells with water. Vision becomes hazy, and in severe cases, painful corneal blisters can occur.

Diseases of the Lens

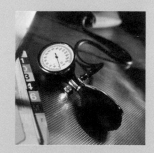

- Cataract is a clouding of the natural lens that results in decreased vision. It is often an age-related process that gradually develops over time. It can also be caused by diabetes, injury, or certain medications. Blurred vision, glare, and halos in one's vision are common symptoms.

- In cataract surgery, the clouded lens is replaced with a clear "plastic" lens.

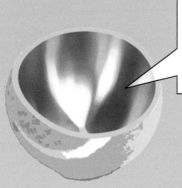

Vitreous Gel: The eye is similar to a tennis ball. It is hollow on the inside.

The vitreous gel is clear and fills the inside of the eye. It is 99% water and 1% collagen and hyaluronic acid.

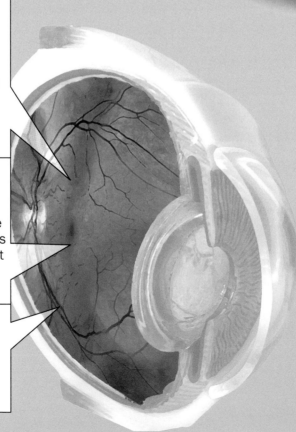

Retina: The light-sensing part of the eye. It is incredibly thin ($1/4$ millimeter) and is comparable to wallpaper that may line the inside of the tennis ball.

Macula: The center of the retina where light is focused and fine images created. It's the most important few millimeters in your body!

Arteries & Veins: Traverse the surface of the retina to provide oxygen and nutrients.

Diseases of the Vitreous

• Over time, the vitreous gel starts to shrivel and shrink. Floaters are visible condensed edges of gel that swirl or "float" in one's vision. They often look like gray dots or spider webs.

• If the vitreous gel shifts positions or shrivels more suddenly, the gel can pull on the retina and cause holes or tears in the retina and can even cause the retina to detach from its normal position. A retinal detachment may result in decreased vision or blindness. Eye surgery and trauma or injury to the eye can also cause retinal detachments, either at the time of the event or many years later.

Diseases of the Retina

• Scar tissue that develops on the surface of the macula is called an epiretinal membrane or macular pucker. This scar tissue can distort one's vision.

• Fluid build-up or swelling in the macula is called macular edema and can cause decreased vision. Macular edema can result from cataract surgery, diabetes, vein occlusions, and other retinal diseases.

• Blockage of the retinal veins (vein occlusion) can cause bleeding, macular edema, and other complications. Decrease in vision can range from mild to severe.

• Blockage of the retinal artery is also called a retinal stroke, and often results in sudden and severe loss of vision.

Diseases of the Retina Continued on Page 13.

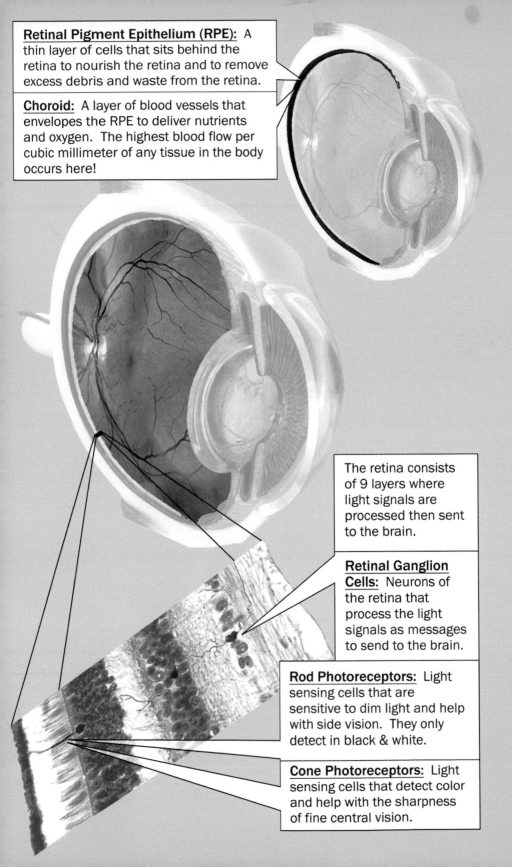

Retinal Pigment Epithelium (RPE): A thin layer of cells that sits behind the retina to nourish the retina and to remove excess debris and waste from the retina.

Choroid: A layer of blood vessels that envelopes the RPE to deliver nutrients and oxygen. The highest blood flow per cubic millimeter of any tissue in the body occurs here!

The retina consists of 9 layers where light signals are processed then sent to the brain.

Retinal Ganglion Cells: Neurons of the retina that process the light signals as messages to send to the brain.

Rod Photoreceptors: Light sensing cells that are sensitive to dim light and help with side vision. They only detect in black & white.

Cone Photoreceptors: Light sensing cells that detect color and help with the sharpness of fine central vision.

Diseases of the Retina   *(Continued from Page 11)*

- Age-related macular degeneration is often simply called macular degeneration. It comes in two forms: dry and wet.

  Dry is more common. 90% of people with macular degeneration have the dry form, which occurs when excess debris called drusen accumulates behind the retina and/or when RPE cells degenerate. Eventually the debris and/or RPE cell loss results in degeneration of photoreceptors. When photoreceptors are lost, vision starts to decrease. The dry form often progresses slowly and vision loss is often not as severe as in the wet form.

  In the wet form, when there are breaks in the RPE, choroidal blood vessels can enter the retina (called choroidal neovascularization). These blood vessels are abnormal and can cause bleeding or fluid leakage in the retina and can distort the architecture of the retina. These abnormal blood vessels can often cause a sudden decrease in vision, which can be quite severe.

- High blood sugars in diabetes can damage the walls of arteries and veins throughout the body, including in the retina. These damaged vessels can easily bleed into the retina or leak fluid, which is called macular edema. In severe cases, bleeding from abnormal blood vessel growth can fill up the entire eye (called a vitreous hemorrhage). Furthermore, abnormal blood vessels can grow and pull on the retina causing it to detach from the back wall of the eye. This type of retinal detachment is called a traction detachment and can result in loss of vision.

- In retinitis pigmentosa and similar hereditary retinal degenerations, abnormal genes in the retina cause the light-sensing cells to degenerate. Many times, children are affected by these retinal degenerations. A variety of symptoms can occur, depending on the gene involved. In retinitis pigmentosa, slowly worsening night-blindness and loss of side vision eventually give way to severe loss of vision.

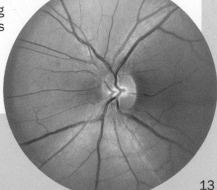

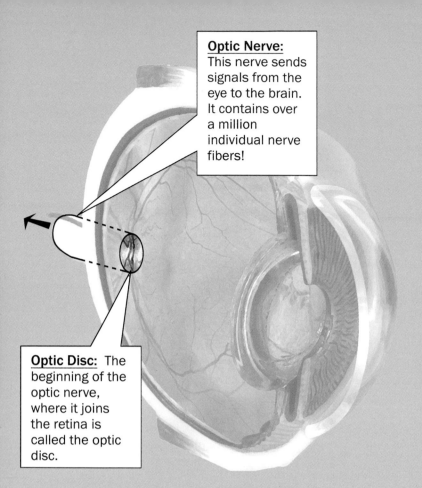

Optic Nerve:
This nerve sends signals from the eye to the brain. It contains over a million individual nerve fibers!

Optic Disc: The beginning of the optic nerve, where it joins the retina is called the optic disc.

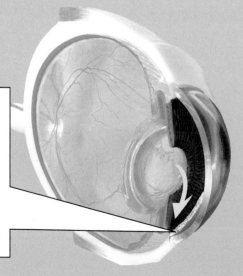

Trabecular Meshwork:
In the angle between the cornea and the iris, there is a mesh of tissue called the trabecular meshwork. This tissue is the main filtration site of the eye, where excess fluid in the eye is removed.

Diseases of the Optic Nerve

- Optic neuritis is an inflammatory disorder of the optic nerve. Often the insulation around the individual nerve fibers becomes damaged, resulting in impaired ability to send light signals to the brain. The result is partial or complete loss of vision. It can be painful at times. Optic neuritis can be associated with multiple sclerosis, a nervous system disease that results in numerous brain and spinal cord impairments including weakness and inability to sense.

- Ischemic optic neuropathy is a stroke of the optic nerve. Blood flow to the optic nerve is compromised and the result is a stroke, with partial or complete loss of vision.

Diseases of the Optic Nerve & Retina

- Glaucoma is a disease of the optic nerve and retina, in which the retinal ganglion cells of the retina degenerate and the nerve fibers that comprise the optic nerve are lost. A very common risk factor for glaucoma is increased eye pressure. The increase in eye pressure can occur when fluid builds up in the eye because the trabecular meshwork becomes clogged and does not filter properly.

Glaucoma is often painless unless the trabecular meshwork becomes suddenly blocked by scar tissue, abnormal blood vessels, or by the iris itself pushing forward. This type of glaucoma is called angle-closure, as opposed to the more common type of glaucoma called open-angle glaucoma.

Diabetes, high blood pressure, and near-sightedness are also risk factors for open-angle glaucoma. The vision loss in open-angle glaucoma often progresses slowly. Side vision is lost at first, and the loss of side vision may not be noticed until the late stages of the disease. If untreated, tunnel vision may develop, and eventually blindness.

Introduction

A common theme in the role of nutrients in eye disease and health is the antioxidant properties of the nutrients. Oxidation is the process whereby chemical compounds lose electrons resulting in potentially toxic modifications to proteins, lipids, and DNA, which can eventually lead to degeneration and even death of cells. An oxidant is any compound that can accept electrons, or remove electrons from another compound. An antioxidant is a compound that donates electrons to prevent oxidation.

Oxygen is a curious molecule. Life depends on oxygen but too much can be harmful. Oxygen byproducts can form reactive oxygen species, or toxic chemicals that result in oxidation. Too much oxygen can tip the balance towards too much oxygen byproducts. These byproducts include chemicals called free radicals, peroxides, and oxygen ions. Metals can also serve as oxidants.

Oxidants can come from sources from within the body as well as outside the body. Ionizing radiation such as gamma-radiation can easily cause ionization of water within cells resulting in formation of oxidants such as hydroxyl radicals and hydrogen peroxide. Non-ionizing radiation such as ultraviolet radiation from sun exposure can produce oxidants such as singlet oxygen and hydrogen peroxide. Exposure to chemicals such as air pollutants from car exhaust or cigarette smoke can produce oxidants such as nitric oxide radicals. Even breathing in transitional metals, such as copper from steel or iron works factories, trash incinerators, or forest fires can lead to excess oxidation. Medicinal drugs such as cancer chemotherapeutic agents can act to produce oxidants to kill off cancer cells. Anesthesia drugs can produce oxidants such as nitric oxide radicals. Pesticides and herbicides are other sources of oxidants. In addition, foods by the nature of cooking or processing them or by their intrinsic composition contain numerous oxidants such as peroxides, aldehydes, oxidized fatty acids, and transitional metals.

In terms of sources from within our own bodies, normal cellular metabolism produces baseline levels of oxidants that the cell can tolerate. Mitochondria, the major energy-producing organelle found within cells of the body, are the major cellular source of oxidants. Almost all, 98%, of the oxygen metabolize in the body is handled by a single enzyme, cytochrome oxidase, within the mitochondria. Other enzyme activities can produce oxidants such as hydrogen peroxide. There are also numerous illnesses in which the body itself produces excess amounts of oxidants.

The damage to lipids, proteins, and DNA caused by oxidants results in numerous diseases, notably retinal disease, cataracts, and cancers. Other diseases are listed in **Table 1**.

The eye is exposed to high levels of oxidants. The retina has the highest oxygen consumption of any tissue in the body and sunlight is concentrated and focused through the lens and on the retina. While much of the sun's ultraviolet radiation is filtered by the cornea (filters shorter wavelength UV-B light less than 295 nm) and the lens (filters longer wavelength UV-B light and UV-A light), simply the energy produced by light itself is toxic. Thermal energy and photochemical changes account for the toxicity of light and participate in producing oxidants.

The retinal pigment epithelium serves to provide nutrition for the photoreceptors and to remove excess debris and waste from the photoreceptors. This debris and waste includes the discs of the photoreceptors, which are shed each day. Photoreceptors contain up to 1000 discs arranged in layers to detect photons, or light particles. Each retinal pigment epithelial cell cleans up by packaging and ingesting 2000 to 4000 discs each day from an average of 30 to 40 adjacent photoreceptor cells. On a cellular level, this task is mammoth and complex, though it can be easily overwhelmed by excess debris. The residue produced is called lipofuscin, which in the presence of light and oxygen results in the production of reactive oxygen species, or toxic chemicals that result in oxidation.

Thus, excess lipofuscin can result in oxidative damage to the retina. Of course light exposure is high in the retina, and the highest amount of oxygen consumption of any tissue in the body occurs in the retina. Therefore, the retina is particularly susceptible to oxidative damage. Similarly, with its high sunlight exposure, the lens is also particularly susceptible to oxidative damage.

There are also diseases that create high levels of oxidants within the eye. The most common of these diseases is diabetes. In diabetes, there are high levels of the sugar glucose in the

Table 1
Some Diseases That Are Associated With Or Exacerbated By Oxidative Damage

Diseases of the Nervous System:
Parkinson's disease
Alzheimer's disease
Huntington's disease
Lou Gehrig's disease
Dementia
Multiple sclerosis

Cancers:
Breast
Colon
Stomach
Ovarian
Cervical
Liver
Lung
Brain
Leukemia

Vasculature Disorders:
Atherosclerosis
Coronary artery disease
Stroke

Other Disorders:
Hepatitis
Diabetes mellitus
Cystic fibrosis
Atopic dermatitis
Psoriasis

circulating blood. High levels of glucose in the presence of oxygen can result in the formation of oxidants such as superoxide radical anion, a reactive oxygen species. Again, because of the high oxygen consumption by the retina, it is particularly susceptible to oxidative damage. Also, in the presence of oxidatively reactive metals, such as copper, glucose can stimulate further oxidative damage. Excess glucose can also alter metabolism in mitochondria, resulting in creation of excess oxidants by the mitochondria.

When its levels are high, glucose attacks proteins resulting in advanced glycation end products, or AGEs, or attacks lipids resulting in advanced lipoxidation end products, or ALEs. Damage from these end products to various structures in the eye, ranging from the cornea to the lens to the retina and retinal pigment epithelium, can lead to eye disease. Early cataracts, for example, may be a result of accumulation of AGEs in lens crystallin proteins. Furthermore, damage from these end products to blood vessels in the eye can also lead to swelling in the retina, a process known as macular edema, or uncontrolled abnormal blood vessel growth, in a process known as proliferative retinopathy, or to lack of blood flow in the center of vision, in a process known as ischemic maculopathy.

These end products also directly increase the rate of production in cells of free radicals and oxidants. These end products can also decrease the antioxidant activity of copper and zinc containing enzymes superoxide dismutase, diminish stores within the cell of glutathione, and activate inflammatory and oxidant producing pathways. This process creates a cycle as these end products then bind to RAGE, a receptor for AGEs, causing signal-mediated changes in gene expression such as pro-inflammatory changes and, importantly, activation of enzymes that result in the production of more oxidants within cells.

This cycle is made worse as oxidation can result in formation of more of these end products which then leads to more oxidative damage. This cycle is found not only in diabetes, but other diseases involving oxidative damage not necessarily with high glucose levels such as diabetes. AGEs are also associated with aging.

The human body's cells are beautifully engineered to defend against oxidative damage _and_ to utilize naturally occurring antioxidants to defend against the damage. The goal of this book is to present information on the naturally occurring antioxidants as well as nutrients so that the reader can better learn to utilize them, as perhaps was intended naturally. Let us understand this remarkable engineering and these amazing nutrients.

The Use of Clinical Studies to Determine Efficacy of a Nutrient for Eye Disease:

How Are Clinical Trials Interpreted?

Clinical trials measure the efficacy and safety of a treatment. With a vast array of constant developments and advancements in the science of new treatments for eye diseases, clinical trials are performed to distinguish which forms of treatments are the most appropriate for a given ailment or condition. A successful clinical trial or series of trials demonstrates that the new treatment under consideration either prevents an undesired condition, minimizes the symptoms of the condition, combats the illness itself, or improves the overall quality of life. However, not all clinical trials can be applied to real life, let alone applied to your life. In fact, there are numerous factors that can undermine the validity of a clinical trial.

Study Subjects: First of all, for a study to be applicable to people with a certain eye disease or to the general community, the participants in the study must be representative of people with that eye disease or of the general community. For example, some trials are very specific in their inclusion criteria, meaning that the subjects studied had specific features of the disease. For example, a study may look only at subjects with specific types of macular degeneration, defined by the number and type of debris spots (drusen) in the retina. Thus, the applicability of the findings to all patients with that disease is limited.

It is vital that the participants be chosen at random in order to increase the validity, and thereby the applicability, of the findings of the study. In an ideal study with broad applicability, participants must represent a broad background and ethnicity. For example, a study of Indonesians with an eye disease may not be applicable to Americans with the same eye disease, because of differences in diet (e.g., nutritional content of diet), lifestyle (e.g., health-conscious lifestyle), geographic and environmental factors (e.g., sun exposure), or even genetic makeup (e.g., ethnic genetic differences that predispose to certain diseases). By having a diverse group of participants, the applicability of the study to the general population is increased.

> The presence or lack of a clinical study does not necessary mean that a nutrient is beneficial or harmful.

Also, even if the same study is performed more than once on similar groups of people, each trial involves a different set of individuals. Accordingly, the people in the different trials presumably hold distinctive qualities as individuals. People who share the same condition or disease may also differ in other areas. For example, some individuals may eat more fruits or others may be smokers. The ways in which smoking damages the body may affect how a nutrient interacts with the body. An ideal study attempts to identify differences and adjust for such differences. However, it is impossible to identify or adjust for all differences.

Study Design: There are many types of study designs. Prospective studies look forwards over time, as opposed to retrospective studies that look at data that has already been collected. It is sometimes difficult to draw conclusions from clinical trials because of differences in study design. Consider for example a retrospective study that looks at the dietary intake of a nutrient and the risk of developing cataract. The study may find that those who had taken a beneficial nutrient had a higher risk of having cataracts. That does not necessarily mean that the nutrient is harmful. It may be that those who had already developed cataracts may have then started the certain nutrient in their diet. Another example is a retrospective study that finds that dietary intake of a nutrient decreased the risk of macular degeneration. However, it may be that those who consumed this nutrient also had a healthier diet and healthier lifestyle and that these factors are what decreased the risk of the disease rather than the nutrient.

Thus, a prospective study has the advantage of being able to randomize or randomly assign subjects to receive either the treatment or a placebo (a sugar-pill that has no nutrient or medication in it). A rigorous randomization enables the researchers to control for differences in study subjects by balancing the groups and preventing biases in selection of subjects.

Researchers have noted that at times patients who are given a placebo but told that it is a medication may show dramatic improvements in their illness or even be "cured." A placebo-controlled clinical study protects against this type of placebo effect. Therefore, it is important to judge the quality and applicability of a study by whether or not it is placebo-controlled.

Some trials are blinded, such that the participant, the researcher, and/or the statistician reviewing the results are all prevented from knowing whether each subject is receiving placebo or treatment. These trials provide an additional level of control against any potential bias.

Number of Participants: Because humans are complex biological creatures, each individual may react differently to a nutrient. Therefore, to increase the validity of the observations of a finding even further, the more participants there are the better. By having many different people 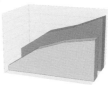 in large samples, more confidence can be placed in the idea that the results of the trials can be applicable to the general population of interest. For example, if a study was conducted on seven people versus a study conducted on one-hundred people for the same treatment, the findings from the study with the larger number of participants would hold more weight and be more applicable to real life. Such large-scale studies therefore increase external validity.

Repeatability & Reproducibility: The clinical trials should also be repeated multiple times with these large, random, and various populations, testing for the same hypothesis every time. The more clinical studies that are present, the better the idea one has of the benefit of a nutrient. The fact that a single study or a few studies show a benefit does not necessarily imply a benefit. The fact that a single study or a few studies find no benefit does not necessarily imply no benefit. The studies must be assessed in the context of the believed or known mechanism(s) of action of the nutrients and in the context of the quality of the clinical study itself.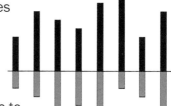

Dosing of Treatment: Also, in efforts to validate whether it is the treatment for which the researcher is testing that is causing the assumed effects on the individual, or whether it is some other factor, the manipulation of the dose of a nutrient that a participant takes could possibly verify whether or not it was the nutrient that caused the change or whether the change in health was caused by something else. Again, in an ideal world, multiple trials should be performed in order to determine the ability of the nutrient to cause the desired change.

Careful Monitoring of Subjects: Clinical trials are more applicable if the volunteers are carefully monitored. If the volunteers are left to administer the experiments themselves, at home, over the internet, or wherever, then the results that arise may prove faulty. The researcher may have no way of verifying whether or not accurate dosages of a nutrient were taken or even if the participant even remembered to take the nutrient every day. Thus, in order to obtain more appropriate data, the participants should be closely monitored—whether it is through them coming into the lab, or at the very least keeping a daily log of their activities and routines.

Length of Study: In diseases with long-term effects or in which the progression of the disease is slow, such as cataracts or age-related macular degeneration, a shorter duration study may not provide enough time for the drug or nutrient of interest to make a measurable impact in the disease. Instead, the duration of years may be more adequate in establishing the true effects of the drug or nutrient of interest. In fact, there are many studies that may not have been run long enough to determine the effects of the drug or nutrient of interest, especially studies that are only a few weeks long or even months.

Unforeseen Interactions: In addition, factors other than what are being monitored in the tests may affect the outcomes. For instance, if a researcher is testing how a nutrient affects an eye condition, the change in the eye condition after treatment may be due to the nutrient of interest, another nutrient already in the diet, or even the interaction of the different nutrients. In other words, a nutrient that is found to be beneficial may be interacting with another nutrient(s) to cause the benefit. The effect of a given nutrient is difficult to isolate often time.

Outcome Measures: The outcomes that are measured and the methods of measuring these outcomes also affect the applicability of the clinical trial. For example, a study that looks at debris in the retina in macular degeneration differs from one that looks prospectively over time at changes in visual acuity. Different results can be obtained from the same group of people depending on how the findings are observed and measured, suggesting that careful interpretation of any result is necessary in order to apply the finding to real life. Finally, the way the statistical analysis is performed may also affect the outcomes of the study.

Summary – An Approximated Scale of Benefit:

Taking into account all of these aspects of clinical trials, it becomes clear that there's a science and an art in evaluating clinical studies. *Invariably, there is no definitive "yes" or "no" answer.* In many sections, a subjective scale of benefit of a nutrient for a specific condition is given. This scale represents a combination of various factors and data from one or more studies to give the reader an approximated sense of what value the nutrient may have on a given disease.

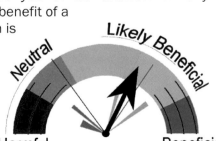

Summary of Nutrients

Nutrient	Selected Benefits: Nutrient Is Good For....	Suggested* Daily Dose Range	Use Caution If You Have / Are...
agaricus	inflammation, scarring after surgery	no dose range established	
alpha-lipoic acid	cataract, glaucoma, retinal disease, diabetes	400–600 mg	diabetic
arginine	blood flow in retina, infection prevention	500–1,500 mg	history of shingles or herpes virus
beta-carotene	macular degeneration, cataracts	10–15 mg	smoker
bioflavonoids	antioxidants for overall eye health	no dose range established	
boron	hormonal balance, macular degeneration	500–3,000 µg	
carnitine	energy production, debris removal from retina	1,000–1,500 mg	epilepsy or Alzheimer's
choline	retina, neural tissue, memory	500–1,000 mg	
chromium	diabetes, debris removal from retina	50–100 µg	
coenzyme Q10	energy production, debris removal from retina	50–200 mg	
coleus	glaucoma, protection of retina	200–500 mg	prone to bleeding, low blood pressure, stomach ulcers
copper	formation of collagen, protection of retina	2–3 mg	high cholesterol
DHA	dry eye, retinal disease, vision in infants	250–500 mg	prone to bleeding
folate	protection of blood vessels in eye, cataract	800–1,000 µg	
genistein	cholesterol regulation, cataract, glaucoma	25–75 mg	
ginkgo	retinal disease, glaucoma, wound healing	15–30 mg	prone to bleeding

*Dosages provided are suggested range. See text for details and specifications.

Nutrient	Selected Benefits: Nutrient Is Good For….	Suggested* Daily Dose Range	Use Caution If You Have / Are…
glutathione	cataract, glaucoma, macular degeneration	0 — 600 mg	
hyaluronic acid	optic nerve, vitreous, retina, fluid filtration	0 — 100 150 mg	
iron	oxygen transportation, energy production	0 — 10 15 mg *	
lutein	immune system, cataract, retinal disease	0 — 6 12 mg	
lycopene	cataract, retinal disease	0 — 4 8 mg	
lysine	collagen formation, diabetes, viral infection	0 — 800 1,200 mg	
magnesium	dry eye, cataract, retinal disease	0 — 300 420 mg *	
manganese	diabetes, cataract, glaucoma, retinal disease	0 — 3 5 mg	
methionine	energy boosting, debris removal from retina	0 — 500 1,000 mg	forms of blood vessel disease
NAC	corneal infections, cataract, retinal disease	0 — 500 750 mg	kidney stones, stomach ulcers
omega-3 oils	dry eye, retinal disease, vision in infants	0 — 2.0 2.5 g	prone to bleeding
phytic acid	binding of metals, debris removal from retina	0 — 1,500 2,000 mg	prone to bleeding
proline	collagen formation, light-sensing in retina	no dose range established	
quercetin	diabetes, inflammation, viral infection	0 — 500 1,200 mg	
SAMe	retinal disease, nerve fiber protection	0 200 — 400 mg	forms of blood vessel disease
selenium	retinal disease, cataract, immune system	0 — 55 100 µg	glaucoma

* Iron dosage varies for women. Magnesium dosage varies by age & gender.

Nutrient	Selected Benefits: Nutrient Is Good For….	Suggested* Daily Dose Range	Use Caution If You Have / Are…
St. John's wort	inflammation, infection, abnormal blood vessels	0 — 300 — mg	light-sensitive skin
sulforaphane	retinal disease, glaucoma, cataract	0 — 200 — 400 μg	
taurine	diabetes, cataract, retinal disease	0 — 1,000 — 1,500 mg	
vanadium	glaucoma, diabetes, cholesterol level	0 — 50 — 100 μg	anemia
vitamin A	immune defense, dry eye, light-sensing in retina	0 — 3,000 — 10,000 IU *	smoker
vitamin B1 (thiamin)	energy production, protection of neural tissue	0 — 1.5 — 3.0 mg	
vitamin B2 (riboflavin)	energy production, neuron signaling	0 — 1.5 — 2.5 mg	
vitamin B3 (niacin)	energy production, protection of neural tissue	0 — 25 — 50 mg	stomach ulcers
vitamin B6 (pyridoxine)	neural signaling, protection of neural tissue	0 — 2 — 4 mg	
vitamin B12 (cobalamine)	DNA protection, nerve tissue insulation	0 — 5 — 20 μg	severe acne
vitamin C	protection of eye surface, blood vessels, collagen	0 — 500 — 800 mg	
vitamin D	bones, immune defense, neuron signaling	0 — 400 — 800 IU	
vitamin E	retinal disease, glaucoma, cataract, dry eye	0 — 150 — 200 IU	prone to bleeding
vitamin K	blood clotting, macular degeneration	0 — 90 — 120 μg	
zeaxanthin	immune system, cataract, retinal disease	0 — 4 — 8 mg	
zinc	DNA formation, retinal disease, corneal disease	0 — 20 — 30 mg	high cholesterol, diabetes

*Vitamin A dosage is best balanced as 1,000 IU vitamin A with beta-carotene.

25

AGARICUS

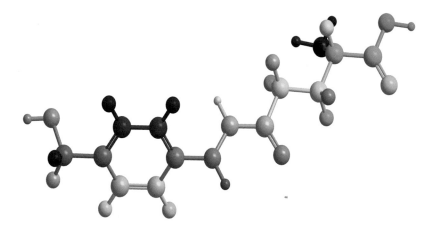

Category

Agaricus is the name for a genus, or group, of mushrooms. This group includes the common button mushroom, which is the white that is that common in many diets and often referred to as the "pizza mushroom." The agaricus group also includes the Portabella mushroom along with other edible and poisonous mushrooms.

The active ingredient of the mushroom is believed to be a lectin, which is a type of protein that binds to types of sugars on sugar-proteins named glycoproteins. These glycoproteins are found on the surface of cells in our bodies.

Cellular Location

Agaricus proteins are distributed through the bloodstream to various organs. Since proteins cannot be stored by the human body, unused proteins are metabolized and excreted.

Structure

Agaricus contains lectin proteins, which are believed to be its active ingredient. Agaricus also contains a chemical called agaritine (N-gamma-L+glutamyl-4-hydroxymethylphenylhydrazine), which is composed of a carbon-based hexagon ring with a long side chain that contains nitrogen and carbon groups.

Mechanisms of Action

The agaricus mushroom lectin binds to a specific sugar-protein (glycoprotein) on the surface of cells to prevent cells from proliferation (an increase in the number of cells). The process of cell proliferation has been shown to be involved in forming scars, in inflammation (the immune system response to infections and irritants), and in cancer.

Biological & Ocular Importance

● **Inhibits scar formation and inflammation in the eye** The agaricus lectin binds to the sugar-protein (glycoprotein) called beta-1,3-N-acetyl-galactosamine. By binding to beta-1,3-N-acetyl-galactosamine, agaricus lectin prevents certain cells from proliferating. These cells have been shown to be involved in scar formation, inflammation, and cancer.

Interestingly, the peanut lectin also binds to the same sugar-protein beta-1,3-N-acetyl-galactosamine. However, instead of preventing proliferation, it turns on the processes involved in inflammation and scar formation. Also, the peanut lectin is believed to be toxic to cells, while the agaricus mushroom lectin is believed to be non-toxic to cells.

● **Role after retinal detachment surgery & glaucoma surgery** Some animal model experiments have shown that the agaricus lectin binds to many different types of cells in the eye. For example, by binding to the glycoprotein on retinal pigment epithelium cells, the agaricus lectin may be involved in blocking the inflammation that causes retinal scarring after retinal detachment surgery. Similarly, by binding to the glycoprotein on inflammatory cells or fibroblast cells (wound-healing cells) under the conjunctiva, the agaricus lectin may be involved in blocking the inflammation that occurs on the surface of the eye that follows any eye surgery. In fact, after glaucoma surgery, this inflammation is believed to be one reason why glaucoma surgery fails to provide a lasting effect.

Human Studies on Utility

There are no human studies on agaricus use in eye disease reported in the scientifically-reviewed medical literature. Nevertheless, the fact that there are no reported clinical studies does not necessarily imply a benefit or lack of benefit. Looking at the mechanism of action, the use of agaricus in moderation may possibly serve some benefit in certain eye diseases, such as inflammatory eye diseases and after eye surgery.

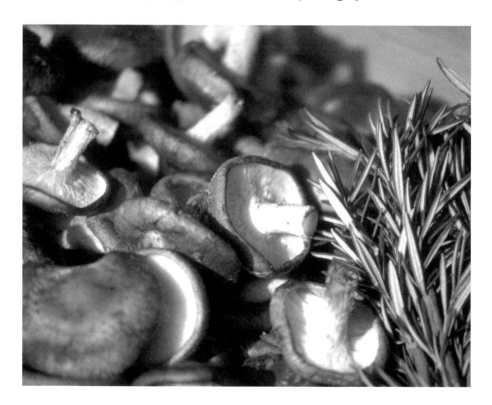

Body Absorption, Metabolism, & Excretion

The agaricus proteins are broken down by the stomach and its acids. Digestive enzymes from the pancreas further break down the agaricus proteins, which are then absorbed into the bloodstream through the intestines.

As proteins are broken down, ammonia is formed. Since ammonia is extremely toxic to cells, it must be converted into a nitrogen-containing chemical known as urea. When ammonia builds up in excess, it can cause poor coordination, difficulties with balance, tremors, seizures, difficulty breathing, swelling of the brain, and can eventually lead to a coma. A normally functioning liver works to remove excess ammonia by creating urea, which is then filtered into the urine by the kidneys.

Deficiency

Deficiency is uncommon. Since agaricus is not an essential nutrient, there are no known consequences of agaricus deficiency.

Toxicity & Side Effects

It is believed that there are no toxicities associated with excess agaricus. However, many things in excess can cause toxicity, so the fact that there are no known toxicities does not provide justification to consume agaricus in excess. As with any protein, agaricus in excess in someone with liver disease or with kidney disease may result in build-up of ammonia or urea in the body, resulting in severe illness (see above).

There is some suggestion that agaricus contains a chemical called agaritine (N-gamma-L+glutamyl-4-hydroxymethylphenyl-hydrazine) that may possibly cause cancers in high doses. Interestingly, there are other reports that suggest that agaricus prevents cancers, possibly through an anti-inflammatory or antioxidant mechanism.

Interactions with Other Nutrients

There are suggestions that agaricus contains high amounts of selenium and selenium-proteins.

Ideal Dosage

No ideal dosage or recommended dosage range has been established.

Sources (Where to Find It)

One whole portabella mushroom or about 10 whole small, white button pizza mushrooms contain an estimated 50 to 200 mg of agaricus lectin.

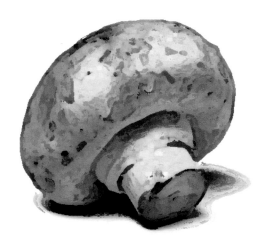

ALPHA-TOCOPHEROL
(SEE VITAMIN E)

ALPHA-LIPOIC ACID
(THIOCTIC ACID)

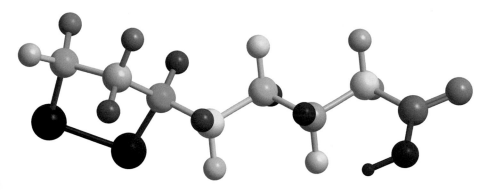

Category

Lipoic acid is a powerful sulfur-containing antioxidant. It was initially considered to be a b-complex vitamin, but when it was found that the body could synthesize lipoic acid, it simply became known as an important vitamin-like nutrient.

Alpha-lipoic acid is also known as thioctic acid, or 6,8-thioctic acid, or 6,8-dithio-octanoic acid, or 1,2-dithiolane-3-pentanoic acid, or 1,2-dithiolane-3-valeric acid.

Cellular Location

Alpha-lipoic acid is a rare nutrient that is soluble in lipids and fats as well as in water. This property enables it to act throughout the cell. By being soluble in lipids, it acts in cell membranes, which are composed of lipids, and in mitochondrial membranes. By being soluble in water, it acts inside the cells themselves as well.

Structure

Alpha-lipoic acid contains two sulfur molecules. These two sulfur molecules form part of a pentagonal ring at one end of the compound. Attached to the ring is a long chain that contains a carboxylic acid at the end.

Mechanisms of Action

Initially alpha-lipoic acid was called "Factor II" and then called "Protogen," based on early discoveries of its function. It acts as an enzyme cofactor (a molecule that assists in a cell's chemical reactions). It also acts as a powerful antioxidant and is known as the "Antioxidant of Antioxidants."

Biological & Ocular Importance

● **Alpha-lipoic acid is the "Antioxidant of Antioxidants"**
Alpha-lipoic acid's two sulfurs allow it to function as an antioxidant by donating electrons or to function in a variety of enzyme reactions as a cofactor that accepts electrons.

Alpha-lipoic acid acts as an antioxidant to scavenge or clear out numerous oxidants such as hydroxyl radicals. However, it is not as effective against some oxidants such as hydrogen peroxide or super-oxide radicals. Nevertheless, alpha-lipoic acid is a particularly strong antioxidant.

When alpha-lipoic acid is free and not bound to any other molecules, it is most effective as an antioxidant. The body can easily convert free lipoic acid into a molecule called dihydrolipoic acid, which is an even more potent antioxidant. Some research suggests dihydrolipoic acid is at least 20 to 30 times more potent than lipoic acid!

When most antioxidants are used up, they either become ineffective or must be recycled in order to function again. When the antioxidant properties of alpha-lipoic acid are used up, it is converted to dihydrolipoic acid. So as alpha-lipoic acid is used up (or "reduced"), it becomes a more powerful antioxidant.

Alpha-lipoic acid is often called the "antioxidant of antioxidants" because it can restore antioxidant properties to other antioxidants, when the antioxidant ability of those molecules is used up. This ability to restore antioxidants is a result of alpha-lipoic acid's excellent electron donating antioxidant ability.

In its form as dihydrolipoic acid, it can provide electrons to antioxidant nutrients, such as vitamin C, glutathione, and coenzyme Q10, in order to assist in recycling these nutrients once they are used up as antioxidants. Since the antioxidants lose electrons as they are used up, a deficiency of electrons is established, which creates the need for electrons. Vitamin C and glutathione can both help recycle vitamin E, so dihydrolipoic acid plays a central role in recycling the antioxidant vitamin E as well (see section on vitamin E).

When the body's converts lipoic acid into dihydrolipoic acid, it produces an important molecule that is necessary for creating an antioxidant called glutathione. This conversion often occurs with the help of the coenzyme (enzyme helper) nicotinamide adenine dinucleo-tide (NAD) or nicotinamide adenine dinucleotide phosphate (NADP). Vitamin B3 is important in producing NAD and NADP (see section on vitamin B3). In the process of converting lipoic acid to dihydrolipoic acid, the amino acid cystine which is oxidized is converted to cysteine. Cysteine can then be recycled in the cell and used to form glutathione (see sections on glutathione and N-acetyl-cysteine). Glutathione is an antioxidant composed of three amino-acid molecules and is called a tri-peptide. One of these amino-acids is cysteine. Throughout the living world, there are numerous occurrences, like this example, of how various nutrients work together.

● **Binds metals to prevent oxidation**   There is evidence that alpha-lipoic acid can chelate (bind and remove) metals such as iron and copper to prevent them from acting as oxidants. Alpha-lipoic can prevent dangerous metals from producing toxic effects. By binding metals, alpha-

lipoic acid is believed to play a role in preventing or reducing many diseases and injuries caused by metals. For example, it is used to bind to the metal mercury to prevent human toxicity from mercury.

Even in its "reduced" (or used up) form, dihydrolipoic acid can act as a metal chelator (an agent that binds the metals to remove them from action). When dihydrolipoic acid chelates iron, however, there is some suggestion that the iron may then act more strongly as an oxidant. Despite this deleterious effect of dihydrolipoic acid, its other antioxidant activities appear to overcome this possible pro-oxidant activity. As noted above, it helps restore antioxidant properties to other antioxidants.

● **Prevents cataract**   Alpha-lipoic acid is known to increase levels of antioxidants such as glutathione and vitamin C in the lens, helping prevent cataract formation. Glutathione is in extremely high concentrations in the lens and is an important antioxidant in protecting the lens (see section on glutathione and vitamin C).

In laboratory research, alpha-lipoic acid's ability to chelate metals has been suggested to be effective in binding metals that cause cataracts. It has also been shown to bind to copper to prevent it from accumulating in the eye, particularly the lens so as to prevent cataract formation.

● Prevents retinal diseases & glaucoma

As an antioxidant, alpha-lipoic acid has been shown in animal models of diabetes to reduce the diabetic retinopathy or retinal disease that occurs during the diabetes. Similarly, in the laboratory, alpha-lipoic acid has been shown to decrease the oxidative damage that occurs in the retinal pigment epithelium in models of macular degeneration. There is evidence that it may also be beneficial to other retinal diseases, where the neurons of the retina are subject to oxidative injury, such as photoreceptor diseases or retinal ganglion cell disease such as glaucoma.

● Blocks ability of sugars to attack proteins in diabetes

In diabetes, there are high levels of the sugar glucose in the circulating blood. High levels of glucose in the presence of oxygen can result in the formation of oxidants (see introduction). In animal models, alpha-lipoic acid has been shown to be beneficial in reducing oxidants formed by diabetes, as well as enhancing the utilization of glucose by the body's cells. In addition, alpha-lipoic acid may also act to prevent the formation of "advanced glycation end products" or AGEs. AGEs are toxic products that damage the retina, the lens, and other ocular structures (see introduction). AGEs are formed when glucose attacks proteins, which occurs during diabetes. The ability of alpha-lipoic acid to block these sugar reactions (or glycation reactions) is believed to be related to its antioxidant abilities, but there also may be other mechanisms that are not well understood.

● May enhance insulin sensitivity in diabetes

There are some studies that suggest that alpha-lipoic acid can also enhance the insulin sensitivity in diabetes. One major problem in diabetes is a decrease in the sensitivity of cells to insulin (the hormone that is the body's usual indicator in signaling cells to decrease the sugar levels). In diabetes, because of the decreased sensitivity of cells to insulin, the same amount of insulin does not function to the same extent in decreasing blood sugars. Therefore, without treatment, blood sugars often go too high.

Alpha-lipoic acid may improve the insulin sensitivity through insulin signaling pathways inside cells. Alpha-lipoic acid may also enhance the role of insulin in transporting sugars by increasing glucose sugar transporters and redistributing these transporters to more beneficial sites.

Therefore, alpha-lipoic acid has been shown to be of benefit for diabetics by reducing blood glucose levels. Furthermore, studies suggest it is of benefit for peripheral nerve disease and kidney disease in diabetes as well.

- **Acts as an enzyme cofactor**   When alpha-lipoic acid is bound to protein it acts as an enzyme cofactor. An enzyme cofactor is a molecule that is necessary to help certain cell reactions occur. Alpha-lipoic acid acts as a cofactor for various enzymes, such as those involved in making DNA and RNA as well as the energy-producing enzymes that function in the mitochondria (the energy-producing organelles in the body's cells). An example is lipoyllysine, which is alpha-lipoic acid bound to lysine, an amino acid (building blocks of proteins).

- **Inactivates a protein that causes blood vessel disease and atherosclerosis, cancer, autoimmune disease, & diabetes**   Alpha-lipoic acid is known to inactivate a protein that is called nuclear factor kappa B. This protein is known as a transcription factor (a protein that turns specific genes on or off). Nuclear factor kappa B turns on the genes (a process called upregulation) involved in inflammation (the immune system response to infections and irritants) and those that play a role in the development of cancer, autoimmune disease, and atherosclerosis (blood vessel cholesterol clots and plaques that can result in heart disease and stroke, as well as artery or vein clots in the retina or optic nerve strokes). So while diabetes increases levels of potentially-harmful nuclear factor kappa B, alpha-lipoic acid inactivates this protein.

  Additionally, alpha-lipoic acid can inhibit the activity of other transcription factors that play roles in cell signaling and cell death.

- **May be beneficial in stroke & Alzheimer's disease**   Some studies suggest that alpha-lipoic acid may be of benefit in protecting the brain after stroke and preliminary findings suggest it may be helpful in Alzheimer's disease as well.

Human Studies on Utility

Currently, there is only one human study on alpha-lipoic use in eye disease reported in the scientifically-reviewed medical literature. Nevertheless, the fact that there is a single, reported clinical study does not necessarily imply a benefit or lack of benefit. Looking at the mechanism of action, the use of alpha-lipoic acid in moderation may be possibly of benefit in many eye diseases.

A 1999 study of over 100 diabetics found that those who took 600 mg of alpha-lipoic acid each day for 3 months developed less oxidative stress, as assessed by oxidative damage to lipids in their bloodstream, than those who did not take the alpha-lipoic acid supplement.[1]

Body Absorption, Metabolism, & Excretion

Most food sources of alpha-lipoic acid contain the amino-acid bound form, lipoyllysine. Lipoyllysine is not broken up in the digestive system and is absorbed in whole as the bound form lipoyllysine.

Lipoic acid is often used up by the body, but excess amounts may either be filtered out by the kidneys for excretion, or dumped back into the intestines for excretion with bile (a green fluid produced by the liver that is stored in the gallbladder to assist in digestion).

Deficiency

The human body is able to make lipoic acid from fatty acids containing 8 carbons. Therefore, a deficiency of alpha-lipoic acid is extremely rare because the body can synthesize its own supply if needed.

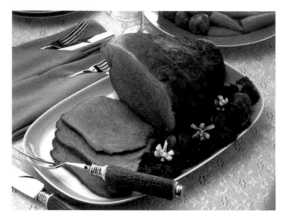

There are some diseases, however, that can cause decreased levels of alpha-lipoic acid. For example, one of many targets for arsenic poisoning is the sulfur groups of lipoic acid in a group of enzymes called dehydrogenase enzymes. Lipoic acid is the key component of dehydrogenase enzymes involved in cellular metabolism, and arsenic can inhibit the function of these enzymes, which would thereby restrain cellular metabolism. Similarly, in a liver disease called primary biliary cirrhosis, antibodies attack the lipoic acid component dehydrogenase enzymes and inhibit cellular metabolism in this way.

Toxicity & Side Effects

There are no known reports of serious toxicity in humans, but allergic skin reactions have been reported.

In diabetics, since alpha-lipoic acid helps improve the body's glucose utilization, people may become hypoglycemic, developing critically low blood sugar levels. This problem can occur as a result of taking a combination of prescribed diabetic medicines with alpha-lipoic acid.

Interactions with Other Nutrients

Nutrients such as alpha-lipoic acid, phytic acid, and bioflavonoids chelate (bind and remove) metals such as copper, aluminum, cadmium, lead, mercury, silver, zinc and iron. Therefore, excess of these nutrients can result in zinc deficiency or iron deficiency. Iron is essential for transport of oxygen in blood cells, and deficiency of iron results in anemia (insufficiency of the red blood cells that carry oxygen) (see sections on zinc and iron).

The nutrient SAMe can participate in the production of alpha-lipoic acid by donating sulfur groups (see section on SAMe).

Glutathione can be made through a pathway that involves alpha lipoic acid, vitamin B3, and cysteine. The conversion of lipoic acid into dihydrolipoic acid involves vitamin B3 (see page 34) and results in conversion of cystine into cysteine. Cysteine can then be recycled into the cell and used to form glutathione (see sections on glutathione and N-acetyl-cysteine).

Alpha-lipoic acid acts with vitamin E, vitamin C, bioflavonoids, and glutathione to form a highly protective antioxidant team. Alpha-lipoic acid and vitamin C protect glutathione from being used up by donating electrons to the oxidized form of glutathione so that it can be reduced to usable glutathione that can act again as an antioxidant (see sections on vitamin C, vitamin E, bioflavonoids, and glutathione).

Increased levels of other sulfur containing nutrients, such as cysteine, taurine, alpha-lipoic acid, and methylsulfonylmethane, also result in increased levels of glutathione, a sulfur-containing tripeptide (see section on glutathione).

Ideal Dosage

The recommended daily dosage of lipoic acid ranges from 200 to 600 mg per day. While some researchers recommend doses as high as 600 mg per day, it may be best to obtain a daily dose of between 400 to 600 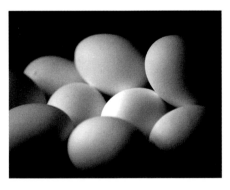 mg per day. Also, rather than a single, larger dose, it is preferable to spread the full amount into smaller doses over the course of the day.

Sources (Where to Find It)

Alpha-lipoic acid was discovered in the laboratory in 1937 as an extract from potatoes that certain bacteria needed so that they could grow. Since then, alpha-lipoic acid has been characterized and found to be present in many sources. Most food sources of alpha-lipoic acid contain the amino-acid bound form, lipoyllysine.

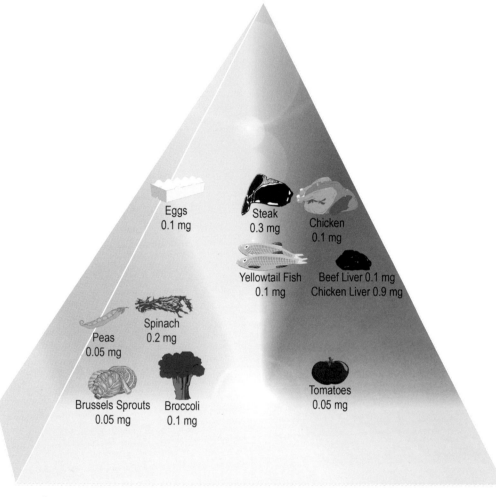

Eggs
0.1 mg

Steak
0.3 mg

Chicken
0.1 mg

Yellowtail Fish
0.1 mg

Beef Liver 0.1 mg
Chicken Liver 0.9 mg

Spinach
0.2 mg

Peas
0.05 mg

Brussels Sprouts
0.05 mg

Broccoli
0.1 mg

Tomatoes
0.05 mg

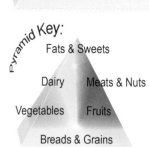

Pyramid Key:

Fats & Sweets

Dairy   Meats & Nuts

Vegetables   Fruits

Breads & Grains

Top sources of alpha-lipoic acid include kidney, heart, and liver (such as from lamb or beef). Spinach and broccoli are also rich in alpha-lipoic acid.

However, dietary supplement pills often contain amounts of alpha-lipoic acid that are several hundred times more, and closer to recommended doses.

ARGININE

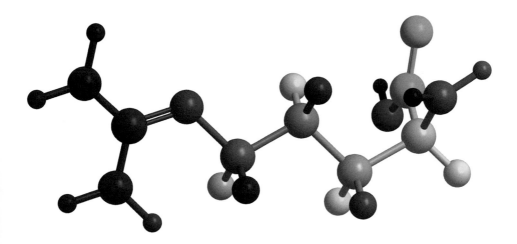

Category

Arginine is an amino acid (building blocks of proteins). It is considered only semi-essential, as the body typically produces enough of its own arginine, except in cases of severe malnutrition or certain metabolic disease states.

Cellular Location

Arginine is distributed through the bloodstream to various organs. Since proteins cannot be stored by the human body, unused proteins are metabolized and excreted.

Structure

Arginine is an amino acid, comprised of a carbon backbone with nitrogen groups. An important feature to note is that at one end there is a structure called a guanidine, which is a tripod-like group containing three nitrogen molecules.

Mechanisms of Action

Arginine assists in the regulation of nitric oxide, a gas that functions as a cell signal to relax or dilate blood vessels in order to increase their blood flow.

Biological & Ocular Importance

● Maintains blood flow & oxygen balance in the eye, particularly in the retina

The highest amount of oxygen consumption of any tissue in the body occurs in the retina. Arginine is essential in maintaining the balance of oxygen. Oxygen is essential for cellular functioning, so the highly metabolic retina requires high amounts of oxygen.

However, excess oxygen can lead to oxidative damage. The presence of light and oxygen with an imbalance in antioxidant mechanisms results in the production of reactive oxygen species (toxic chemicals that result in oxidation). Due to the high oxygen consumption by the retina, it is particularly susceptible to oxidative damage.

Arginine is a precursor for the formation of nitric oxide. When nitric oxide is released from cells, it helps maintain the proper dilation of blood vessels and helps prevent the development of hypertension (high blood pressure).

Nitric oxide is also believed to be important in maintaining blood flow in the retina in diseases such as diabetic retinopathy and glaucoma.

When nitric oxide resides inside the cell for too long, however, it can form peroxy-nitrites (chemicals that cause oxidation or damage to the cells).

● Prevents infections

Nitric oxide also helps prevent infections in our bodies, particularly in our throats, sinuses, and lungs.

● Prevents osteoporosis

Nitric oxide, along with other agents, also helps block the bone-eating cells called osteoclasts that are involved in the development of osteoporosis.

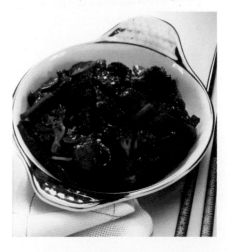

Human Studies on Utility

Currently, there is only one human study on arginine use in eye disease reported in the scientifically-reviewed medical literature. This study involves a retinal disease called gyrate atrophy.

Gyrate atrophy is a rare inherited disorder of cellular metabolism of ornithine (an amino acid that plays a role in the formation of arginine, another amino acid involved in building proteins). Ornithine also plays a significant role in the removal of excess nitrogen from cells through a process called the urea cycle. Deficiency of the enzyme involved in the cellular metabolism of ornithine results in excess build-up of ornithine and a disease called gyrate atrophy. Gyrate atrophy is a retinal disease resulting in night-blindness and loss of peripheral (or side) vision.

One of the enzymes in the metabolism of ornithine works with vitamin B6, a cofactor, or substance that helps in the enzymatic process (see section on vitamin B6). Increasing dietary intake of vitamin B6 results in more metabolism of ornithine and decreased build-up of ornithine in the bloodstream and tissues of concern. Also, these people are asked to decrease their intake of the amino acid arginine, which is a precursor in the ornithine metabolism pathway.

Restriction in arginine along with the use of vitamin B6 has been reported to be helpful in people with gyrate atrophy.

Body Absorption, Metabolism, & Excretion

Arginine is digested by the stomach with the help of stomach acids. Digestive enzymes from the pancreas further break down proteins, which are then absorbed into the bloodstream through the intestines.

As proteins are broken down, ammonia is formed. Since ammonia is extremely toxic to cells, it must be converted into a nitrogen-containing chemical known as urea. When ammonia builds up in excess, it can cause poor coordination, difficulties with balance, tremors, seizures, difficulty breathing, swelling of the brain, and can eventually lead to a coma. A normally functioning liver works to remove excess ammonia by creating urea, which is then filtered into the urine by the kidneys.

Deficiency

Arginine deficiency is not common, but the rare instances can occur in cases of severe protein deficiency. Deficiency of arginine can cause hair loss, skin rash, difficulties with healing of wounds, constipation, and liver disease.

Also, excess ammonia is believed to result in arginine deficiency.

Toxicity & Side Effects

Arginine supplementation has been reported to cause allergic reactions, and should be avoided in people who may be prone to severe allergies.

Excess arginine, like other amino acids, is often broken down and converted into sugars or fats, and either used for energy, or stored as fat in the body's fat stores. Excess amino acids can stress the kidneys and the bloodstream and cause dehydration. Furthermore, excess amino acids can cause the kidneys to lose calcium resulting in weakened bones. As with any amino acid, excess arginine in someone with liver disease or with kidney disease may result in build-up of ammonia or urea in the body, resulting in severe illness (see above under body absorption, metabolism, & excretion).

In diabetics, excess amino acids can result in an increased sugar load on the body, or increased fat deposits in the body!

For reasons unknown, excess arginine can trigger the release of herpes virus in people that have it "harbored", or hidden and sequestered in their bodies. Likewise, arginine can cause additional complications in people who are experiencing herpes virus disease.

Interactions with Other Nutrients

Excess lysine is believed to induce the breakdown of arginine (see section on lysine).

Ideal Dosage

The recommended daily dose of arginine is 500 to 1,500 mg. Some researchers have suggested doses well above 2,000 mg, up to 20,000 mg per day. However, no supplemental arginine is necessary if one's diet is well-balanced. With higher doses, spreading the full amount into smaller doses over the course of the day is preferable to a single larger dose.

Sources (Where to Find It)

Fruits & Vegetables:

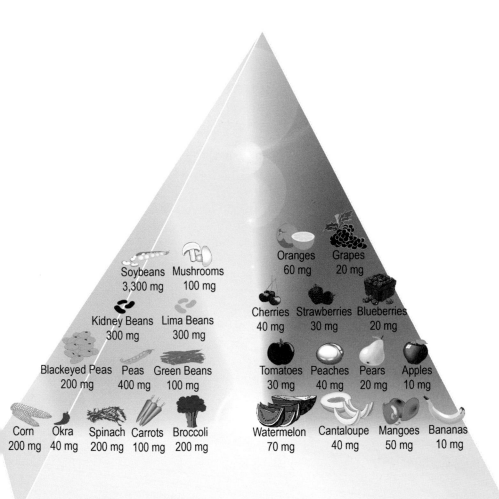

Soybeans 3,300 mg
Mushrooms 100 mg

Kidney Beans 300 mg
Lima Beans 300 mg

Blackeyed Peas 200 mg
Peas 400 mg
Green Beans 100 mg

Corn 200 mg
Okra 40 mg
Spinach 200 mg
Carrots 100 mg
Broccoli 200 mg

Oranges 60 mg
Grapes 20 mg

Cherries 40 mg
Strawberries 30 mg
Blueberries 20 mg

Tomatoes 30 mg
Peaches 40 mg
Pears 20 mg
Apples 10 mg

Watermelon 70 mg
Cantaloupe 40 mg
Mangoes 50 mg
Bananas 10 mg

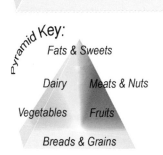

Pyramid Key:

Fats & Sweets

Dairy   Meats & Nuts

Vegetables   Fruits

Breads & Grains

*See Guides on Pages 467-468.

Dairy, Meats, & Grains:

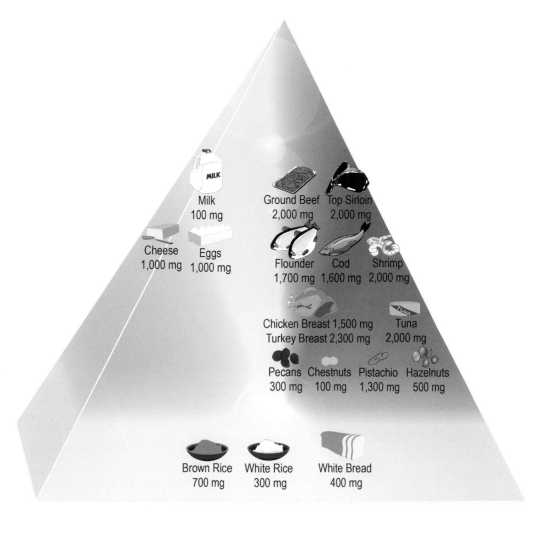

Milk
100 mg

Ground Beef
2,000 mg

Top Sirloin
2,000 mg

Cheese
1,000 mg

Eggs
1,000 mg

Flounder
1,700 mg

Cod
1,600 mg

Shrimp
2,000 mg

Chicken Breast 1,500 mg
Turkey Breast 2,300 mg

Tuna
2,000 mg

Pecans
300 mg

Chestnuts
100 mg

Pistachio
1,300 mg

Hazelnuts
500 mg

Brown Rice
700 mg

White Rice
300 mg

White Bread
400 mg

Arginine is found in any foods that contain proteins, particularly meats (including beef, chicken, and fish) and dairy products. Some nuts such as pistachio and beans such as soybeans are especially high in arginine. Among the fruits and vegetables, peas, broccoli, spinach, and corn contain somewhat high amounts of arginine, though much lower than that of meats, dairy products, nuts, and beans.

ASCORBATE
(SEE VITAMIN C)

ASCORBIC ACID
(SEE VITAMIN C)

BETA-CAROTENE

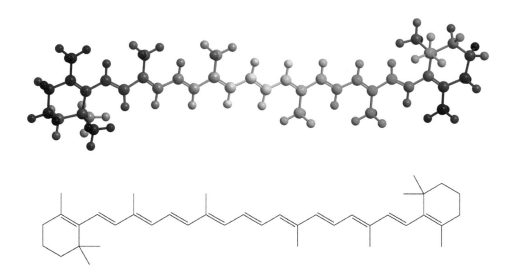

Category

Beta-carotene is a type of molecule known as a carotenoid. Carotenoids are organic pigments that occur naturally in plants, but cannot be made by animals (see section on carotenoids).

Beta-carotene is a precursor of vitamin A, meaning that beta-carotene can be converted into vitamin A. This conversion can occur in the liver and in the retinal pigment epithelium.

Cellular Location

Beta-carotene is carried in the bloodstream by fat-protein carriers and is stored in the liver and converted to vitamin A when needed. Other storage sites include body fat.

Structure

Beta-carotene is composed of two rings connected by a very long chain. In fact, the long chain contains many double bonds that give it its characteristic orange color. Because its structure causes it to be insoluble in water, it prefers to be in the presence of oils and fats.

Mechanisms of Action

See section on vitamin A.

Biological & Ocular Importance

See section on vitamin A.

Human Studies on Utility

Summary of Studies for Macular Degeneration: Over a dozen clinical trials have been performed looking at the role of beta-carotene in both preventing and treating macular degeneration. These clinical trials are of various types, some of which are very well-designed and well-performed studies.

As a whole, the clinical studies provide no definitive answer as to whether beta-carotene is beneficial, and, in fact, the majority of studies found no benefit to beta-carotene for macular degeneration. However, there is some evidence from the studies that it may be beneficial, particularly in combination with other antioxidant nutrients. Looking at the mechanisms of action, there is good reason to use beta-carotene in moderation for macular degeneration.

The studies can be summarized as follows: several large, well-performed studies found no benefits from the past use of beta-carotene on the risk of macular degeneration, while one study did find a benefit in the past use of beta-carotene in decreasing the risk of macular degeneration. Several smaller studies have found no link (neither protective nor harmful) between levels of beta-carotene in the blood and macular degeneration, though one study found that higher levels of beta-carotene in the blood are associated with a decrease in the risk of macular degeneration.

In following people over time, several large, well-performed studies found that those who took beta-carotene did not have any benefit compared to those who did not take beta-carotene.

Beta-Carotene for
Macular Degeneration
Scale of Benefit

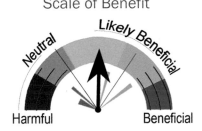

Another study also found that beta-carotene by itself did not have any benefit in preventing macular degeneration. However, this study did find that in combination with other nutrients, beta-carotene decreased the risk of macular degeneration by one-half! Similarly, another study also found that the use of a multivitamin with beta-carotene decreased the future risk of macular degeneration over time.

> Looking at the mechanisms of action, there is good reason to use beta-carotene in moderation for macular degeneration and cataract.

● **In large studies: no benefits in past use of beta-carotene found on risk of macular degeneration** A study of over 3,500 people age 49 and over found no link (neither protective nor harmful) between the risk of developing macular degeneration over a 5 year period and people who took the following nutrients, alone or in combination, in the past: beta-carotene, lutein and zeaxanthin, lycopene, vitamin A, or zinc. Surprisingly, however, the study found, that those who took vitamin C supplements combined with a diet high in vitamin C had a 2-fold increase in their risk of developing macular degeneration.[2] This finding is quite surprising, as one would expect vitamin C to protect against macular degeneration, as opposed to increasing the risk of macular degeneration. However, the finding highlights the problems associated with these types of studies: namely, that the findings may occur coincidentally and other true findings may be missed. It is sometimes difficult to explain the findings or apply them to real life.

Looking at a group of nearly 2,000 people from a study population of nearly 5,000 people, researchers found no link (neither protective nor harmful) between the risk of developing macular degeneration and a diet high in carotenoids, vitamin C, or vitamin E. However, they did find a decreased risk of early-stage macular degeneration for those who consumed diets high in zinc.[3]

● **In one large study: no benefits in past use of *higher amounts* of beta-carotene found on risk of macular degeneration** A study of nearly 3,000 people age 49 and over found no link (neither protective nor harmful) between the risk of having macular degeneration a diet with higher amounts of beta-carotene, vitamin A, vitamin C, or zinc in the past.[4]

● **Though the several studies above found no link, one large study found a benefit: past use of beta-carotene associated with decreased risk of macular degeneration** A study of over 1,000 people age 55 to 80 found that those who consumed a diet high in beta-carotene had a 40% decrease in the risk of having wet macular degeneration compared to those who did not consume a diet high in beta-carotene. Similarly, dietary carotenoids as well as dietary vitamin A decreased the risk by over 40%, while dietary lutein and zeaxanthin decreased the risk by nearly 60%. The authors found no link (neither protective nor harmful) between macular degeneration and a diet high in vitamin C or E.[5]

● In several studies: no link between blood levels of beta-carotene and macular degeneration

Another study of nearly 100 people found no difference in the blood levels of carotenoids, beta-carotene, lutein and zeaxanthin, lycopene, vitamin A, vitamin C, zinc, or selenium between those with or without macular degeneration (looking at both early and severe or advanced macular degeneration). However, the study found that those who had severe or advanced macular degeneration had lower blood levels of vitamin E compared to those without macular degeneration. They found no differences in the blood levels of vitamin E between those with or without early macular degeneration.[6]

A study of over 300 people from a group of nearly 5,000 people found no difference in the blood levels of beta-carotene, lycopene, or lutein and zeaxanthin between those with or without macular degeneration. They also found that those who had macular degeneration had lower blood levels of vitamin E compared to those without macular degeneration. Interestingly, they also found that fewer people with macular degeneration use vitamin C than people without macular degeneration.[7]

A study of 300 people from a group of nearly 4,000 people found no link (neither protective nor harmful) between the risk of having macular degeneration and higher blood levels of beta-carotene or of vitamin E.[8]

A study of 130 people also found no difference in the blood levels of beta-carotene, lutein, lycopene, vitamin A, or vitamin E between those with or without macular degeneration.[9]

A study of 500 people age 40 and over found no link (neither protective nor harmful) between higher blood levels of beta-carotene, vitamin A, or vitamin C, and macular degeneration. However, the study also found that those with higher blood levels of vitamin E had an over 50% decrease in the risk of having macular degeneration when compared to those who had lower blood levels of vitamin E.[10]

● Though the several studies above found no link, one large study found a benefit: decreased risk of macular degeneration in those with higher blood levels of beta-carotene

A study of over 1,000 people age 55 to 80 found that having higher blood levels of carotenoids decreased the risk of having wet macular degeneration by 60% compared to those who had lower blood levels of carotenoids.[11] Looking at specific carotenoids, the study found that having higher blood levels of beta-carotene decreased the risk of having macular degeneration by 70%. Higher blood levels of lutein and zeaxanthin also decreased the risk by 70% and higher blood levels of lycopene decreased the risk by

60%. Also, higher blood levels of a combination of three or more of four nutrients (carotenoids, vitamin C, vitamin E, and selenium) decreased the risk by 70%. The study found no link (neither protective nor harmful) between higher blood levels of vitamin C, vitamin E, or selenium by themselves and macular degeneration.[12]

● **In several large studies: no benefits from the use of beta-carotene on the future risk of macular degeneration over time** Looking forward over time, a study of nearly 3,000 people age 49 and over found no link (neither protective nor harmful) between the risk of having macular degeneration and taking any of the following nutrients (alone or in combination) in the past: beta-carotene, vitamin A, vitamin B1, vitamin B2, vitamin B3, vitamin B6, vitamin B12, vitamin C, vitamin E, folate or zinc.[13]

Looking over a 5-year period, a study of 2,000 people from a group of nearly 5,000, found no link (neither protective nor harmful) between macular degeneration and a diet high in beta-carotene, carotenoids, lutein and zeaxanthin, vitamin C, vitamin E, or zinc.[14]

A study of over 75,000 people (nurses and health professionals) followed over time for up to 18 years found no link (neither protective nor harmful) between the risk of developing macular degeneration (wet or dry) and a diet high in any of the following nutrients: beta-carotene, carotenoids, lutein and zeaxanthin, lycopene, vitamin A, vitamin C, or

vitamin E. The study did find that those who consumed more than 3 servings of fruit each day were $1/3$ less likely to develop *wet* macular degeneration over time compared to those who consumed less than $1\frac{1}{2}$ servings of fruit each day. No link (neither protective nor harmful) was found when looking at increased fruit consumption for dry macular degeneration, nor when looking at increased vegetable consumption for dry or wet macular degeneration.[15]

One study of over 29,000 smokers looked at whether or not supplements of vitamin E (70 IU) and/or beta-carotene (20 mg) taken daily for 6 years could prevent cancer. The study also looked at macular degeneration and found no link (neither protective nor harmful) between taking beta-carotene, vitamin E, or the two together and the risk of developing macular degeneration. Because the study looked only at smokers, its applicability to the general population is limited. Such limitations are always concerns of clinical trials.[16]

A small study of 71 people with macular degeneration found no benefit to the macular degeneration or to vision in those who took a daily antioxidant combination, for over $1\frac{1}{2}$ years, that consisted of beta-carotene (20,000 IU), vitamin B2 (25 mg), vitamin C (750 mg), vitamin E (200 IU), chromium (100 µg), selenium (50 µg), zinc (12.5 mg), taurine (100 mg), N-acetyl cysteine (100 mg), glutathione (5 mg), and selected bioflavonoids, compared to placebo.[17] It is impossible, however, to ascertain the individual effect of beta-carotene from this type of study.

● **In one study: no benefits from the use of beta-carotene by itself on the future risk of macular degeneration over time, but use of beta-carotene with multiple nutrients decreases future risk of macular degeneration** A study of nearly 4,000 people, looking forward over an average of 8 years, found no link (neither protective nor harmful) between macular degeneration and a diet high in beta-carotene, lutein and zeaxanthin, lycopene, vitamin A, vitamin C, iron, or zinc. However, a diet high in vitamin E decreased the risk of having macular degeneration by 20%. A diet high in multiple nutrients (beta-carotene, vitamin C, vitamin E, and zinc together) decreased the risk of having macular degeneration by about ½![18]

● **Similarly, another large study found a benefit: use of multi-vitamin with beta-carotene decreases the future risk of macular degeneration over time** A recent 10-year study of over 3,000 people age 55 and over found that taking a daily antioxidant combination of vitamin C (500 mg), vitamin E (400 IU), and beta-carotene (15 mg), with or without zinc (80 mg) and copper (2 mg) reduced the risk of developing severe or wet macular degeneration, in people with certain features of dry macular degeneration within their retinas. The risk of developing severe or advanced macular degeneration decreased by 34% in people taking the antioxidant combination with zinc and copper, by 24% in people taking the antioxidant combination alone without zinc and copper, and by 30% in people taking the zinc and copper without the antioxidant combination. Looking at vision, the antioxidant combination with zinc and copper decreased the risk of losing vision from macular degeneration by 25% in these people with certain features of dry macular degeneration. There was no benefit to vision for people who took the antioxidant combination alone, without the zinc and copper, or the zinc and copper alone. This study has been used widely to recommend the multivitamin combination for macular degeneration, though the results are only applicable to people with certain features of macular degeneration in their retinas. Moreover, what confounds the interpretation of the data is the use of multivitamins in two-thirds of the people.[19]

Summary of Studies for Cataract: Over a dozen clinical trials have been performed looking at the role of beta-carotene in both preventing and treating cataract. These clinical trials are of several different types, some of which are very well-designed and well-performed studies.

As a whole, the studies provide no definitive answer that beta-carotene is beneficial. Many of the studies found no benefit to beta-carotene for cataract. However, there is some suggestion that it may be beneficial, as 4 out of the 16 studies found a benefit.

Beta-Carotene for
Cataract
Scale of Benefit

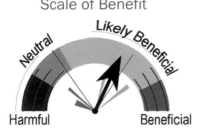

Looking at the mechanisms of action, there is reason to use beta-carotene in moderation for cataract.

The studies can be summarized as follows: three studies found no benefits from the past use of beta-carotene on the risk of cataract, while two studies did find a benefit in the past use of beta-carotene in decreasing the risk of cataract. Two studies have found no link (neither protective nor harmful) between levels of beta-carotene in the blood and cataract, though one study found that higher levels of beta-carotene in the blood are associated with a decrease in the risk of cataract.

In following people over time, several large, well-performed studies found that those who took beta-carotene did not have any benefit compared to those who did not take beta-carotene. However, one smaller study did find that beta-carotene with vitamin C and vitamin E

decreased the future risk of cataract over time.

● **In three studies: no benefits in past use of beta-carotene found on risk of cataract** A study of nearly 500 people age 53 to 73 found no link (neither protective nor harmful) between the intake of beta-carotene, carotenoids, lutein and zeaxanthin, or lycopene and the risk of having cataracts. However, the study did show that the past intake of *higher* amounts of vitamin C decreased the risk of having cataracts by nearly 70%. It also found that long-term intake of vitamin C for over 10 years decreased the risk of having cataracts by nearly 65%. Similarly, past intake of *higher* amounts of vitamin B2 decreased the risk of having cataracts by over 60%, and past intake of *higher* amounts of folate decreased the risk by about 10%. It also found that long-term intake of vitamin E for over 10 years decreased the risk of having cataracts by over 50%, even though the study found no link (neither protective nor harmful) between the past intake of *higher* amounts of vitamin E and the risk of having cataracts. The finding of no beneficial link with higher doses of vitamin E may be related to increased risks associated with the higher doses. Furthermore, the use of a multivitamin for over 10 years reduced the risk of having cataract by over 40%.[20]

Another study of 400 people age 50 to 86 found no link (neither protective nor harmful) between the past use of beta-carotene, lutein, lycopene, vitamin A, or vitamin E and the risk of having cataract.[21]

An Italian study of over 900 people also found no link (neither protective nor harmful) between intake of higher levels of beta-carotene, methionine, vitamin A, or vitamin D and the risk of having cataracts. However, this study found that those who consumed higher dietary levels of folate and vitamin E had a lower risk of developing cataracts that required surgery.[22]

● **Though the three studies above found no link, two studies found a benefit: past use of beta-carotene associated with decreased risk of cataract**   A study of 300 women age 56 to 71 from a group of over 120,000 people found that in non-smokers, the past use of beta-carotene in higher doses reduced the risk of having cataracts by over 70%. In fact, carotenoids, as a group, in higher doses reduced the risk of having cataracts by over 80%. The study also found that folate in higher doses reduced the risk of having cataracts by nearly 75%. In addition, past use of higher doses of vitamin C decreased the risk of having cataract by nearly 60% and the use of vitamin C for over 10 years decreased the risk by 60%. However, the study found no link (neither protective nor harmful) between the use of vitamin E or B2 and cataract.[23]

A study of over 5,000 people found that the past intake of higher amounts of beta-carotene reduced the risk of having cataract by 75 to 90% (depending on the type of cataract). The past intake of higher amounts of vitamin E decreased the risk of having certain types of cataracts by about 80%, and the use of vitamin E for greater than 5 years also decreased the risk by about 80%. Similarly, the past intake of higher amounts of vitamin C decreased the risk of having certain types of cataracts by about 90%, and the use of vitamin C for greater than 5 years reduced the risk by about 85%.[24]

● **In two studies: no link between blood levels of beta-carotene and cataract**   A study of over 1,000 people found no link (neither protective nor harmful) between higher levels of beta-carotene, vitamin A, or glutathione in the blood and the risk of having cataracts. However, the study did find that higher levels of vitamin C in the blood decreased the risk of one type of cataract by nearly 50%. Of concern, the study found that higher levels of vitamin E in the blood increased the risk by nearly twice of having cataracts (this finding may be related to increased risks associated with higher doses of vitamin E)![25]

Another study of 400 people found no link (neither protective nor harmful) between higher blood levels of beta-carotene, lutein, or lycopene and the risk of having cataracts. However, unlike the other study, this study found that higher blood levels of vitamin E decreased the risk of having cataracts by 60%.[26] The study also looked at gender differences in this same group of people and found that some nutrients, such as lycopene, are more beneficial in women and other nutrients, such as vitamin A, are more beneficial in men. These results, however, are much more difficult to interpret.[27]

● **Though the two studies above found no link, one study found a benefit: decreased risk of cataract in those with higher blood levels of beta-carotene** A study of nearly 400 people age 66 to 75 found that higher levels of beta-carotene and alpha-carotene in the blood decreased the risk of having one type of cataract but not another. Similarly, higher levels of lutein in the blood decreased risk of having one type of cataract, whereas higher levels of lycopene in the blood decreased risk of having another type of cataract. However, the study found no link (neither protective nor harmful) between higher levels of vitamin C or vitamin E or zeaxanthin and the risk of having any type of cataract.[28]

● **In several large studies: no benefits from the use of beta-carotene on the future risk of cataract over time** A recent 10-year study of over 3,000 people found that taking an antioxidant combination of beta-carotene (15 mg), vitamin C (500 mg), and vitamin E (400 IU), with or without zinc and copper each day reduced the risk of macular degeneration over time, but found no link (neither protective nor harmful) to the risk of cataracts over time.[29]

Another study of nearly 2,000 people randomly sampled from a study of over 20,000 people found no link (neither protective nor harmful) between taking 20 mg of beta-carotene each day for 5 to 8 years and the risk of cataracts over time. Also, there was no link between taking 20 mg of beta-carotene with vitamin E, or taking vitamin E alone, each day for 5 to 8 years and the risk of cataracts over time.[30]

A large study of over 20,000 men found no link (neither protective nor harmful) between taking 25 mg of beta-carotene each day for 12 years and the risk of developing cataract.[31]

A large study of nearly 40,000 women also found no link (neither protective nor harmful) between the risk of developing cataract and a daily intake of 25 mg of beta-carotene for about 2 years.[32]

A study of over 2,000 people given a multivitamin or a placebo for 5 years found a 36% decrease in the risk of developing cataracts in those people who were age 65 to 74. Of note, there was no difference in risk in the younger group age 45 to 64. These results exemplify the positive benefit of multivitamins; however, it is difficult to apply these results to a healthy population, as the study was performed on somewhat nutritionally-deprived people in rural China.[33]

The researchers also looked at specific nutrients in a group of over 3,000 people from the same population. They found no link (neither beneficial nor harmful) over the 5-year period between the risk of cataract and those who took selenium with beta-carotene and vitamin E, or those who took vitamin A and zinc, or those who took vitamin C and molybdenum. In contrast, in those who took vitamin B2 (5.2 mg) and vitamin B3 (40 mg) daily for 5 years had a 41% decrease in the risk of developing cataracts, compared to those who took placebo.[33]

● **Though the several large studies above found no link, one smaller study found a benefit: use of multi-vitamin with beta-carotene decreases the future risk of cataract over time** A combined British and U.S. study of nearly 300 people found a mild benefit of taking 18 mg beta-carotene, 750 mg vitamin C, and 600 IU of vitamin E each day in reducing the risk of cataract, compared to taking placebo. Interestingly, the results showed that the vitamins were more beneficial to those who lived in the U.S. as compared to those who lived in England, possibly because of genetic, environmental, or dietary differences.[34]

Body Absorption, Metabolism, & Excretion

Digestion of fruits and vegetables occurs in the stomach with the assistance of stomach acids that help break down the fruits and vegetables to release the carotenoids. The carotenoids are not soluble in water, and so they need to be dissolved in fat micelles (spherical soap-bubble-like conglomerates of fat) that can carry the carotenoids into the bloodstream from the intestines. Accordingly, eating a small quantity of fat with the carotenoids assists in the absorption of the carotenoids and greatly increases the amount that is delivered to the bloodstream.

Beta-carotene is split by enzymes into vitamin A. Much of this splitting occurs in the liver (see section on vitamin A).

Beta-carotene is also carried to the eye and can be converted into vitamin A in a regulated manner by the retinal pigment epithelium that nourishes the retina. A recent study has found the presence of enzymes in the retinal pigment epithelium that can convert beta-carotene into vitamin A. These enzymes in the eye can be carefully regulated by molecular mechanisms to ensure the appropriate levels of conversion occur. What this means is that while intake of high amounts vitamin A can cause toxicity in the eye, intake of high amounts of beta-carotene may not cause toxicity in the eye because the eye regulates the conversion of beta-carotene.

Excretion of vitamin A occurs mostly through the kidneys. Some excretion occurs through the digestive tract, whereby excess carotenoids are dumped back into the digestive tract through bile (a green fluid produced by the liver that is stored in the gallbladder to assist in digestion).

Deficiency

There are no known disorders of pure beta-carotene deficiency. Instead, the deficiency that ensues is from vitamin A deficiency (see section on vitamin A).

Toxicity & Side Effects

In and of itself, beta-carotene is not toxic in excess. Though beta-carotene is converted into vitamin A, excess beta-carotene does not result in excess vitamin A and vitamin A toxicity. Beta-carotene is metabolized by the liver in a regulated manner such that only the amount of vitamin A needed by the body is produced while excess beta-carotene is stored.

The storage of extra beta-carotene occurs in the skin and is commonly known to produce an orange discoloration of the palms and soles that sometimes mistaken for jaundice, though it is not jaundice. Jaundice can be distinguished from beta-carotene storage by the fact that beta-carotene storage does not occur in the whites of the eyes, while jaundice causes discoloration of the whites of the eyes as well. The beta-carotene discoloration is called carotenodermia or xanthosis cutis. It is harmless and can be reversed upon cessation of the supplementation.

High levels of beta-carotene and/or vitamin A supplementation may be associated with increased risk of lung cancer in both smokers and people with increased exposure to second-hand smoke. The effect is believed to be mediated by the consequences of high levels of vitamin A in the lung. Smoking and second-hand smoke, in the lung, can cause proliferation of cells (an increase in the number of cells) that react to the toxic effects of smoke. Vitamin A can exacerbate this proliferation within the lung, possibly resulting in cancer. A study of over 29,000 smokers, called the "Alpha Tocopherol (Vitamin E), Beta-carotene Cancer Prevention Study," showed that those smokers who took 20 mg per day beta-carotene supplement were nearly 20% more likely to develop lung cancer, compared to those smokers who did not take the beta-carotene supplement. Another study of over 18,000 smokers, called the "Beta-carotene and Retinol Efficacy Trial," also found that those smokers who took 30 mg per day of beta-carotene and 25,000 IU per day of vitamin A supplementation, were nearly 30% more likely to develop lung cancer, as compared to those who did not take the beta-carotene and vitamin A supplements. These numbers are staggering!

Smoking in itself creates high levels of oxidative stress and injury throughout the body. There is also evidence that vitamin A or beta-carotene supplementation also places smokers, and those who drink alcohol—whether moderately or excessively—at risk for other forms of cancer, such as colon cancer. However, there is conflicting evidence that these nutrients can be beneficial in smokers, especially when obtained from natural sources such as fruits and vegetables. Therefore, for anyone who smokes or is exposed to second hand smoke, it is best avoid high levels of beta-carotene and/or vitamin A supplementation. The best option, of course, is to avoid smoking or second-hand smoke altogether.

Interactions with Other Nutrients

It is important to note that beta-carotene can compete with lutein for absorption in the digestive tract, so that excess beta-carotene can result in lutein deficiency. While high amounts of beta-carotene can decrease lutein absorption, high amounts of lutein do not decrease beta-carotene absorption.

There is also suggestion that high levels of beta-carotene result in decreases in levels of vitamin E in the bloodstream.

Ideal Dosage

A daily consumption of 2 mg or less of beta-carotene is often enough to maintain sufficient vitamin A levels in the body. A more ideal dose of beta-carotene is 10 to 15 mg per day. In smokers, 20 mg per day is possibly unsafe. In non-smokers, dosages up to 300 mg per day have been reported safe, though it is recommended that a daily dosage not exceed 30 mg.

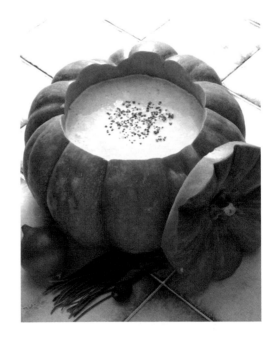

Sources (Where to Find It)

Vegetables:

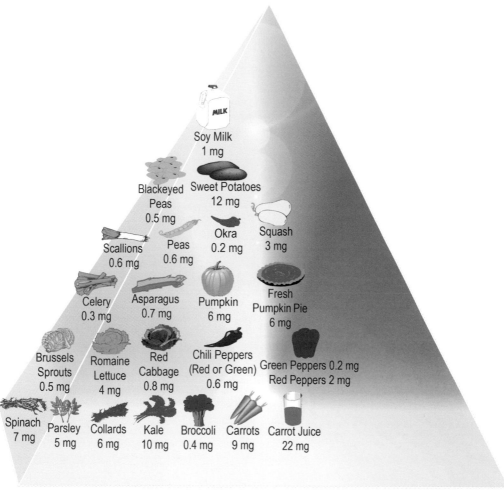

Soy Milk 1 mg
Blackeyed Peas 0.5 mg
Sweet Potatoes 12 mg
Squash 3 mg
Scallions 0.6 mg
Peas 0.6 mg
Okra 0.2 mg
Celery 0.3 mg
Asparagus 0.7 mg
Pumpkin 6 mg
Fresh Pumpkin Pie 6 mg
Brussels Sprouts 0.5 mg
Romaine Lettuce 4 mg
Red Cabbage 0.8 mg
Chili Peppers (Red or Green) 0.6 mg
Green Peppers 0.2 mg
Red Peppers 2 mg
Spinach 7 mg
Parsley 5 mg
Collards 6 mg
Kale 10 mg
Broccoli 0.4 mg
Carrots 9 mg
Carrot Juice 22 mg

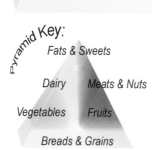

Pyramid Key:
Fats & Sweets
Dairy
Meats & Nuts
Vegetables
Fruits
Breads & Grains

Fruits:

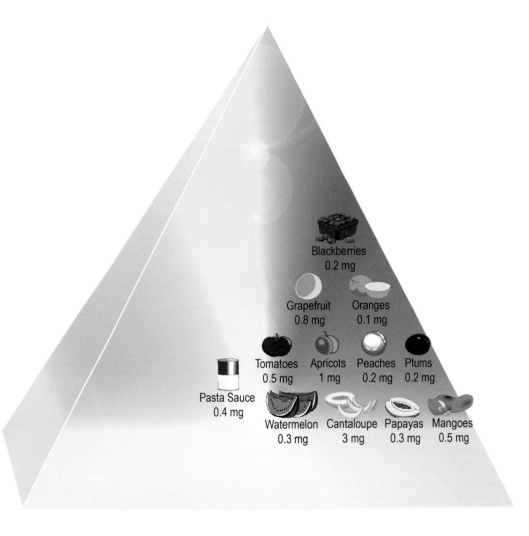

Blackberries
0.2 mg

Grapefruit   Oranges
0.8 mg   0.1 mg

Tomatoes   Apricots   Peaches   Plums
0.5 mg   1 mg   0.2 mg   0.2 mg

Pasta Sauce
0.4 mg
Watermelon   Cantaloupe   Papayas   Mangoes
0.3 mg   3 mg   0.3 mg   0.5 mg

Beta-carotene is found in fruits and vegetables, particularly those that are orange-colored. It is not found in meats as it cannot be made by animals.

Top sources include the orange-colored vegetables: sweet potato, pumpkin, and carrots. Some greens such as collards, kale, and spinach are particularly high in beta-carotene.

BIOFLAVONOIDS

Category

Bioflavonoids are ring shaped nutrients derived from plant sources.

Currently, there are about 5,000 identified bioflavonoids. Those that are most important to eye disease and health are listed in separate sections (see sections on quercetin, genistein, and the flavonoid glycoside component of ginkgo). Bioflavonoids can be divided into several categories including:

Flavonols: Rutin, Quercetin, Quercetrin, Kaempferol, Kaempferide, Myricetin, Myricitrin, Galangin, Spirenoside, Robinin, Rhamnetin, Isorhamnetin, Fisetin, Morin

Flavanols (Flavan-3-ols): Catechin, Gallocatechin, Epicatechin, Epigallocatechin, Epicatechin 3-gallate, Epigallocatechin 3-gallate, Theaflavin, Theaflavin 3-gallate, Theaflavin 3'-gallate, Theaflavin 3,3' digallate, Thearubigins

Flavones: Luteolin, Apigenin, Apigetrin, Tangeretin, Eupafolin, Eupatilin, Baicalein, Chrysin, Techtochrysin, Diosmin, Diosmetin, Hispidulin

Flavanones: Hesperetin, Neohesperidin, Naringenin, Naringin, Eriodictyol, Pinocembrin, Likvirtin, Liquiritin, Liquiritigenin, Eriocitrin, Poncirin, Isosakuranetin

Isoflavones: Genistein, Daidzein, Glycitein

Flavylium Salts (Anthocyanidins): Cyanidin, Delphinidin, Malvidin, Pelargonidin, Peonidin, Petunidin

Cellular Location

Bioflavonoids are a large group of nutrients, and since they are not required for cellular function, they are concentrated in the bloodstream and delivered to the tissues and organs that need their actions.

Structure

They are nutrients with ring shaped chemical structures that are in the group of chemicals called polyphenols.

Mechanisms of Action

Bioflavonoids are very powerful antioxidants. They also have various other actions, including anticancer, antimicrobial, anti-inflammatory, anti-allergic, and anti-clotting.

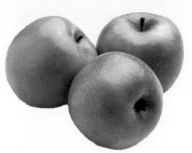

Biological & Ocular Importance

● Powerful antioxidants

Bioflavonoids have hydroxyl groups and double bonds in combination with ring groups that are very effective as antioxidants by donating electrons. They can also act as antioxidants by limiting the effects of enzymes that end up generating reactive oxygen species (toxic chemicals that result in oxidation).

In fact, some bioflavonoids are believed to be more potent antioxidants against lipid peroxidation than vitamin C or vitamin E! Lipids are the major component of cell membranes, and bioflavonoids can alter the membrane fluidics (the mobility of lipids in the membranes). By playing a role within cell membranes, bioflavonoids act as lipid antioxidants right at the target: lipids. By altering the membrane fluidics, they prevent membranes from becoming disrupted and subject to further oxidative stress. Furthermore, they alter the composition of the membranes preventing pro-oxidant components from increasing in proportion along with other harmful components. This alteration of membrane fluidics overall plays a beneficial role, such as prevention of cancer. It is believed that this increased membrane rigidity is beneficial to cells; however, it has yet to be determined if there is a harmful effect of increasing membrane rigidity, especially in cells that depend on the increased membrane fluidics.

● Additional antioxidant effect by binding metals

Bioflavonoids act as antioxidants by chelating (binding to) metals that are toxic or cause oxidative damage, such as iron, copper, cadmium, lead, and mercury. They can bind to these metals to prevent them from accepting electrons and acting as oxidants. They can also help remove these metals to prevent their toxicity. In fact, in nature, some of the most beautiful colors of flowers, such as the wide range of blues, are the result of bioflavonoids bound to metals that acting as pigments.

Additionally, by binding metals, some bioflavonoids become stronger antioxidants as a bioflavonoid-metal complex than the bioflavonoid by itself. In effect, these bioflavonoids are providing double the action! They are binding the metals to prevent the metal toxicity and also acting as stronger antioxidants (more effectively donating electrons to reduce oxidants).

● Protect the eye from oxidative damage

Bioflavonoids are believed to protect the retina from oxidative damage, thus decreasing the risk of many eye diseases, ranging from retinal diseases such as macular degeneration to glaucoma.

Similarly, the lens has high light exposure, as light is collected by the lens to be focused on the retina, and bioflavonoids are believed to play an antioxidant role in protecting the lens from cataract formation. There are several animal studies demonstrating the role of bioflavonoids in protecting the lens from oxidative damage and preventing cataracts. Furthermore, numerous bioflavonoids have been shown to reduce enzymes that are associated with cataract formation, particularly in diseases such as diabetes.

● Powerful anti-inflammatory & anti-allergic agents

Bioflavonoids can also act as anti-inflammatory and anti-allergic agents. Some bioflavonoids have been found to exhibit the ability to block enzymes involved in sending signals within cells. Some of these signals are involved in inflammation and allergic effects. The anti-inflammatory activity of bioflavonoids is believed to be due to inhibition of inflammatory pathways through blocking inflammatory enzymes, such as lipoxygenase and cyclo-oxygenase, popularly known as COX, the target of many new anti-inflammatory COX-inhibitor drugs. There is belief that inflammatory proteins may play a role in numerous eye diseases, ranging from retinal diseases to glaucoma to cataract.

● Prevent inflammation and leakage from blood vessel capillaries

Bioflavonoids strengthen blood vessel capillaries and prevent leakage of fluid leading to swelling in the retina as well as leakage of inflammatory proteins. Bioflavonoids may be beneficial in retinal disease in which new capillaries grow, such as wet macular degeneration, or in retinal diseases in which capillaries are broken and lead to leakage, such as macular edema or central serous chorio-retinopathy. There is no evidence of any beneficial effect of bioflavonoids in any of these conditions, though there is sufficient reason to believe that these nutrients can help decrease the inflammation and leakage in macular edema.

● Prevent or fights off infections

Bioflavonoids often act as plant phytoalexins, or products that function as antimicrobial agents by attacking viral or bacterial organisms. They may also act as plant phyto-anticipins, or chemicals that function in the day-to-day defense barrier mechanism of healthy plants. They can also function to inhibit enzymes involved in the formation of DNA by microbes, in the formation of energy by microbes, or in a microbe's cell wall protective function. For this reason, bioflavonoids have been used to prevent or fight off infections.

● **Used for cancer prevention**
Bioflavonoids are not required for cellular function and the body can survive without any bioflavonoids. However, there are numerous beneficial effects of bioflavonoids. In addition to their antioxidant effects, bioflavonoids have an anti-inflammatory and anti-allergic effect as well as an anti-cancer effect. Through these effects as well as inactivation of certain enzymes in the cell, bioflavonoids can act to prevent mutation of DNA. This DNA mutagenesis is thought to be a precursor of cancer. For this reason, bioflavonoids have been suggested as cancer prevention agents.

Isoflavones, particularly genistein, have estrogenic activity and can affect transcription factors (proteins that turn specific genes on or off). One such transcription factor that is blocked by genistein is known as CCAAT and blocking it can help starve cancer cells of nutrients that allow them to grow (see section on genistein).

● **Improve blood circulation**
Bioflavonoids can help decrease clotting of blood that interferes with blood circulation in the heart, brain, and eyes. Bioflavonoids are believed to block unhealthy platelet dysfunction that results from oxidative damage. They can also change platelet function through cell signaling pathways, possibly by interfering or altering enzymes or proteins involved in the processes. Furthermore, bioflavonoids can block inflammation and oxidation in vessels that eventually result in atherosclerosis (blood vessel cholesterol clots and plaques that can result in heart disease and stroke, as well as artery or vein clots in the retina or optic nerve strokes).

Many bioflavonoids have been found to improve retinal blood flow in animal models. As a matter of fact, in doing so, they have been shown to improve retinal function in disease.

Bioflavonoids can also relax smooth muscle involved in spasm. One theory of migraines is that smooth muscle spasm of blood vessels occurs, so there is thought that bioflavonoids can help in the treatment of migraines.

● **Prevent growth of abnormal blood vessels in the eye** Another vascular process that bioflavonoids help regulate is called angiogenesis (the formation of abnormal new blood vessels). Angiogenesis is particularly harmful in the retina, cornea, and trabecular meshwork (filtration site of the eye) and can cause loss of vision. The problems that result are called choroidal neovascularization (seen in wet macular degeneration), or retinal neovascularization (seen in severe diabetic retinopathy or retinal disease), or corneal neovascularization (seen in corneal injury or disease), or iris neovascularization (seen in angle-closure glaucoma and inflammatory eye disease). Bioflavonoids act to inhibit the expression of enzymes and cellular growth factors that stimulate new blood vessel growth, in order to prevent angiogenesis in the eye.

Human Studies on Utility

Currently, there are only a handful of human studies on bioflavonoid use in eye disease reported in the scientifically-reviewed medical literature. These studies are summarized below. Nevertheless, the fact that there are only few reported clinical studies does not necessarily imply a benefit or lack of benefit. Looking at the mechanism of action, the use of bioflavonoids in moderation may be possibly of benefit in many eye diseases.

● **The "French paradox" of lower heart disease**   The powerful activities of bioflavonoid are believed to explain why grape- and berry-derived drinks are known to have such a beneficial effect on the heart. In some regions in France, where consumption of cheese and high-fat foods is commonplace, one would expect soaring heart disease rates. However, the so-called "French paradox" is that in these areas, heart disease is actually lower! Some studies have suggested that it is likely due to their high consumption of grape- and berry-derived beverages. Grapes and berries have extremely high levels of bioflavonoids and other antioxidants.

● **In one small study: improves blood vessel capillaries in diabetes**   A small study of 25 people with diabetes found that blood vessel capillary fragility decreased with use of bioflavonoids.

● **In one small study: improves vision in retinal vein occlusions**   A study of over 50 people with vein occlusions in their retinas found that taking a bioflavonoid derivative of rutin

Looking at the mechanisms of action, there is good reason to use bioflavonoids in moderation for the health of the eye.

(called troxerutin) results in improved visual acuity, improved retinal vascular circulation, and decreased fluid build-up in the retina, as compared with those who did not take the bioflavonoid derivative.[35]

● **In one small study: no benefits from the use of bioflavonoids on the future risk of macular degeneration over time**   A small study of 71 people with macular degeneration found no benefit to the macular degeneration or to vision in those who, over 1½ years, took a daily antioxidant combination consisting of selected bioflavonoids along with beta-carotene (20,000 IU), vitamin B2 (25 mg), vitamin C (750 mg), vitamin E (200 IU), chromium (100 μg), taurine (100 mg), selenium (50 μg), N-acetyl cysteine (100 mg), zinc (12.5 mg), and glutathione (5 mg), when compared to placebo.[17] It is impossible, however, to ascertain the individual effect of bioflavonoids from this type of study.

● **In one study: past use of bioflavonoids associated with decreased risk of cataract**   A study of over 300 people age 55 or over found that the past use of higher quantities of tea, which contains high amounts of bioflavonoids, reduced the risk of having cataract by over 60%, and that the past use of vitamin E decreased the risk by nearly 50%.

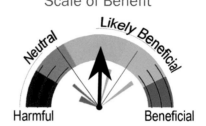

Bioflavonoids for Cataract
Scale of Benefit

However, there was no link (neither beneficial nor harmful) between the use of vitamin C and the risk of having cataracts.[36]

Body Absorption, Metabolism, & Excretion

Digestion of fruits, vegetables, herbs and other sources of bioflavonoids occurs in the stomach with the assistance of stomach acids that help break down the fruits, vegetables, and herbs to release the bioflavonoids. In the intestines, though, enzymes often further break down the bioflavonoids. Some bioflavonoids, particularly those bound to sugars, are absorbed in the small intestines, while most bioflavonoids pass to the large intestines where they are further broken down.

Overall, a small amount of the bioflavonoids are absorbed in the digestive tract and then into the bloodstream. The majority of bioflavonoids are not absorbed and remain in the digestive tract, where they are either broken down by enzymes or are excreted.

Of the bioflavonoids absorbed in the bloodstream, excretion occurs mostly through the kidneys.

Deficiency

There are no known disorders of bioflavonoid deficiency, as bioflavonoids are non-essential nutrients. Instead, any deficiency that ensues is often from a widespread nutritional deficiency.

Toxicity & Side Effects

There are no known toxicities associated with bioflavonoids since the body absorbs relatively little of the bioflavonoids in the digestive tract.

Nevertheless, there are some reports of nausea or headaches associated with excess intake of specific bioflavonoids.

Interactions with Other Nutrients

Bioflavonoids were initially called vitamin P ("P" for protection) based on a 1936 report of the role in protecting vitamin C. In fact, just as vitamin C can donate electrons to vitamin E to recycle the vitamin E, bioflavonoids can donate electrons to both vitamin C and E when they are used up and recycle them. In fact, some researchers suggest that a daily dosage of vitamin C should be associated with ingestion of about three-quarters of that amount of bioflavonoids.

Bioflavonoids act with vitamin E, vitamin C, glutathione, and alpha-lipoic acid to form a highly protective antioxidant team. Vitamin C and alpha-lipoic acid protect glutathione from being used up by donating electrons to the oxidized form of glutathione so that it can be reduced to usable glutathione that can act again as an antioxidant (see sections on vitamin C, alpha-lipoic acid, and glutathione).

Bioflavonoids and phytic acid can help stabilize levels of hyaluronic acid, a water-holding support compound of the eye (see section on hyaluronic acid).

Nutrients such as alpha-lipoic acid, phytic acid, and bioflavonoids chelate (bind and remove) metals, such as copper, aluminum, cadmium, lead, mercury, silver, zinc and iron. Therefore, excess of these nutrients can result in zinc deficiency or iron deficiency. Iron is essential for transport of oxygen in blood cells, and deficiency of iron results in anemia (insufficiency of the red blood cells that carry oxygen) (see sections on zinc and iron).

Ideal Dosage

There is no established ideal dosage since the bioflavonoids are non-essential and the body absorbs relatively little of the bioflavonoids in the digestive tract.

Sources (Where to Find It)

Fruits:

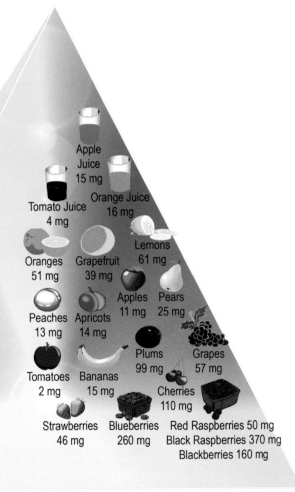

Apple Juice 15 mg
Orange Juice 16 mg
Tomato Juice 4 mg
Lemons 61 mg
Oranges 51 mg
Grapefruit 39 mg
Apples 11 mg
Pears 25 mg
Peaches 13 mg
Apricots 14 mg
Plums 99 mg
Grapes 57 mg
Tomatoes 2 mg
Bananas 15 mg
Cherries 110 mg
Strawberries 46 mg
Blueberries 260 mg
Red Raspberries 50 mg
Black Raspberries 370 mg
Blackberries 160 mg

Pyramid Key:
Fats & Sweets
Dairy   Meats & Nuts
Vegetables   Fruits
Breads & Grains

*See Guides on Pages 467-468.

Vegetables, Nuts, & Sweets:

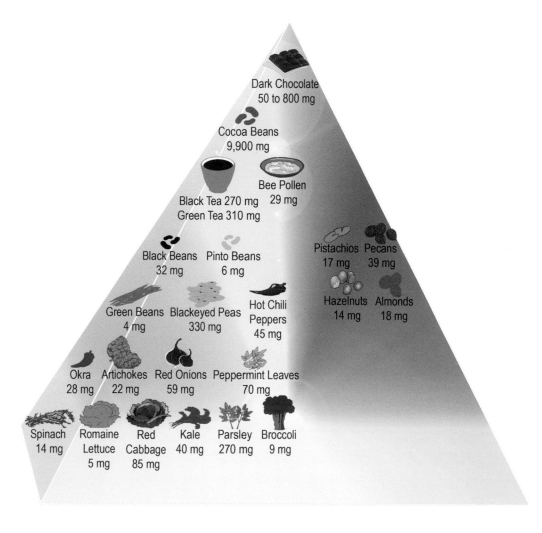

Dark Chocolate
50 to 800 mg

Cocoa Beans
9,900 mg

Bee Pollen
29 mg

Black Tea 270 mg
Green Tea 310 mg

Black Beans   Pinto Beans
32 mg   6 mg

Pistachios Pecans
17 mg   39 mg

Green Beans Blackeyed Peas   Hot Chili
4 mg   330 mg   Peppers
                              45 mg

Hazelnuts Almonds
14 mg   18 mg

Okra   Artichokes   Red Onions Peppermint Leaves
28 mg   22 mg   59 mg   70 mg

Spinach   Romaine   Red   Kale   Parsley   Broccoli
14 mg   Lettuce   Cabbage   40 mg   270 mg   9 mg
          5 mg   85 mg

   Top sources of bioflavonoids include berries, particularly black raspberries and blueberries and, to a lesser extent, blackberries and cherries. Plums are also moderately high sources.
   Other top sources include tea and cocoa beans, including certain cocoa-rich chocolates.
   Out of the vegetables, blackeyed peas, parsley, and red cabbage are good sources.

BORON

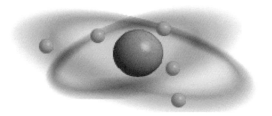

Category

Boron is an ultra-trace, semi-metallic element.

Cellular Location

Most of the boron found in the body is located in the bones, teeth, nails, and hair.

Structure

Boron is a metalloid, meaning that it is sometimes found as a metal and sometimes as a powder. Its symbol on the periodic table of elements is B, and its atomic number is 5. It is found next to carbon on the periodic table.

Mechanisms of Action

Boron works to enhance the activity of many enzymes in the body as well as enhance the availability of hormones. Some of its actions may be a result of its effects on cell membranes.

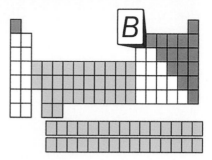

Biological & Ocular Importance

● **Maintains hormonal balance**   Boron is essential in hormonal balance, especially in the balance of estrogen in women and testosterone in men. It also helps increase levels of other hormones and steroids in the blood, and is often used by athletes as a dietary supplement.

● **Hormonal balance plays a role in preventing eye disease** Estrogen is important in raising the levels of high-density lipoproteins, also known as HDL (the good type of cholesterol). Balanced cholesterol helps prevent atherosclerosis (blood vessel cholesterol clots and plaques that can result in heart disease and stroke, as well as artery or vein clots in the retina or optic nerve strokes).

In addition, HDL is important in the transport of lutein and zeaxanthin to the retina, two essential carotenoids. In fact, in animal models, boron deficiency has been associated with abnormalities of the light-sensing photoreceptors of the retina.

Estrogen may also help prevent cataract formation.

● **Decrease the risk of macular degeneration** Women who develop menopause early have reduced estrogen levels and more often develop macular degeneration. Similarly, people who use a class of cholesterol lowering drugs, known as statins, have decreased HDL (the good type of cholesterol). With decreased HDL, these people may more often develop macular degeneration.

● **Maintains bone density** Boron helps in maintenance of bone density and prevention of arthritis by playing a role in many enzymes involved in the upkeep of bones.

● **Regulates of glucose and prevents of diabetes**   Boron is also believed to play a role in regulating glucose use. When glucose use is not regulated properly, diabetes may develop.

● **Decreases inflammation** Boron may also affect enzymes in inflammatory response, decreasing inflammation.

Human Studies on Utility

Currently, there are no human studies directly on boron use in eye disease reported in the scientifically-reviewed medical literature. Nevertheless, the fact that there are no reported clinical studies does not necessarily imply a benefit or lack of benefit. Looking at the mechanism of action, the use of boron in moderation may be possibly of benefit in certain eye diseases.

Body Absorption, Metabolism, & Excretion

Most of the ingested boron rapidly diffuses into the bloodstream. The kidneys filter out most of the excreted boron.

Deficiency

Boron deficiency is likely to cause subtle abnormalities in various areas of bodily function, including the eyes. In the past, boron was believed to be essential for animals, yet not as essential for humans; but now there is growing evidence of the role of boron in human cellular function.

Toxicity & Side Effects

Short-term excess of boron has been reported to cause severe lack of energy, as well as nausea, vomiting, and diarrhea.

Long-term excess of boron also has been associated with nausea and decreased appetite and weight loss. In addition, dry skin and seizures have been reported. Long-term excess of boron may also cause anemia (insufficiency of the red blood cells that carry oxygen). Some of the symptoms of anemia include fatigue, shortness of breath, increased heart rate, mouth sores or ulcers, tongue soreness, pale skin, and brittle nails.

Interactions with Other Nutrients

Excess boron has been shown to cause excess filtration of vitamin B2 out of the body by the kidneys.

Since boron is essential in balancing estrogen levels, and because estrogen levels help increase levels of hyaluronic acid, boron plays an important role in maintaining appropriate levels of hyaluronic acid. Hyaluronic acid is a water-holding support compound of the eye that is important for the health of the eye (see section on hyaluronic acid).

Ideal Dosage

A recommended daily allowance of boron is estimated to be around 3,000 μg. The average intake is 500 to 2,500 μg per day. Some suggest intakes up to 10,000 μg per day to be safe and beneficial, but a dose of 20,000 μg per day should not be exceeded.

Sources (Where to Find It)

Fruits & Vegetables:

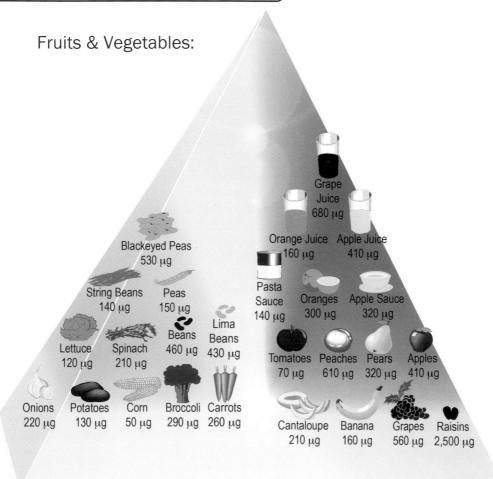

Grape Juice 680 μg

Orange Juice 160 μg   Apple Juice 410 μg

Blackeyed Peas 530 μg

String Beans 140 μg   Peas 150 μg

Pasta Sauce 140 μg   Oranges 300 μg   Apple Sauce 320 μg

Lima Beans 430 μg

Beans 460 μg

Lettuce 120 μg   Spinach 210 μg

Tomatoes 70 μg   Peaches 610 μg   Pears 320 μg   Apples 410 μg

Onions 220 μg   Potatoes 130 μg   Corn 50 μg   Broccoli 290 μg   Carrots 260 μg

Cantaloupe 210 μg   Banana 160 μg   Grapes 560 μg   Raisins 2,500 μg

Pyramid Key:

Fats & Sweets

Dairy   Meats & Nuts

Vegetables   Fruits

Breads & Grains

*See Guides on Pages 467-468.

Dairy, Meats, & Grains:

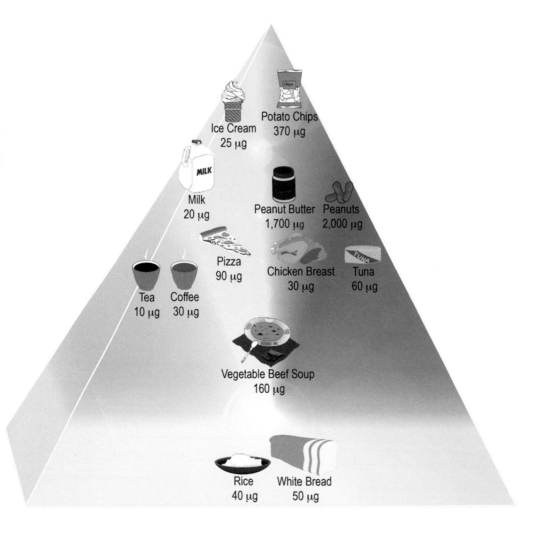

Ice Cream
25 µg

Potato Chips
370 µg

Milk
20 µg

Peanut Butter
1,700 µg

Peanuts
2,000 µg

Pizza
90 µg

Chicken Breast
30 µg

Tuna
60 µg

Tea
10 µg

Coffee
30 µg

Vegetable Beef Soup
160 µg

Rice
40 µg

White Bread
50 µg

Top sources of boron are raisins and peanuts. Other high sources of boron include apples, grapes, peaches, beans, broccoli, and carrots.

CALCIFEROL
(SEE VITAMIN D)

CALCITRIOL
(SEE VITAMIN D)

CARNITINE

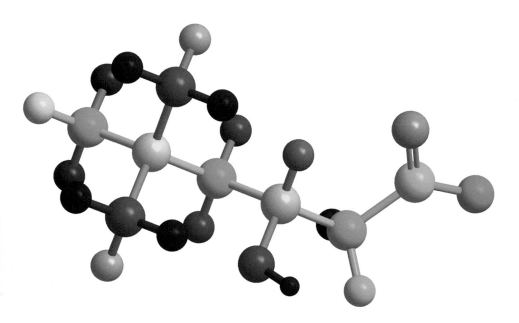

Category

Carnitine is a compound derived from lysine, an amino acid (building blocks of proteins). It is also known as beta-hydroxy-gamma-trimethylaminobutyric acid. It was originally called vitamin BT, for its original name, but it was discovered that carnitine was neither an essential nutrient, nor a vitamin.

Cellular Location

95% of all the body's carnitine is located in the heart and skeletal muscles. In the eye, carnitine levels are the highest in the lens.

Structure

Carnitine is an ammonium compound, as it contains nitrogen. Structurally, it bears some resemblance to an amino acid since it is derived from the amino acid lysine.

Mechanisms of Action

Carnitine often acts as a co-factor to help enzymes in cellular activities.

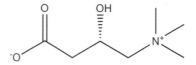

Biological & Ocular Importance

● **Helps cells produce energy**
Carnitine helps transport long-chain fatty acids, or fatty oils, into the mitochondria (the energy-producing organelles in the body's cells). These long-chain fatty acids act as fuel to produce energy inside cells.

When oxygen and sugar-energy levels are low, carnitine assists in producing more ATP, or energy packets that our cells use, by transporting these fatty acids into the mitochondria in order to form energy. This process of forming energy helps cells that are deprived of appropriate energy sources, such as when blood supply and oxygen become low in disorders of the retina like diabetic retinopathy.

Carnitine also helps remove the shorter-chain fatty acids out of the mitochondria.

● **Energy for muscle & heart function**   Carnitine, found in the highest concentrations in the body's muscles and heart, plays an important role in providing the appropriate amount of energy for muscle function and for heart function. Maintaining appropriate carnitine levels is thought to play a role in preventing heart attacks and heart failure. It is also thought to improve athletic performance as well.

● **Helps prevent oxidation & preserve cell membranes**
Carnitine can also help preserve membranes and repair membrane lipids that are damaged by excess oxidation. By doing so, it may enhance the antioxidant capabilities of our cells, either directly or indirectly, by sparing other antioxidants.

In the lens, carnitine has been shown to decrease the formation of advanced glycation end products, or AGEs, produced when glucose attacks proteins. Early cataracts, for example, may be a result of accumulation of AGEs in lens crystallin proteins.

● **Helps remove debris from behind retina**   Carnitine can assist in removal of lipofuscin from the body. Lipofuscin is a residue debris, which, in the presence of light and oxygen, results in the production of reactive oxygen species (toxic chemicals that result in oxidation). Thus, excess lipofuscin can result in oxidative damage to the retina. Of course light exposure is high in the retina, and the highest amount of oxygen consumption of any tissue in the body occurs in the retina. Therefore, the retina is particularly susceptible to oxidative damage.

Lipofuscin results from the accumulation of debris behind the rod and cone photoreceptors, in a layer of tissue called the retinal pigment epithelium. This layer of tissue serves to provide nutrition for the photoreceptors and to remove excess debris and waste from the photoreceptors. This debris and waste includes the discs of the photoreceptors, which are shed each day.

Digestion of debris is an important component of the action of the retinal pigment epithelium (the layer of cells behind the retina that serve to nourish the retina and remove the excess debris from the retina). Debris accumulation is one mechanism that retinal diseases, such as age-related macular degeneration and childhood-inherited retinal disease like Stargardt's disease (see hereditary retinal degenerations on page 13), unfortunately develop.

Human Studies on Utility

Currently, there is only one human study on carnitine use in eye disease reported in the scientifically-reviewed medical literature. However, there are several studies that show that carnitine can remove lipofuscin from the brain, but there are not any such studies in the retina. Nevertheless, the fact that there is only one reported clinical study does not necessarily imply a benefit or lack of benefit. Looking at the mechanism of action, the use of carnitine in moderation may be possibly of benefit in certain eye diseases.

● **One study found a benefit: use of carnitine improves vision over time in macular degeneration and decreases debris accumulation** A recent

Looking at the mechanisms of action, there is good reason to use carnitine in moderation for macular degeneration and several other retinal diseases.

study in Italy looked at over 100 people with early macular degeneration. The study divided participants into two groups: one that took a cocktail of 3 supplements, consisting of 200 mg of carnitine, 1060 mg of omega-3 oils, and 20 mg of coenzyme Q10 daily for one year, and another that took placebo. The study found that those who took the supplement cocktail were less likely to develop worsening of their macular degeneration, as assessed by visual acuity and visual fields. In fact, on average, people who took the supplement cocktail showed an improvement in vision, compared to the average decline in vision in those who did not take the supplement cocktail! This finding is quite remarkable in that it is rare for macular degeneration to improve! Furthermore, the study found that the amount of drusen (damaging debris) that accumulates behind the retina in macular degeneration, actually decreased in people who took the supplement cocktail in comparison to those who did not. In those who took the supplement cocktail, the amount of drusen *decreased* by an average of 15% to 23%, while, in those who took the placebo, the amount of drusen *increased* by an average of 11% to 13%. This improvement in drusen is also unheard of![37] The same authors found similar results in their earlier pilot study involving 14 people taking a somewhat higher dose cocktail consisting of 500 mg of carnitine, 1320 mg of omega-3 oils, and 30 mg of coenzyme Q10.[38]

Body Absorption, Metabolism, & Excretion

Carnitine is digested by the stomach with the help of stomach acids. Digestive enzymes from the pancreas further break down proteins, which are then absorbed into the bloodstream through the intestines. Afterward, carnitine is distributed to the muscles for use and storage.

A lot of the carnitine is filtered directly by the kidneys only to be recycled by the kidneys and sent back into the bloodstream.

When carnitine levels are low, the body can make its own carnitine. The liver and kidneys play a role in making carnitine.

As proteins are broken down, ammonia is formed. Since ammonia is extremely toxic to cells, it must be converted into a nitrogen-containing chemical known as urea. When ammonia builds up in excess, it can cause poor coordination, difficulties with balance, tremors, seizures, difficulty breathing, swelling of the brain, and can eventually lead to a coma. A normally functioning liver works to remove excess ammonia by creating urea, which is then filtered into the urine by the kidneys.

Deficiency

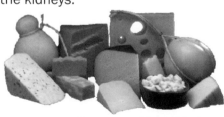

Deficiency of carnitine is rare, because the body can make its own carnitine. However, when carnitine levels are low, cells may not be able to produce energy as efficiently. As a result, symptoms may include fatigue, muscle weakness and muscle aches, heart disease with irregular heart beating, or neurologic disease with impaired sensation in arms and legs. In more severe cases, coma can occur.

Toxicity & Side Effects

There are reports of having a fishy body odor in those who intake doses of more than 3,000 mg per day.

Some reports suggest that high doses of carnitine can cause excess agitation in some people with Alzheimer's disease or cause increased seizures in some people with epilepsy (seizure disorder).

Excess carnitine, like other proteins, is often broken down and converted into sugars or fats, and either used for energy or stored as fat in the body's fat stores. Excess protein can stress the kidneys, stress the bloodstream, and cause dehydration. Furthermore, excess protein can cause the kidneys to lose calcium resulting in weakened bones. As with any protein, carnitine in excess in someone with liver disease or with kidney disease may result in build-up of ammonia or urea in the body, resulting in severe illness (see page 79).

In diabetics, excess amino acids can result in an increased sugar load on the body, or increased fat deposits in the body!

Interactions with Other Nutrients

Lysine is required in the pathway of making carnitine, as lysine forms the backbone of carnitine. Therefore, lysine deficiency may result in carnitine deficiency, though the carnitine deficiency that ensues is often only a minimal deficiency.

Vitamin C is also required in the process of making carnitine, as it plays an important role in two of the steps of formation of carnitine. Vitamin C deficiency results in a more severe carnitine deficiency. Vitamins B3 and B6 and iron also play roles in the pathway.

SAMe plays a role in providing methyl groups to methionine, an amino acid (building blocks of proteins), which follows a pathway into carnitine.

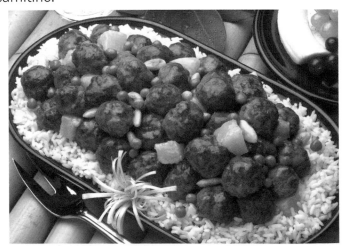

Ideal Dosage

A recommended daily dose of carnitine is 1,000 to 1,500 mg, but a dose of 200 to 500 mg per day may be sufficient. With higher doses, spreading the full amount into smaller doses over the course of the day is preferable to a single, larger dose.

Sources (Where to Find It)

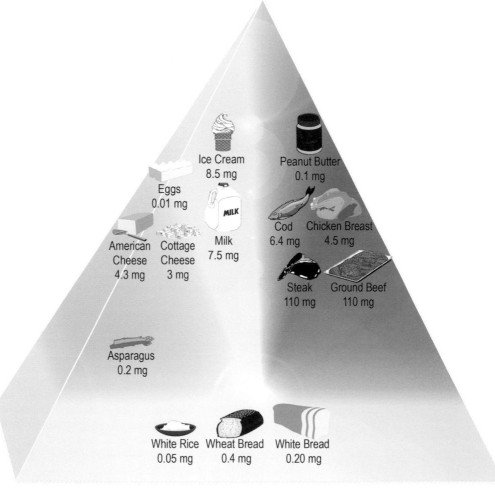

Ice Cream
8.5 mg

Peanut Butter
0.1 mg

Eggs
0.01 mg

MILK

Cod   Chicken Breast
6.4 mg   4.5 mg

American   Cottage   Milk
Cheese   Cheese   7.5 mg
4.3 mg   3 mg

Steak   Ground Beef
110 mg   110 mg

Asparagus
0.2 mg

White Rice   Wheat Bread   White Bread
0.05 mg   0.4 mg   0.20 mg

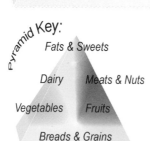

Pyramid Key:
Fats & Sweets

Dairy   Meats & Nuts

Vegetables   Fruits

Breads & Grains

The top source of carnitine is meat, particularly steak and ground beef. Chicken contains smaller amounts of carnitine. Dairy products such as milk and cheese also contain smaller amounts of carnitine.

*See Guides on Pages 467-468.

CAROTENOIDS

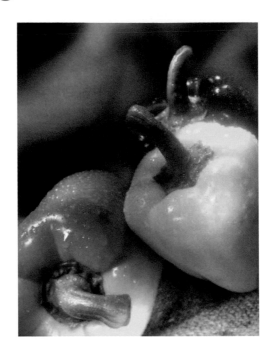

Category

Carotenoids are organic pigments that occur naturally in plants, algae, and some photosynthetic bacteria. However, they cannot be made by animals. Many hundred carotenoids are known. They include: alpha-carotene, beta-carotene, beta-cryptoxanthin, lycopene, lutein, and zeaxanthin, which are the most important known carotenoids in the human diet.

They play an essential role in the energy transfer process during plant photosynthesis and protect the photosynthetic reaction center from excess oxidation. They are long-chain carbon compounds often with rings on the end. This long chain with double bonds gives these pigments their color, by absorbing light of various wavelengths. The yellow carotenoids are lutein and zeaxanthin, both also known as xanthophylls (see sections on lutein and on zeaxanthin). Beta-carotene and alpha-carotene are yellow-to-orange carotenoids, beta-cryptoxanthin is a darker orange-to-red carotenoid, and lycopene is a red carotenoid, and these groups of carotenoids are known as carotenes, as opposed to the xanthophylls.

Beta-carotene, alpha-carotene, and beta-cryptoxanthin are the carotenes that are able to be converted by the body into vitamin A (for details on mechanisms of action, biological and ocular activities, and dietary sources and recommendations, see sections on vitamin A, beta-carotene, lutein, lycopene, and zeaxanthin).

Human Studies on Utility

Many reports on carotenoids study the particular carotenoids individually rather than as a group. These reports are discussed in this book according to the particular carotenoids used.

Some reports discuss carotenoids as a group, rather than individually. These are reported in this chapter.

 Summary of Studies for Macular Degeneration: Over a half-dozen clinical trials have been performed looking at the role of carotenoids in both preventing and treating macular degeneration. These clinical trials are of various types, some of which are very well-designed and well-performed studies.

As a whole, the clinical studies provide no definitive answer as to whether carotenoids are beneficial. Some of the studies found no benefit while others found a benefit to carotenoids for macular

Carotenoids for
Macular Degeneration
Scale of Benefit

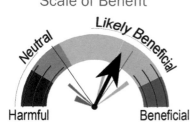

degeneration. Looking at the mechanisms of action, there is good reason to use carotenoids in moderation for macular degeneration.

The studies can be summarized as follows: one large, well-performed study found no benefits from the past use of carotenoids on the risk of macular degeneration, while one large, well-performed study did find a benefit in the past use of carotenoids in decreasing the risk of macular degeneration. Several smaller studies have found no link (neither protective nor harmful) between levels of carotenoids in the blood and macular degeneration, though one study found that higher levels of carotenoids in the blood are associated with a decrease in the risk of macular degeneration.

In following people over time, two large well-performed studies found that those who took carotenoids did not have any benefit in preventing macular degeneration compared to those who did not take carotenoids.

● **In one large study: no benefits in past use of carotenoids found on risk of macular degeneration**
Looking at a group of nearly 2,000 people from a study population of nearly 5,000 people, researchers found no link (neither protective nor harmful) between the risk of developing macular degeneration and a diet high in carotenoids, vitamin C, or vitamin E. However, they did find a decreased risk of early-stage macular degeneration

for those who consumed diets high in zinc.[3]

● **Another large study found a benefit: past use of carotenoids associated with decreased risk of macular degeneration**

Looking at the mechanisms of action, there is good reason to use carotenoids in moderation for macular degeneration and cataract.

A study of over 1,000 people age 55 to 80 found that those who consumed a diet high in carotenoids had a greater than 40% decrease in the risk of having wet macular degeneration compared to those who did not consume a diet high in carotenoids. Similarly, dietary beta-carotene decreased the risk by 40% and dietary vitamin A decreased the risk by over 40%, while dietary lutein and zeaxanthin decreased the risk by nearly 60%. The authors found no link (neither protective nor harmful) between macular degeneration and a diet high in vitamin C or E.[5]

● **In several studies: no link between blood levels of carotenoids and macular degeneration** A study of over 300 people from a group of nearly 5,000 people found no difference in the blood levels of beta-carotene, lycopene, or lutein and zeaxanthin between those with or without macular degeneration. They also found that those who had macular degeneration had lower blood levels of vitamin E compared to those without macular degeneration. Interestingly, they also found that fewer people with macular degeneration use vitamin

C than people without macular degeneration.[7]

Another study of nearly 100 people found no difference in the blood levels of beta-carotene, carotenoids, lutein and zeaxanthin, lycopene, vitamin A, vitamin C, zinc, or selenium between those with or without macular degeneration (looking at both early and severe or advanced macular degeneration). However, the study found that those who had severe or advanced macular degeneration had lower blood levels of vitamin E compared to those without macular degeneration. They found no differences in the blood levels of vitamin E between those with or without early macular degeneration.[6]

A study of over 100 people, found no difference in the blood levels of carotenoids, vitamin A, vitamin C, vitamin E, or selenium between those with or without macular degeneration. However, the study did find that those who had macular degeneration had lower blood levels of zinc compared to those without macular degeneration.[39]

● **Though the several studies above found no link, one large study found a benefit: decreased risk of macular degeneration in those with**

higher blood levels of carotenoids   A study of over 1,000 people age 55 to 80 found that having higher blood levels of carotenoids decreased the risk of having wet macular degeneration by 60% compared to those who had lower blood levels of carotenoids.[11] Looking at specific carotenoids, the study found that having higher blood levels of beta-carotene decreased the risk of having macular degeneration by 70%. Higher blood levels of lutein and zeaxanthin also decreased the risk by 70% and higher blood levels of lycopene decreased the risk by 60%. Also, higher blood levels of a combination of three or more of four nutrients (carotenoids, vitamin C, vitamin E, and selenium) decreased the risk by 70%. The study found no link (neither protective nor harmful) between higher blood levels of vitamin C, vitamin E, or selenium by themselves and macular degeneration.[12]

● **In two large studies: no benefits from the use of carotenoids on the future risk of macular degeneration over time**   Looking over a 5-year period, a study of 2,000 people from a group of nearly 5,000, found no link (neither protective nor harmful) between macular degeneration and a diet high in carotenoids, beta-carotene, lutein and zeaxanthin, vitamin C, vitamin E, or zinc.[14]

A study of over 75,000 people (nurses and health professionals) followed over time for up to 18 years found no link (neither protective nor harmful) between the risk of developing macular degeneration (wet or dry) and a diet high in any of the following nutrients: carotenoids, lutein and zeaxanthin, beta-carotene, lycopene, vitamin A, vitamin C, or vitamin E. The study did find that those who consumed more than 3 servings of fruit each day were 1/3 less likely to develop *wet* macular degeneration over time compared to those who consumed less than 1½ servings of fruit each day. No link (neither protective nor harmful) was found when looking at increased fruit consumption for dry macular degeneration, nor when looking at increased vegetable consumption for dry or wet macular degeneration.[15]

Summary of Studies for Cataract: 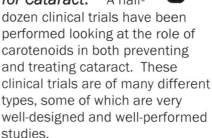 A half-dozen clinical trials have been performed looking at the role of carotenoids in both preventing and treating cataract. These clinical trials are of many different types, some of which are very well-designed and well-performed studies.

As a whole, the clinical studies provide no definitive answer as to whether carotenoids are beneficial, though the majority of the studies found a

Carotenoids for
Cataract
Scale of Benefit

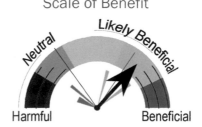

benefit to carotenoids for cataract. Furthermore, looking at the mechanism of action, there is good reason to use carotenoids in moderation for cataract.

The studies can be summarized as follows: two studies found no benefits from the past use of carotenoids on the risk of having cataract, while one study did find a benefit in the past use of beta-carotene in decreasing the risk of cataract. Two additional studies found that higher levels of beta-carotene in the blood are associated with a decrease in the risk of cataract.

In following people over time, one large study found a diet high in carotenoids decreased the risk of developing cataracts.

● In two studies: no benefits in past use of carotenoids found on risk of cataract

A study of nearly 500 people age 53 to 73 found no link (neither protective nor harmful) between the intake of carotenoids, beta-carotene, lutein and zeaxanthin, or lycopene and the risk of having cataracts. However, the study did show that the past intake of *higher* amounts of vitamin C decreased the risk of having cataracts by nearly 70%. It also found that long-term intake of vitamin C for over 10 years decreased the risk of having cataracts by nearly 65%. Similarly, past intake of *higher* amounts of vitamin B2 decreased the risk of having cataracts by over 60%, and past intake of *higher* amounts of folate decreased the risk by about 10%. It also found that long-term intake of vitamin E for over 10

years decreased the risk of having cataracts by over 50%, even though the study found no link (neither protective nor harmful) between the past intake of *higher* amounts of vitamin E and the risk of having cataracts. The finding of no beneficial link with higher doses of vitamin E may be related to increased risks associated with the higher doses. Furthermore, the use of a multivitamin for over 10 years reduced the risk of having cataract by over 40%.[20]

A study of over 100 people age 40 to 70 found no link (neither beneficial nor harmful) between cataract and the past use of carotenoids or vitamin E. However, the past use of vitamin C in high amounts decreased the risk of having cataract by 75%. This study also found that a diet with at least 3½ servings of fruits and vegetables each day reduced risk of having cataracts by over 80%![40]

● Though the two studies above found no link, two studies found a benefit: past use of carotenoids associated with decreased risk of cataract

A study of 300 women age 56 to 71 from a group of over 120,000 people found that in non-smokers, the past use of beta-carotene in higher doses reduced the risk of having cataracts by over 70%. In fact, carotenoids, as a group, in higher doses reduced the risk of having cataracts by over 80%. The study also found that folate in higher doses reduced the risk of having cataracts by nearly 75%. In addition, past use of higher doses of vitamin C decreased the risk of having cataract by nearly 60% and the use of vitamin C for over 10 years decreased the risk by 60%. However, the study found no link (neither protective nor harmful) between the use of vitamin E or B2 and cataract.[23]

● Two studies found a benefit: decreased risk of cataract in those with higher blood levels of carotenoids

A study of 165 people found that those who had cataracts had lower levels of carotenoids and vitamin D in their blood compared to those who did not have cataracts. However, the study found no link (neither beneficial nor harmful) between cataracts and vitamin A, vitamin E, zinc, copper, and magnesium levels in the blood. On the other hand, the study found that those who had cataracts had higher levels of selenium in their blood.[41]

A study of over 100 people age 40 to 70 found that higher blood levels of carotenoids decreased risk of having cataracts by over 80%. Similarly, higher blood levels of vitamin C decreased risk of having certain types of cataracts.[40]

● One large study found a benefit: use of carotenoids decreases the future risk of cataract over time

Looking over an 8-year period into the future, a year study of over 50,000 women from a group of over 120,000 participants age 45 to 67 found that a diet with higher amounts of carotenoids decreased the risk of developing cataracts by over 25%. Similarly, a diet with higher amounts of vitamin A decreased the risk by nearly 40%. No such links (neither beneficial nor harmful) were found between diets high in vitamin B2, vitamin C, or vitamin E and cataract. However, the study did find that the duration of vitamin C intake mattered. Those who consumed vitamin C supplements for 10 or more years had a 45% decreased chance of developing cataracts.[42]

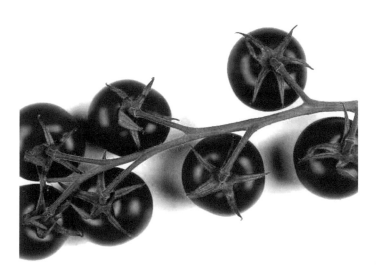

CHOLINE
(CITICHOLINE)

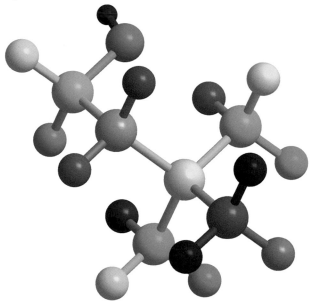

Category

Choline is an amine type of chemical compound and considered an essential nutrient.

Citicholine is a form of choline that, as a nutrient, can more easily travel from the bloodstream to the retina and brain. Citicholine is also known as CDP-choline, and its chemical name is cytidine-5'-diphosphocholine. It acts to increase cellular levels of choline and of cell membrane components, called phospholipids (unique fatty compounds, see page 228), composed of choline. Phosphatidyl-choline is a phospholipid membrane molecule that contains choline.

Cellular Location

Most of the body's choline is found in the membrane fat components, called phospholipids.

Structure

Choline is a relatively simple nutrient, consisting of an amine, which is an organic compound that contains nitrogen and bears a resemblance to ammonia.

Mechanisms of Action

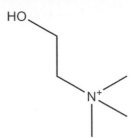

Choline works as a cell membrane component as well as making other chemical signaling agents.

Biological & Ocular Importance

● Forms signaling molecules
Choline is used to make acetylcholine, which is formed from choline and vitamin B5 (pantothenic acid). Acetylcholine is a neurotransmitter, or a communication signal that is used to send messages between neurons or brain cells. It acts as a neurotransmitter in the retina.

Choline also forms other chemicals that act as cell signaling molecules that send signals to different areas within a single cell. These cell signaling molecules play many roles in the health and activities of the cell.

● Improves memory
Animal studies have suggested that choline can help improve memory as well as learning, by increasing the rate of synthesis, or creation, of neurotransmitters.

● Present in nerve-endings in the cornea
Because the cornea is the most highly innervated tissue of the body, having more nerve ends than any other part of the body, the surface of the cornea has a very high concentration of acetylcholine and the acetylcholine-producing enzyme choline acetyltransferase.

● Protects against over-stimulation in the retina
Higher levels of acetylcholine may protect against over-stimulation of neural cells such as the cells of the retina and optic nerve. The over-stimulation is a process called excitotoxicity and can cause degeneration and death of the neural cells.

● Helps form & protect retinal cell membranes
Choline is also involved in the creation of cell membrane components, called phospholipids, and can help protect neurons whose cell membranes have been damaged. In the retina, choline serves as a membrane phospholipid component.

Photoreceptor cells are believed to accumulate high amounts of choline for use in their membranes, as each photoreceptor cell has a high amount of membrane that forms its discs and the turnover of these disc membranes is high (see introduction).

- **Involved in cholesterol transport**   Choline also plays an important role in the fat and cholesterol transporters, called chylomicrons, which are composed of proteins and fats and require phospholipids.

- **Decreases vessel-damaging toxin homocysteine**   Choline also forms a chemical called betaine in the body, and betaine works in the liver to convert homocysteine to methionine, in order to decrease levels of homocysteine in the body. Homocysteine is an amino acid (protein building block) known to cause atherosclerosis (blood vessel cholesterol clots and plaques that can result in heart disease and stroke, as well as artery or vein clots in the retina or optic nerve strokes). Homocysteine can cause damage by signaling stress in the protein building organelles and causes proteins to be misfolded. Elevated levels of homocysteine are associated with vascular disease including blood clots, heart disease, stroke, and vein occlusions in the retina, as well as Alzheimer's disease.

- **Helps kidneys maintain water balance**   The chemical betaine formed from choline also helps the kidney maintain water balance. Improper water balance can cause fluid build-up and swelling in different parts of the body.

Human Studies on Utility

Currently, there are only a handful of human studies on choline use in eye disease reported in the scientifically-reviewed medical literature. These studies involve the eye disease, glaucoma, and are summarized below. Of note, the studies involve only small numbers of people, so the benefits found may be found by chance, and it is difficult to assess the broad applicability of the findings.

- **Four small studies suggest possible benefit in glaucoma**
A recent 2003 study of 11 people with glaucoma looked at the effect of citicholine (1 g of citicholine each day for 2 weeks, followed by a 2-week break, then again 2 weeks of citicholine, followed by a 2-week break) on the functioning of the optic nerve. The study found that the signals sent through the optic nerve to the brain were quicker and stronger following the treatment than before the treatment.[43] The findings were very interesting, yet there was no control group to compare.

Another study of 40 people with glaucoma found that compared to placebo, citicholine (1 g daily for a 60-day period followed by a 120-day break, then again 1 g daily for a 60-day period followed by a 120-day break) over a 1-year period improved retinal function, as measured by electrical signals generated by the retina. The study also found that the signals sent through the optic nerve to the brain were quicker and stronger in the group receiving citicholine compared to the group receiving placebo.[44]

A study of 30 people found that taking citicholine 1 g per day for 10 days resulted in improved visual field testing. These findings are also interesting, but again there was no control group to compare, raising the possibility that the same effect may have been found if people were given a placebo. There is also concern that the effect may not be related to an improvement in eye functioning but rather another type of effect, such as improved attention.[45]

Finally, another study of 23 people with glaucoma found that taking citicholine (1 g daily for a 15-day period once every 6 months) over a period of 10 years prevented visual fields deterioration and retinal sensitivity worsening, as compared with receiving no citicholine over 10 years.[46]

Body Absorption, Metabolism, & Excretion

While the human body can make its own choline, it is not enough and most of the choline used by the body comes from the diet. In the digestive tract, choline is broken down into cytidine and choline, and then absorbed into the bloodstream. Excretion of choline occurs mostly through the kidneys.

Deficiency

Choline deficiency is uncommon, but is more prevalent in strict vegans who avoid dairy products such as milk and eggs.

Because choline also plays an important role in the fat and cholesterol transporters, called chylomicrons, deficiency of choline results in low amounts of the fat and cholesterol transporters. As a result, fats start to accumulate in the liver, causing a disease called fatty liver. There are also reports that choline deficiency is associated with an increase in liver cancer in animals.

Muscle damage is also known to occur in choline deficiency.

Toxicity & Side Effects

Choline in excess can cause dizziness or lightheadedness from lowered blood pressure. In extremely high doses, it can cause sweating, salivation, and vomiting.

High doses of choline can also affect liver function.

There are reports that excess choline can cause a fishy body odor.

Some preparations of choline have been associated with body itching as well as ringing in the ears.

Interactions with Other Nutrients

In the process of creating phospholipids, choline requires the assistance of nutrients, such as SAMe, to provide chemical methyl groups.

Betaine, the chemical that helps reduce the vessel-damaging toxin homocysteine (see above), is found in vegetables such as beets. Increased dietary intake of betaine allows choline to be more available for the beneficial choline activities. This increased availability may be because when betaine is low, the body converts some of the dietary choline to use as betaine.

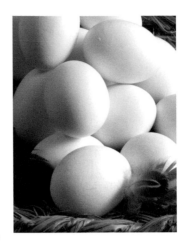

Ideal Dosage

A minimum intake of 425 to 550 mg per day has been recommended. For boys and men over the age of 13, a minimum intake of 550 mg per day has been recommended, and for women over the age of 18, a minimum intake of 425 mg per day has been recommended. For girls age 14 to 18 and for pregnant women, the minimum recommendation increases to 450 mg per day, and for lactating women, it increases to 550 mg per day. A dose of 1,000 mg per day may be considered a reasonable balanced recommendation. The upper limit of what is considered safe is 3,500 mg per day.

Supplements that contain phosphatidyl-choline, a phospholipid membrane molecule, provide about 13% choline. So 1,000 mg of phosphatidyl-choline provides 130 mg of choline. Supplements that contain lecithin contain phosphatidyl-choline, though anywhere from one-quarter to 90% of the lecithin is phosphatidyl-choline. Thus, 1,000 mg of lecithin provides between 30 to 120 mg of choline.

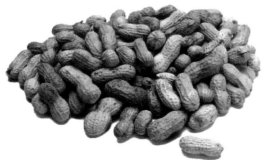

Fruits & Vegetables:

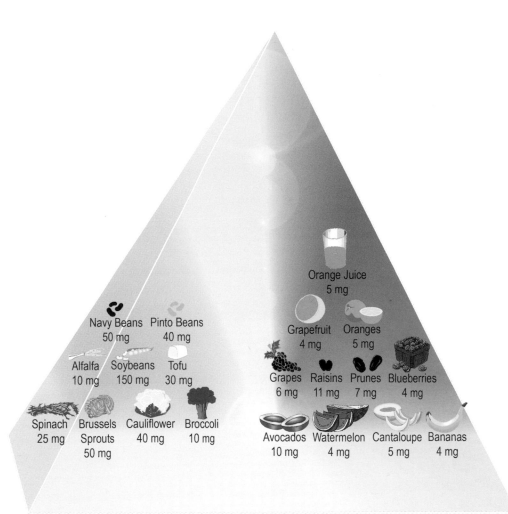

Navy Beans
50 mg

Pinto Beans
40 mg

Alfalfa
10 mg

Soybeans
150 mg

Tofu
30 mg

Spinach
25 mg

Brussels
Sprouts
50 mg

Cauliflower
40 mg

Broccoli
10 mg

Orange Juice
5 mg

Grapefruit
4 mg

Oranges
5 mg

Grapes
6 mg

Raisins
11 mg

Prunes
7 mg

Blueberries
4 mg

Avocados
10 mg

Watermelon
4 mg

Cantaloupe
5 mg

Bananas
4 mg

Pyramid Key:

Fats & Sweets

Dairy   Meats & Nuts

Vegetables   Fruits

Breads & Grains

*See Guides on Pages 467-468.

Dairy, Meats & Grains:

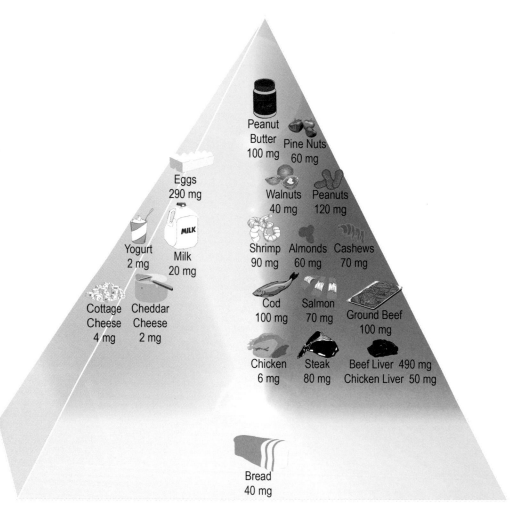

Eggs 290 mg

Peanut Butter 100 mg

Pine Nuts 60 mg

Walnuts 40 mg

Peanuts 120 mg

Yogurt 2 mg

Milk 20 mg

Shrimp 90 mg

Almonds 60 mg

Cashews 70 mg

Cottage Cheese 4 mg

Cheddar Cheese 2 mg

Cod 100 mg

Salmon 70 mg

Ground Beef 100 mg

Chicken 6 mg

Steak 80 mg

Beef Liver 490 mg

Chicken Liver 50 mg

Bread 40 mg

Top sources of choline include meats, fish, and nuts. Beef liver and eggs are particularly high sources of choline. Among the vegetables, soybeans are a top source. Other high sources include beans, Brussels sprouts, and cauliflower.

CHROMIUM

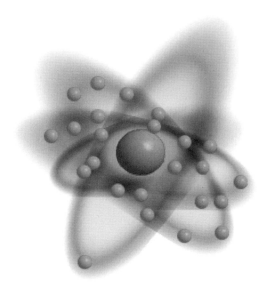

Category

Chromium is an essential element.

Cellular Location

Chromium is found in its highest concentrations in the kidneys, followed by the spleen, liver, lungs, heart, skeletal muscles, pancreas, and bones.

Structure

Chromium is a metallic element. Its symbol on the periodic table of elements is Cr, and its atomic number is 24. It is found between vanadium and manganese on the periodic table.

Mechanisms of Action

Little is known about the mechanisms of action of chromium. It is believed to interact with proteins that activate cell signaling messengers on the surface of cells. These cell signaling messengers then act inside cells to stimulate cellular pathways, such as pathways involved in insulin activity.

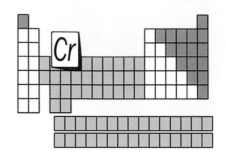

Biological & Ocular Importance

● **Regulates of insulin & handling of blood sugars**
Chromium is believed to play an important role in conjunction with insulin in regulating the use of glucose by cells. As such, some small studies have shown a benefit of chromium in preventing diabetes or in helping diabetics better handle sugars. However, there is much controversy regarding such claims, and the FDA in 2005 advised against claims that chromium may be beneficial in diabetes.

Chromium may also play a role in weight loss and balancing cholesterol levels as well.

● **Removes debris from behind the retina** One study has shown that, in the presence of methionine, chromium can assist in removal of lipofuscin from the body. Lipofuscin is a residue debris, which in the presence of light and oxygen results in the production of reactive oxygen species (toxic chemicals that result in oxidation). Therefore, excess lipofuscin can result in oxidative damage to the retina. Of course light exposure is high in the retina, and the highest amount of oxygen consumption of any tissue in the body occurs in the retina. Thus, the retina is particularly susceptible to oxidative damage. Lipofuscin results from the accumulation of debris from shedding of the discs of photoreceptors in a layer of tissue called the retinal pigment epithelium (the layer of cells behind the retina that serve to nourish the retina and remove excess debris from the retina).

Digestion of debris is an important component of the action of the retinal pigment epithelium. Debris accumulation is one mechanism that causes retinal disease, such as age-related macular degeneration and childhood inherited retinal disease like Stargardt's disease (see page 13), to develop.

Human Studies on Utility

Currently, there is only one human study on chromium use in eye disease reported in the scientifically-reviewed medical literature. This study involves macular degeneration. Nevertheless, the fact that there is only one reported clinical study does not necessarily imply a benefit or lack of benefit. Looking at the mechanism of action, the use of chromium in moderation may be possibly of benefit in certain eye diseases.

● In one small study: no benefits from the use of chromium with other antioxidants on the future risk of macular degeneration over time   A small study of 71 people with macular degeneration found no benefit to the macular degeneration or to vision in those who took a daily antioxidant combination, for over 1½ years, that consisted of chromium (100 µg), beta-carotene (20,000 IU), vitamin B2 (25 mg), vitamin C (750 mg), vitamin E (200 IU), selenium (50 µg), zinc (12.5 mg), taurine (100 mg), N-acetyl cysteine (100 mg), glutathione (5 mg), and selected bioflavonoids, in comparison to taking placebo.[17] It is impossible, however, to ascertain the individual effect of chromium from this type of study.

Body Absorption, Metabolism, & Excretion

About 99% of the chromium intake is not absorbed and is excreted in the digestive tract. The 1% that is absorbed goes into the bloodstream and is sent by protein carriers to various organs. It is thought that there are certain binding agents in our diets that bind chromium in the stomach in order to deliver it to the intestines for absorption and to prevent it from precipitating (forming solid chunks that are incapable of being absorbed by the intestines). Vitamin C may also help in the process of chromium absorption.

Some grain products and vegetables actually increase the precipitation of chromium in the stomach, thus preventing its absorption.

Most of the chromium is excreted directly into the digestive tract, while the chromium that goes into the bloodstream is used by the body and is filtered out by the kidneys and excreted in the urine.

Deficiency

Historically, chromium was recognized as an essential nutrient when people who consumed chromium-deficient diets began to develop diabetes. It was found that the diabetes that develops with chromium deficiency was reversed with appropriate chromium intake.

Chromium deficiency is also associated with abnormal growth and increased fat.

A greater loss of chromium in the urine is often associated with stress as well.

With respect to the eye, some animal studies have shown that a diet deficient in chromium, particularly when associated with low protein intake as well, results in scarring of the cornea that does not reverse with improved chromium intake. There is also some suggestion that chromium deficiency can affect the eye pressure.

Toxicity & Side Effects

It is believed that chromium in its dietary trivalent form is quite safe, even at high doses. There is very little known toxicity that has been reported, though there are a couple of reports of kidney failure, one of which occurred with liver failure. These reports suggest the kidney failure occurred after ingesting doses of 600 µg or more on a daily basis for several weeks.

Although dietary chromium is in the trivalent form, there are other forms of chromium. Chromium in its form with 6 less electrons is called hexavalent chromium, which is extremely toxic at any dose. Hexavalent chromium can cause skin irritation as well as severe eye irritation. In fact, a half teaspoon of hexavalent chromium is lethal. Its ingestion is associated with gastrointestinal bleeding and liver and kidney failure. Breathing of hexavalent chromium is associated with severe lung disease. It is also a carcinogen (a cancer-causing chemical). Hexavalent chromium was made popular in a movie portraying a cover up of industrial poisoning of a town's drinking water.

Interactions with Other Nutrients

Excess iron may prevent the normal transport of chromium whereas vitamin C may help in the process of chromium absorption (see above).

Ideal Dosage

The minimum recommended intake of chromium is 25 to 30 µg per day, and many researchers believe that doses in the range of 50 to 100 µg per day are ideal. The National Academy of Sciences has established a range of 50 to 200 µg to be adequate and safe.

Additionally, there is some suggestion that diabetics may often need more chromium each day, but these dosages should be carefully worked out with an internist or endocrinologist in order to prevent serious glucose imbalances and comas.

Sources (Where to Find It)

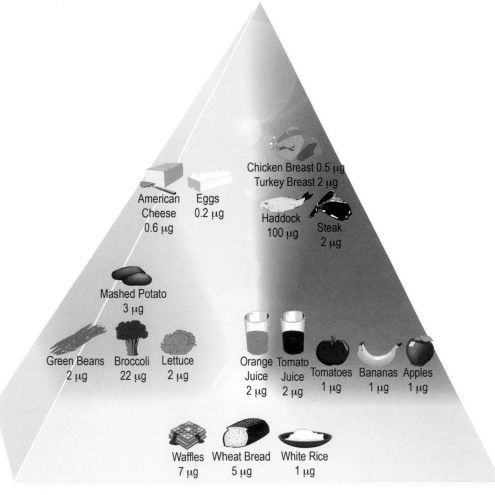

Chicken Breast 0.5 µg
Turkey Breast 2 µg

American Cheese 0.6 µg

Eggs 0.2 µg

Haddock 100 µg

Steak 2 µg

Mashed Potato 3 µg

Green Beans 2 µg

Broccoli 22 µg

Lettuce 2 µg

Orange Juice 2 µg

Tomato Juice 2 µg

Tomatoes 1 µg

Bananas 1 µg

Apples 1 µg

Waffles 7 µg

Wheat Bread 5 µg

White Rice 1 µg

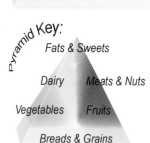

Pyramid Key:
Fats & Sweets
Dairy   Meats & Nuts
Vegetables   Fruits
Breads & Grains

The top source of chromium is fish, particularly haddock. Another top source is broccoli. Other meats, vegetables, and fruits contain smaller amounts of chromium.

*See Guides on Pages 467-468.

COBALAMINE
(SEE VITAMIN B12)

COENZYME Q10
(UBIQUINONE OR UBIQUINOL)

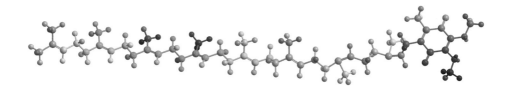

Category

    Coenzyme Q10 is a ubiquitous quinone, and hence it received the name ubiquinone. It is sometimes referred to as vitamin Q.

Cellular Location

    Coenzyme Q10 is located in the membranes of mitochondria, endoplasmic reticulum, peroxisomes, and lysosomes. Mitochondria are the major energy-producing organelle found within cells of the body; accordingly, coenzyme Q10 plays an essential role in energy production. Most of the initial digestion of coenzyme Q10 is taken to the liver.

Structure

    Coenzyme Q10 is a quinone (ring shaped compound) with a long side chain, called an isoprenoid side chain (similar to vitamin E and vitamin K). It has 10 side chain units in a row, hence the name Q10. It is also known by its formal chemical name 2,3 dimethoxy-5 methyl-6 decaprenyl benzoquinone.
    Ubiquinol is ubiquinone that is chemically altered, or reduced by what is termed "two equivalents" in chemistry.

Mechanisms of Action

Coenzyme Q10 acts as an antioxidant and plays an essential role in energy production within cells of the body.

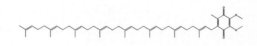

Biological & Ocular Importance

● **Helps mitochondria produce energy**   Mitochondria can produce energy by passing electrons along an electron transport chain. Coenzyme Q10 is an essential part of this process as it accepts electrons to push forward the energy production. Coenzyme Q10 also transfers protons across the inner mitochondrial membrane to produce a proton-gradient that is an essential component of the energy production by mitochondria.

Coenzyme Q10 is often used by athletes to enhance performance and long-term endurance. It may also be used by people with muscle disease, such as muscular dystrophy or those with diseases of the mitochondria that may also affect muscle functioning.

There is also evidence that coenzyme Q10 improves the performance of the heart and, as a result, may be used in heart disease and during heart surgery.

● **Helps in production of energy required to keep cornea clear**   Also, coenzyme Q10 may be essential to the function of certain highly-metabolic ocular structures as well. For example, the clarity of the cornea depends on the ability of the cells that line its back surface (the endothelial cells) to pump water out of the cornea to make sure that the inner layers of the cornea remain clear and dry. This pump function requires a lot of energy and is therefore dependent on mitochondrial function and coenzyme Q10.

● **Helps in production of energy in retina**   Similarly, the retina is an extremely highly metabolic tissue, so coenzyme Q10 plays an essential role in energy production in photoreceptor cells and the retinal pigment epithelium.

● **Helps cells digest debris** Lysosomes are organelles within cells that function to digest extra debris that is produced. Coenzyme Q10 plays a role by transferring hydrogen protons across the membrane of the lysosomes. The protons accumulate within the lysosome, making the lysosome more acidic so that it can more effectively digest debris.

Digestion of debris is an important component of the action of the retinal pigment epithelium (the layer of cells behind the retina that serve to nourish the retina and remove the excess debris from the retina). Debris accumulation is one mechanism that causes retinal diseases, such as age-related macular degeneration and childhood inherited retinal diseases like Stargardt's disease, to develop (see page 13).

Certain types of debris result from the shedding of the discs of photoreceptors (see introduction). Certain types of debris in the presence of light and oxygen can cause the production of reactive oxygen species (toxic chemicals that result in oxidation). Thus, excess debris can result in oxidative damage to the retina. Moreover, because light exposure is high in the retina, and the highest amount of oxygen consumption of any tissue in the body occurs in the retina, the retina is therefore particularly susceptible to oxidative damage.

● **Acts as a powerful antioxidant to prevent eye disease** Coenzyme Q10 is a powerful antioxidant that plays an important role in preventing oxidation in mitochondria. It also plays an antioxidant role in other cell membranes, and as such, it helps preserve the antioxidant vitamin E in cell membranes. In fact, coenzyme Q10 has similar antioxidant characteristics as vitamin E (see section on vitamin E).

As an antioxidant, it is believed to be beneficial to retinal diseases, such as macular degeneration and childhood hereditary photoreceptor diseases, in which oxidative damage plays a role in the disease. It may also be beneficial in diseases, such as glaucoma or optic nerve diseases, in which oxidative damage plays a role as well. Furthermore, it may also help prevent cataract formation or corneal disease, again by preventing or decreasing oxidative damage.

As such, coenzyme Q10 has been found to be helpful in healing of wounds, such as after laser corneal surgery for refractive procedures, such as lasik. In experimental animal models of lasik, coenzyme Q10 can decrease injury to or death of cells of the cornea, in what is believed to be its antioxidant capacity.

Also in the photoreceptors, coenzyme Q10 has been described as an "electron sink" or "miniature capacitor" with the ability to remove excess electrons that form during the chemical cascade when light triggers a photoreceptor cell. Excess electrons attack oxygen in mitochondria to form a superoxide anion. The superoxide anion then acts to take away electrons from compounds, or donates electrons to other reactions to create oxidants, such as hydrogen peroxide. This creation of oxidants is how superoxide anion causes cell damage.

● **Prevents eye disease associated with atherosclerosis** Coenzyme Q10 plays a role in preventing oxidation of cholesterol and, thus, may play a role in the prevention of atherosclerosis (blood vessel cholesterol clots and plaques that can result in heart disease and stroke, as well as artery or vein clots in the retina or optic nerve strokes). Coenzyme Q10 also helps decrease blood pressure in people with hypertension (high blood pressure). There is also evidence that it may slow down the progression of Alzheimer's disease.

Atherosclerosis is believed to play a role in many eye diseases, ranging from retinal diseases such as vein occlusions and macular degeneration, to optic nerve diseases such as optic nerve strokes and glaucoma.

● **Other activities: strengthens immune defense, helps against cancer, decreases migraines** There is suggestion that coenzyme Q10 helps the immune defense system function better and, thus, may decrease the risk of infections. There is also suggestion that it may decrease the risk of cancers, such as breast cancer.

Interestingly, some studies have also shown that coenzyme Q10 can help prevent or minimize the effects of migraines.

Human Studies on Utility

Currently, there are only a handful of human studies on coenzyme Q10 use in eye disease reported in the scientifically-reviewed medical literature. These reports involve retina and optic nerve disease, and are summarized below. Of note, the studies involve only small numbers of people, so the benefits found may be by chance, and it is difficult to assess the broad applicability of the findings.

● **One study found a benefit: use of coenzyme Q10 improves vision over time in macular degeneration and decreases debris accumulation** A recent study in Italy looked at over 100 people with early macular degeneration. The study divided participants into

Looking at the mechanisms of action, there is good reason to use coenzyme Q10 in moderation for macular degeneration and several other retinal diseases.

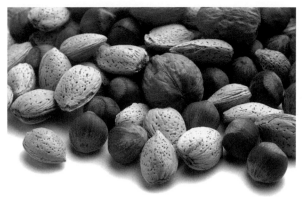

average of 11% to 13%. This improvement in drusen is also unheard of![37] The same authors found similar results in their earlier pilot study involving 14 people taking a somewhat higher dose cocktail consisting of 30 mg of coenzyme Q10, 1320 mg of omega-3 oils, and 500 mg of carnitine.[38]

two groups: one that took a cocktail of 3 supplements, consisting of 20 mg of coenzyme Q10, 1060 mg of omega-3 oils, and 200 mg of carnitine daily for one year, and another that took placebo. The study found that those who took the supplement cocktail were less likely to develop worsening of their macular degeneration, as assessed by visual acuity and visual fields. In fact, on average, people who took the supplement cocktail showed an improvement in vision, compared to the average decline in vision in those who did not take the supplement cocktail! This finding is quite remarkable in that it is rare for macular degeneration to improve! Furthermore, the study found that the amount of drusen (damaging debris) that accumulates behind the retina in macular degeneration, actually decreased in people who took the supplement cocktail in comparison to those who did not. In those who took the supplement cocktail, the amount of drusen *decreased* by an average of 15% to 23%, while, in those who took the placebo, the amount of drusen *increased* by an

● **Report that coenzyme Q10 may help in people with Leber's hereditary optic neuropathy** Coenzyme Q10 has been reported, anecdotally, to help improve vision in people with Leber's hereditary optic neuropathy (a disease of the mitochondria in which vision suddenly decreases due to optic nerve disease). Based on the mechanism of disease, it makes sense for coenzyme Q10 to be helpful in such diseases, but the anecdotal reports are far from any convincing proof of its benefit.

● **Report that coenzyme Q10 may help in people with retinitis pigmentosa** In a 1994 study, 3 people with retinitis pigmentosa were each given 100 mg of coenzyme Q10 each day for 2½ months. Two of the 3 people found improvement in one measure of energy production in their brains.[47] The relevance of this study to retinal energy production or visual functioning, however, is unknown.

Body Absorption, Metabolism, & Excretion

Most of the coenzyme Q10 that is ingested is not absorbed into the bloodstream. Some studies have shown that only about 2% of the coenzyme Q10 ingested is absorbed into the bloodstream. The coenzyme Q10 that is absorbed is absorbed with fats, so eating small amounts of fat with coenzyme Q10 assists in its absorption.

When in the bloodstream, coenzyme Q10 is carried around in fats. Most of the initial digestion of coenzyme Q10 is taken to the liver.

Coenzyme Q10 is excreted by being dumped back into the digestive tract through bile (a green fluid produced by the liver that is stored in the gallbladder to assist in digestion).

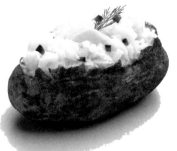

Deficiency

Most people, particularly the young and healthy, are able to produce sufficient amounts of coenzyme Q10 on their own, so deficiency of coenzyme Q10 does not often occur. However, the elderly or those who are ill or have diabetes, heart disease, or cancer may not be able to make enough coenzyme Q10.

Certain cholesterol medications may lower coenzyme Q10 levels by blocking the pathway of cholesterol synthesis as well as the pathway of coenzyme Q10 synthesis by the body. A precursor to cholesterol is formed from a chemical side chain called isoprene, which is also the side chain of coenzyme Q10. One class of cholesterol lowering medications, called statins, block an enzyme called acetyl CoA, which is involved in the process of synthesizing the isoprene side chains. Therefore, these statin drugs can reduce cholesterol levels but also reduce coenzyme Q10 levels.

Toxicity & Side Effects

High amounts of coenzyme Q10 intake can result in a variety of gastrointestinal symptoms, such as upset stomach, heartburn, nausea, vomiting, and diarrhea. These gastrointestinal symptoms may be decreased if the daily amount of coenzyme Q10 is taken as several divided doses throughout the day.

Other side effects include headaches and dizziness, rashes and itching, as well as fatigue. There are also reports that coenzyme Q10 has lowered peoples' blood sugar levels, which may be dangerous in certain scenarios. Coenzyme Q10 can lower blood pressure, which may be beneficial in some people, but harmful in others.

Although athletes use coenzyme Q10 to enhance performance, coenzyme Q10 may also cause damage to the organs when the organs receive an inadequate supply of oxygen during vigorous exercise or athletic activities. Proper exercise with proper breathing and oxygenation is recommended to avoid organ damage when using high doses of coenzyme Q10.

In the eyes, increased light sensitivity has been reported with high intake of coenzyme Q10.

Interactions with Other Nutrients

When the body is producing its own coenzyme Q10, vitamin B6 is required in the first step.

Alpha-lipoic acid is able to assist in reforming coenzyme Q10 when it is used up as an antioxidant. When coenzyme Q10 is used up, it becomes oxidized having lost electrons. Alpha-lipoic acid can donate electrons to coenzyme Q10 to regenerate it (see section on alpha-lipoic acid).

Similarly, coenzyme Q10 is able to assist in reforming vitamin E when it is used up as an antioxidant. Coenzyme Q10 can donate electrons to oxidized vitamin E to reform it (see section on vitamin E). Coenzyme Q10 often plays such an antioxidant role in cell membranes, where vitamin E is also present.

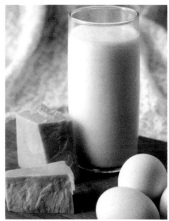

Sulforaphane can help in recycling coenzyme Q10 back into its active form when its antioxidant ability is used up (see section on coenzyme Q10).

Ideal Dosage

A recommended daily dosage of coenzyme Q10 is 50 to 200 mg. Some researchers suggest doses up to 300 mg per day. Others have recommended doses up to 1200 mg per day.

Because so little of coenzyme Q10 is absorbed into the bloodstream, it is best ingested in divided doses.

Sources (Where to Find It)

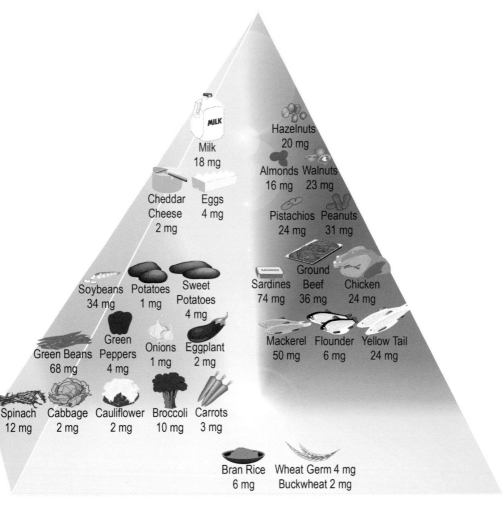

Milk
18 mg

Cheddar
Cheese
2 mg

Eggs
4 mg

Hazelnuts
20 mg

Almonds Walnuts
16 mg 23 mg

Pistachios Peanuts
24 mg 31 mg

Soybeans Potatoes
34 mg 1 mg

Sweet
Potatoes
4 mg

Sardines
74 mg

Ground
Beef
36 mg

Chicken
24 mg

Green Beans Green
68 mg Peppers
4 mg

Onions
1 mg

Eggplant
2 mg

Mackerel Flounder Yellow Tail
50 mg 6 mg 24 mg

Spinach Cabbage Cauliflower Broccoli Carrots
12 mg 2 mg 2 mg 10 mg 3 mg

Bran Rice Wheat Germ 4 mg
6 mg Buckwheat 2 mg

Pyramid Key:
Fats & Sweets
Dairy   Meats & Nuts
Vegetables   Fruits
Breads & Grains

Top sources of coenzyme Q10 include meats, such as ground beef and chicken, as well as fish, such as sardines and mackerel. Nuts are also a particularly good source of coenzyme Q10.

*See Guides on Pages 467-468.

COLEUS

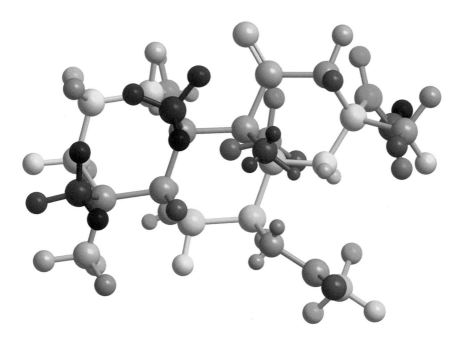

Category

Coleus forskohlii is a mint family nutrient. It is often called forskolin, named after the Finnish scientist who discovered it. The mint family is known by its scientific name, Lamiaceae. This family contains some 200 subgroups or genera. One of these subgroups is the coleus genera. In addition to coleus forskohlii, other plants in the mint family include spices such as basil, oregano, sage, rosemary, thyme, and lavender. Many of the plants in the mint family are known for their beautifully colored leaves.

Cellular Location

Because coleus is not required for cellular function, it is not stored in any particular location.

Structure

The compound known as forskolin is composed of several hexagonal rings and its structure is of the category called terepenes. It is an organic compound composed of carbon, hydrogen, and oxygen molecules.

Mechanisms of Action

Coleus assists certain enzymes that increase levels inside cells of the molecule cyclic adenosine monophosphate, also known as cAMP. The molecule cAMP acts as a signaling molecule within cells and often acts to signal the effects of hormones or other chemical messengers that send signals to the cells. When these messages are received by the cell, the cAMP molecule is activated and takes the message inside the cell to activate the specific chemical pathways requested by the original chemical messenger.

Biological & Ocular Importance

● **Plays a role in a variety of conditions: asthma, obesity, skin disease, blood vessel disease, platelet clotting, & heart disease** Coleus plays an important role in preventing blood vessel disease particularly in the heart, hypertension (high blood pressure), asthma, and skin disease such as psoriasis.

By increasing the breakdown of fat, it may prevent or decrease obesity. However, in doing so, it effectively increases the amount of sugars in the bloodstream as well.

Coleus is thought to block some of the activity of platelet clotting, by blocking the effects of a platelet-activating enzyme.

● **Prevents fluid build-up & glaucoma** By activating cAMP, coleus is thought to decrease the production of fluid in the eye and, thus, decrease the pressure build-up in the eye that may occur in some forms of glaucoma.

● **Protects neural cells in the retina from injury** Numerous studies in animal models have demonstrated that coleus can protect the neural cells of the retina, such as retinal ganglion cells that are injured in glaucoma, or the photoreceptors that are injured in diseases such as macular degeneration or childhood hereditary retinal disease, such as retinitis pigmentosa. By activating cAMP, coleus triggers these neural cells to become responsive to protectant factors that are secreted by supporting cells and other neural cells. These protectant factors are proteins that are often called neurotrophic factors. They act on receptors of the neural cells to promote the survival and rescue of the cells. cAMP can increase the amount in these cells of receptors for the trophic factors, making them more amenable to stimulation by trophic factors.

110

Human Studies on Utility

There are no human studies on coleus use in eye disease reported in the scientifically-reviewed medical literature. Nevertheless, the fact that there are no reported clinical studies does not necessarily imply a benefit or lack of benefit. Looking at the mechanism of action, the use of coleus in moderation may be possibly of benefit in certain eye diseases.

Body Absorption, Metabolism, & Excretion

Most of the coleus digestion is believed to occur in the stomach with the assistance of stomach acids while absorption occurs in the intestines. However, it is likely that most of the coleus is not absorbed, and instead remains in the digestive tract, either being broken down by enzymes or excreted. The excretion of coleus that does get absorbed occurs mostly through the kidneys.

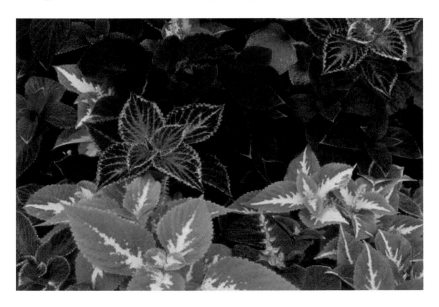

Deficiency

There are no known disorders of coleus deficiency, as coleus is a non-essential nutrient. Instead, any deficiency that ensues is often from a widespread nutritional deficiency.

Toxicity & Side Effects

Since coleus affects the ability of platelets to clot, in excess it can result in bleeding complications, particularly in people who are already taking blood thinners or aspirin.

Given that it can lower blood pressure, coleus also has been noted to cause low blood pressure, both in high doses or in people already taking blood pressure medications.

Additionally, coleus has been reported to increase the risk of stomach ulcers in those who may be predisposed to stomach ulcers.

Interactions with Other Nutrients

There is limited knowledge of the interaction of coleus with other nutrients.

Ideal Dosage

Some researchers recommend divided doses of up to 200 to 500 mg per day. There are no established ideal doses as coleus is non-essential, and the body likely absorbs relatively little of the coleus in the digestive tract.

Sources (Where to Find It)

Coleus is often grown in the subtropical climates in Southeast Asia. The nutrient portion is derived from the root of the plant.

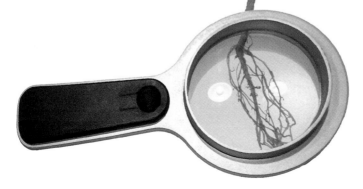

COPPER

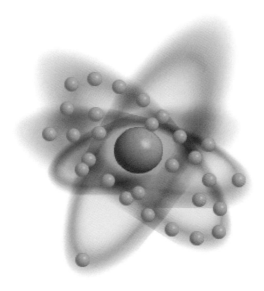

Category

An essential trace element.

Cellular Location

Most of the copper absorbed goes into the bloodstream and is stored in the liver. Other tissues that have high concentrations of copper are muscle, brain, kidney, and connective tissue.

Structure

Copper is a metallic element that comes in two forms: cuprous (Cu^{1+}) and cupric (Cu^{2+}). The cupric form is in higher concentrations in the body. Its symbol on the periodic table of elements is Cu, and its atomic number is 2. It is found between nickel and zinc on the periodic table.

Mechanisms of Action

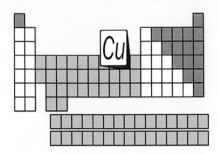

Copper can both donate and accept electrons, and thus plays a role in oxidation, both as an antioxidant and as a pro-oxidant.

Copper plays an essential role in various enzymes in cells.

Biological & Ocular Importance

● **Activates many genes**
Copper plays an important role in transcription factors (proteins that turn specific genes on or off). Therefore, changes in copper levels within cells can change the molecular makeup of these cells through activation of genes. Copper is also essential for other protein enzymes.

● **Involved in energy production in cells**   Copper is the central metal in an enzyme called cytochrome c oxidase that helps mitochondria (the energy-producing organelles in the body's cells) produce energy by transferring electrons.

● **Helps form nerve fiber insulation**   Furthermore, cytochrome c oxidase plays an important role in the formation of myelin sheaths (the insulation around nerves fibers that enables the signals to be sent efficiently).

● **Helps balance neurotransmitters**   Copper is found in the enzyme monoamine oxidase, which plays an important role in metabolism of the neurotransmitters epinephrine, norepinephrine, and dopamine, as well as in the degradation of the neurotransmitter serotonin.

● **Plays a central role in antioxidant enzymes**   Copper plays a central role in the enzyme superoxide dismutase, a powerful antioxidant enzyme. One form of superoxide dismutase works within cells and requires both copper and zinc. A second form of the enzyme works outside of cells and requires only the copper. As such, copper is important for its role in the antioxidant enzyme.

By itself, copper can both donate and accept electrons, and thus act as both an antioxidant and a pro-oxidant. As a pro-oxidant, it can cause oxidative damage to cells if it is in excess. Excess copper is associated with retinitis pigmentosa and retina dysfunction, presumably from its role as an oxidant. Therefore, it is believed that excess copper may be as harmful as copper deficiency, since both states result in oxidation.

As an antioxidant booster, it is believed to play a role in

preventing many types of eye diseases (see introduction).

● Essential for pigment (color formation) in the eye, which protects against light damage
Copper is also found in the enzyme tyrosinase, which plays an important role in the formation of melanin (a pigment, which plays a major role in retinal pigment epithelium by absorbing excess light in order to protect against the light toxicity). Melanin is also found in skin and hair, as well as the iris and the retinal pigment epithelium in the eyes. More melanin pigmentation in the retinal pigment epithelium is associated with higher levels of light absorption and less light toxicity and oxidative damage. At particularly high levels, though, melanin can actually cause oxidation of cellular compounds, particularly lipids or membrane oils.

● Involved in iron transport enzymes
Copper functions in ceruloplasmin, also known as ferroxidase I, and in ferroxidase II, two enzymes that are involved in oxidation of iron so that it can be mobilized out of storage sites and transported.

● Helps enzymes that regulate blood vessel dilation
Copper is involved in helping enzymes that regulate the proper dilation of blood vessels by promoting those that dilate the blood vessels while decreasing the activity of those that constrict blood vessels.

● Required for collagen support for the cornea, vitreous, retina, eye filtration site, and optic nerve support site
Copper is a central metal in the enzyme lysyl oxidase (an enzyme that is required for cross-linking of collagen and elastin). The lysyl oxidase enzymes convert the lysine amino acid (building blocks of proteins) in collagen and in elastin into allysine, which condenses to form cross-links that provide a great deal of mechanical strength to collagen and the rubber-like elasticity of elastin.

Collagen is an important component of many parts of the eye, as well as other parts of the body, including bones. Collagen is formed with the help of vitamin C as well as amino acids, lysine and proline (see section on vitamin C).

Collagen is the major protein of the cornea and its uniformity and pattern of arrangement is essential in maintaining the clarity of the cornea. Along with elastin, it forms the layers of Bruch's membrane, a support layer that separates the retinal pigment epithelium from the underlying choroidal blood vessels. In wet macular degeneration as well as in extremely high myopia (near-sightedness), cracks can develop in Bruch's membrane through which new blood vessels grow that can lead to bleeding and scarring as well as detachment and distortion of the retina.

Collagen maintains the trabecular meshwork, the main filtration site of the eye and a target of damage in glaucoma. The trabecular meshwork is the site of filtration of fluid from the eye, making it a critical component in the fluid balance of the eye. Malfunction of this filtration site is a common mechanism of glaucoma.

Collagen also forms the lamina cribrosa, a structure that supports individual nerve fibers as they pass from the retina into the optic nerve. One mechanism of glaucoma is damage to these nerve fibers when the lamina cribrosa is unable to support them.

Collagen is also the major structural component of the vitreous. The vitreous gel is water supported by collagen and hyaluronic acid (see section on hyaluronic acid). In fact, the vitreous is 99% water supported in this collagen and hyaluronic acid meshwork. Vitreous floaters, which appear as cobwebs or spiders or spots floating in one's vision, occur when the vitreous begins to shrink. The vitreous shrinks at different ages for different people, often ranging from age 20 to age 70, though more commonly in the elderly. Decrease in collagen is associated with earlier shrinking of the vitreous. Vitreous shrinking is associated with tears in the retina as well as detachments of the retina.

Excess copper, as well as excess iron and vitamin B2, when released into the vitreous, however, may result in early or accelerated liquefaction of the vitreous gel by increasing hyaluronidase. Hyaluronidase is an enzyme that breaks down hyaluronic acid, the major water-holding matrix compound in the vitreous gel, and also increases the liquefaction of the vitreous gel (see section on hyaluronic acid).

Finally, collagen is also an important protein that forms skin, tendons, ligaments, and blood vessels as well. Capillaries are where the arteries thin to the point of supplying tissue with nutrients and oxygen from the blood supply, in exchange for waste materials and carbon dioxide that must be transported out in veins. Capillary malfunction can result in tissue swelling, bleeding, and inappropriate control of tissue nutrition and oxygenation.

Human Studies on Utility

Currently, there are only a handful of human studies on copper use in eye disease reported in the scientifically-reviewed medical literature. These studies involve cataract, glaucoma, and retinal diseases. The studies are summarized below. Of note, the studies involve only small numbers of people, so the benefits found may be by chance, and it is difficult to assess the broad applicability of the findings.

Looking at the mechanisms of action, there is good reason to use copper in careful balance for the health of the eye, as high doses may cause or exacerbate eye disease.

● In small studies: possible link between high copper levels and retinitis pigmentosa

Some studies have shown elevated blood levels of copper in people with retinitis pigmentosa, while other studies have shown no difference. In 1981, a small study of 7 people with retinitis pigmentosa (a night-blinding retinal disease), found that adhering to a copper-restricted diet and taking a copper-removing pill, penicillamine actually improved visual acuity and peripheral vision over a period of 2 years. Another study with people who had retinitis pigmentosa associated with deafness found that taking a copper-removing pill improved their hearing but not their vision.

● One large study found benefit: use of multi-vitamin with copper decreases the future risk of macular degeneration over time

A recent 10-year study of over 3,000 people age 55 and over found that taking a daily antioxidant combination of vitamin C (500 mg), vitamin E (400 IU), and beta-carotene (15 mg), with or without zinc (80 mg) and copper (2 mg) reduced the risk of developing severe or wet macular degeneration, in people with certain features of dry macular degeneration within their retinas. The risk of developing severe or advanced macular degeneration decreased by 34% in people taking the antioxidant combination with zinc and copper, by 24% in people taking the antioxidant combination alone without zinc and copper, and by 30% in people taking the zinc and copper without the antioxidant combination. Looking at vision, the antioxidant combination with zinc and copper decreased the risk of losing vision from macular degeneration by 25% in these people with certain features of dry macular degeneration. There was no benefit to vision for people who took the antioxidant combination alone, without the zinc and copper, or the zinc and copper alone. This study has been used widely to recommend the multivitamin combination for macular degeneration, though the results are only applicable to people with certain features of macular degeneration in their retinas. Moreover, what confounds the interpretation of the data is the use of multivitamins in two-thirds of the people.[19]

● **One large study found no benefits from use of multi-vitamin with copper on the future risk of cataract over time** The same recent 10-year study of over 3,000 people that found that taking an antioxidant combination of beta-carotene (15 mg), vitamin C (500 mg), and vitamin E (400 IU), with or without zinc and copper each day reduced the risk of macular degeneration over time, found no link (neither protective nor harmful) to the risk of cataracts over time.[29]

● **One study: no link between blood levels of copper and cataract** A study of 165 people found no link (neither beneficial nor harmful) between cataracts and copper, zinc, magnesium vitamin A, and vitamin E levels in the blood. However, the study found that those who had cataracts had lower levels of carotenoids and vitamin D in their blood compared to those who did not have cataracts. On the other hand, the study found that those who had cataracts had higher levels of selenium in their blood.[41]

● **One study: decreased risk of cataract in those with higher blood levels of copper** A study of over 1,400 people in India found that those who had higher blood levels of copper had a 56% higher risk of having certain types of cataracts. Similarly, the study found that those who had higher blood levels of vitamin C also had an 87% higher risk of having certain types of cataracts.[48]

● **One study: decreased risk of glaucoma in those with higher blood levels of copper** A small study suggested that people with glaucoma have higher copper levels in their aqueous fluid (the fluid behind the cornea that bathes the natural lens). Perhaps in these people, excess copper acts as an oxidant resulting in glaucoma. However, the implications of this study are not clear and the number of people studied too small to draw any definitive conclusion one way or the other.[49]

Body Absorption, Metabolism, & Excretion

Typically about half of the copper ingested is absorbed. However, when the amount of copper ingested is increased, the amount absorbed decreases to about a quarter. It is absorbed in the intestines, carried to the liver, and then carried in the bloodstream on a protein called ceruloplasmin. Once in the bloodstream, copper goes to the liver for storage, and excess copper is dumped out of the liver back into the intestines for excretion.

Deficiency

Because of copper's role in enzymes of iron oxidation and transport, copper deficiency is associated with anemia (insufficiency of the red blood cells that carry oxygen). Some of the symptoms of anemia include fatigue, shortness of breath, increased heart rate, mouth sores or ulcers, tongue soreness, pale skin, and brittle nails. However, copper-deficiency anemia does not improve by iron supplementation. It requires treatment with copper supplementation. Copper deficiency may also cause low levels of white blood cell (cells that are involved in fighting off infections).

Because of copper's role in formation of neurotransmitters and myelin sheaths of nerve fibers, pigmentation of the skin and eyes, and creation of energy within cells, copper deficiency may cause neurological disease, loss of pigmentation, and impaired growth.

There is conflicting evidence on whether copper deficiency or copper excess causes atherosclerosis, coronary artery disease, and heart disease. The justification for deficiency as a cause is based on the decreased antioxidant enzyme activity, such as superoxide dismutase, while the underlying principle for copper excess as a cause is based on it role as an oxidant (see below, under toxicity).

Nevertheless, copper deficiency is associated with increased oxidative damage. The lack of copper may cause improper constriction of blood vessels by blocking enzymes that favor dilation and by promoting enzymes that favor constriction. In animal models, copper deficiency has been associated with abnormalities of blood vessel activity and inflammation.

More uncommon signs of copper deficiency are loss of skin and hair pigmentation.

Menkes' disease, also known as kinky hair disease, is a genetic copper deficiency disease resulting from impaired copper transport, and can cause neurological impairments and seizures in addition to hair, skin, and bone changes. It can also cause droopy eyelids as well as thinning and loss of color of the iris. Cases of retinal degeneration have been reported to be associated with this disease as well.

There is some thought that infants who are born premature may have copper deficiency, and this copper deficiency may predispose them or increase their risk for developing retinopathy of prematurity.

Toxicity & Side Effects

Sudden excess in copper can result in stomach pains, nausea and vomiting, diarrhea, a metallic taste in the mouth, headaches and dizziness, and weakness. Severe copper toxicity is rare but can lead to liver disease, kidney failure, coma, and death.

While low levels of copper can be associated with oxidation, high levels of copper also can be associated with oxidation, as copper itself can be an oxidant. In addition, copper can bind with glutathione to prevent its antioxidant action and it can disrupt other metabolic and essential cellular activities.

As such, long-term high copper levels have been associated with cataract formation in the lens. Similarly, in some cases, high copper levels have been associated with retinitis pigmentosa. In fact, in these people, decreasing the copper levels through diet and medicines can result in improvement in visual acuity and visual fields. Furthermore, high serum copper levels have been associated with low serum zinc levels in some cases of retinitis pigmentosa (see section on zinc).

Long-term excess copper, resulting in excess oxidation, is associated with atherosclerosis, coronary artery disease, and heart disease. A study of blood copper levels in over 4,000 people found that those with higher copper levels were more likely to die from heart disease than those with "normal" copper levels. However, this and other studies are controversial because it is difficult to truly measure copper levels in the blood, since inflammation from atherosclerosis can cause measured blood copper levels to appear very high. Basically, atherosclerosis, coronary artery disease, and heart disease may cause elevated levels of the copper carrier protein ceruloplasmin, which results in higher measured copper levels. Thus, it is difficult to determine whether the high copper levels caused the disease or the disease caused the high copper levels.

Excess copper can result in high cholesterol levels. Copper works with zinc to balance cholesterol levels (see below, under interaction with other nutrients).

Liver and gallbladder disease can also be associated with high copper levels when copper is unable to be dumped back into the intestines for excretion.

Wilson's disease is a genetic excess copper disease resulting from a defect in a copper transport gene similar to the gene that causes Menkes' disease. While copper levels are low in Menkes' disease, they are high in Wilson's disease. Furthermore, in Wilson's disease, the high copper levels result in liver disease as well as neurologic diseases that including tremors, gait difficulty, seizures, and psychiatric disorders. A ring of copper accumulation appears in at the edges of the cornea.

Interactions with Other Nutrients

There are numerous interactions between copper and other nutrients. The important concept is that a balance should be achieved between intake of copper and other nutrients.

Copper works with zinc to balance cholesterol levels. An imbalance in the ratio between copper and zinc can result in higher cholesterol levels because of improper absorption of either the zinc or the copper. This ratio should be one-fold copper to ten-fold zinc. Zinc and copper compete with each other for absorption in the digestive system. Deficiency of zinc can lead to excess copper, whereas, excess zinc can lead to low copper levels because zinc produces an enzyme, known as metallothionein, which can bind copper inside the intestines to prevent its absorption.

A balance is needed between copper and iron. Low copper levels are associated with low availability of iron for use by the body, because copper functions in iron transport enzymes. On the other hand, high iron levels can interfere with copper intake and decrease copper levels.

There is also some controversial evidence that high doses of vitamin C can result in copper deficiency. This finding has been observed in animals, though it has not been demonstrated in humans. Nevertheless, balancing vitamin C intake with appropriate mineral intake is necessary.

There is also thought that alpha-lipoic acid can chelate (bind and remove) metals like copper and iron to prevent them from acting as oxidants. This data comes from test tubes and has not been demonstrated in cells. It has, however, been shown to bind to copper to prevent it from accumulating in the eye, particularly to the lens to prevent cataract formation.

In addition, excess copper, zinc, iron, and magnesium may inhibit the absorption of vitamin B2.

Ideal Dosage

The recommended daily intake of copper is about 1.5 to 3 mg each day in adults. In children age 11 to 18, the recommended daily intake of copper is about 1.5 to 2.5 mg each day. It is recommended that the daily intake not exceed 10 mg (or 10,000 µg).

It may be best to obtain a dose of about 2 to 3 mg per day. It is imperative, however, that, care must be taken to consume copper in a proper ratio with zinc in order to maintain proper cholesterol levels (see section on zinc). This ratio should be ten-fold zinc to one-fold copper. Thus, it may be best to match with a dose of zinc of about 20 to 30 mg per day.

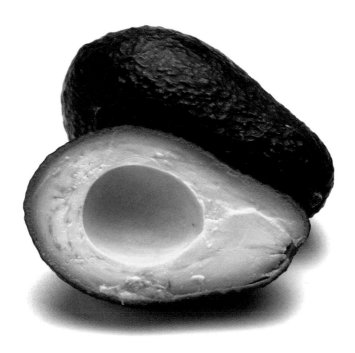

Sources (Where to Find It)

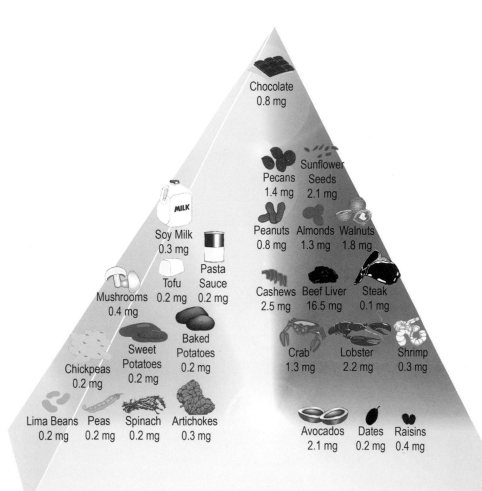

Chocolate
0.8 mg

Pecans 1.4 mg
Sunflower Seeds 2.1 mg

Soy Milk 0.3 mg

Peanuts 0.8 mg Almonds 1.3 mg Walnuts 1.8 mg

Tofu 0.2 mg Pasta Sauce 0.2 mg

Mushrooms 0.4 mg

Cashews 2.5 mg Beef Liver 16.5 mg Steak 0.1 mg

Sweet Potatoes 0.2 mg Baked Potatoes 0.2 mg

Crab 1.3 mg Lobster 2.2 mg Shrimp 0.3 mg

Chickpeas 0.2 mg

Lima Beans 0.2 mg Peas 0.2 mg Spinach 0.2 mg Artichokes 0.3 mg

Avocados 2.1 mg Dates 0.2 mg Raisins 0.4 mg

Pyramid Key:

Fats & Sweets

Dairy   Meats & Nuts

Vegetables   Fruits

Breads & Grains

The top source of copper is beef liver. Other high sources include lobster, crab, nuts, and avocadoes.

*See Guides on Pages 467-468.

CYANOCOBALAMIN

Category

Cyanocobalamin is a commonly found form of vitamin B12 (see section on vitamin B12). The common active form of vitamin B12 is methylcobalamin.

DOCOSAHEXAENOIC ACID
(DHA)

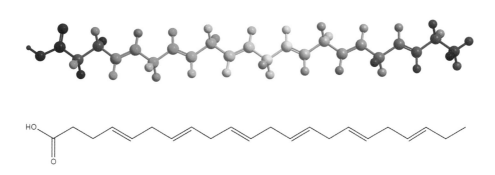

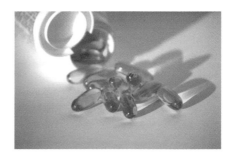

Category

Docosahexaenoic acid (DHA) is a member of the omega-3 fatty acids (see section on omega-3 oils).

Structure

DHA is an Omega-3 oils. It is a long-chain fatty acid, with 22 carbons forming its chain. It is an unsaturated fatty acid, with numerous double bonds. DHA contains a double bond at the third carbon position.

Sources (Where to Find It)

Seafood is the top source of DHA. The approximate amount of DHA in a 4 ounce serving of common types of seafood is listed below:

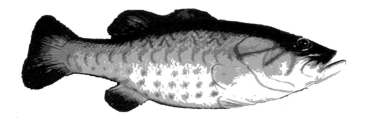

Mackerel (Atlantic)..............1.8 g
Mackerel (King)...................1.4 g
Salmon (Atlantic) ....1.4 g
Tuna (Bluefin) ....1.4 g
Tuna (Albacore)..................1.3 g
Anchovy ....1.0 g
Trout (Rainbow) ....1.0 g
Herring (Atlantic)................1.0 g
Herring (Pacific) ....0.8 g
Salmon (Sockeye)..............0.8 g
Sardines ....0.7 g
Rockfish.............................0.6 g
Bass...................................0.5 g
Swordfish ....0.5 g
Trout (Farm) ....0.5 g
Catfish ....0.4 g
Halibut...............................0.4 g
Cod ....0.3 g
Red Snapper......................0.3 g
Haddock ....0.2 g
Shrimp...............................0.2 g
Crab ....0.1 g
Lobster ....0.1 g
Scallop..............................0.1 g
Flounder ....0.1 g
Sole...................................0.1 g

FOLATE
(FOLIC ACID)

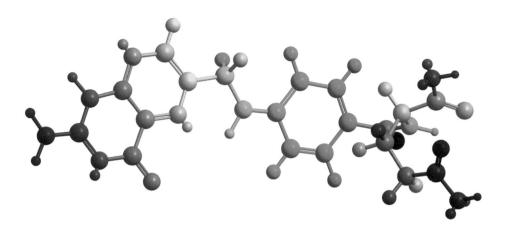

Category

Folate is a member of the vitamin B family, also known as vitamin B9. It is also known as pteroyl-glutamate or pteroyl-monoglutamic acid. Folate was originally known as Vitamin M before being reclassified as a B-complex vitamin.

Cellular Location

Most of the body stores of folate are in the liver, though folate is sent through the bloodstream to all organs for constant use in cellular activities.

Structure

Folate is a complex compound consisting of three main components. On one end, there is a double ring structure comprised of two adjacent nitrogen-containing hexagonal rings. In the middle is a structure called PABA, which is a very important organic compound that is made of a hexagonal ring. On the other end is attached a compound called glutamate. Of note, glutamate is an amino acid (building blocks of proteins) that serves in many roles, including as a neurotransmitter signaling molecule.

Mechanisms of Action

Folate acts as an enzyme used for making proteins and DNA.

Biological & Ocular Importance

● **Essential for making proteins & DNA** Folate plays an important role in the ability of cells to synthesize or manufacture proteins and DNA. It is required for the formation of SAMe, which donates chemical methyl groups to form DNA and amino acids (building blocks of proteins) (see section on SAMe).

● **Decreases risk of birth defects, cancer, and Alzheimer's** Folate has been shown to decrease the risk of birth defects during pregnancy.

It can also decrease the risk of certain types of cancer; this effect is believed to be a result of folate's ability to form SAMe in order to donate methyl groups to DNA to prevent DNA damage. Research suggests that DNA damage is an important precursor to cancer formation.

There is some suggestion that folate can help in Alzheimer's disease.

There is also some suggestion that folate helps reduce chronic fatigue.

● **Decreases vessel-damaging toxin homocysteine** Folate acts as an indirect antioxidant by decreasing stress on protein-building organelles within cells by reducing the activity of homocysteine, a toxic amino acid (protein building block) known to cause atherosclerosis (blood vessel cholesterol clots and plaques that can result in heart disease and stroke, as well as artery or vein clots in the retina or optic nerve strokes).

The amino acid homocysteine signals stress in the protein building organelles and causes proteins to be misfolded. High levels of homocysteine are associated with vascular disease including blood clots, heart disease, stroke, and vein occlusions in the retina, as well as Alzheimer's disease. Taurine, betaine, vitamin B2, and vitamin B12 also help reduce homocysteine levels. As such, folate is also believed to be important in preventing vein occlusions in the retina.

The retina is an extremely highly metabolic tissue, and as such the cells of the retina, particularly the photoreceptor cells, have a high demand for manufacturing or synthesizing proteins and DNA. There is a particularly high concentration of folate receptors in the retinal pigment epithelium (the layer of cells behind the retina that serve to nourish the retina and remove the excess debris from the retina). There is also an exceptionally high concentration of folate transporter proteins in the retinal pigment epithelium. These transporters are found only in a few tissues, such as intestines, liver, kidneys, and retinal pigment epithelium.

Human Studies on Utility

Currently, there are only a handful of human studies on folate use in eye disease reported in the scientifically-reviewed medical literature. These studies are summarized below. Of note, four clinical trials have been performed, looking at the role of folate in both preventing and treating cataract. These clinical trials are of different types, some of which are very well-designed and well-performed studies. However, there is no definitive answer from these studies. Overall, studies suggest that there may be good reason to use folate in moderation for decreasing the risk of cataract.

● **In a large study: no benefits in past use of folate found on risk of macular degeneration** Looking forward over time, a study of nearly 3,000 people age 49 and over found no link (neither protective nor harmful) between the risk of having macular degeneration and taking any of the

● **Decreases formation of cataracts** Folate can decrease the formation of cataracts. It is believed to act in this role via its indirect antioxidant activities, by decreasing stress on protein-building organelles within cells by reducing the activity of homocysteine.

> Looking at the mechanisms of action, there is good reason to use folate in moderation for cataract.

following nutrients (alone or in combination) in the past: folate, beta-carotene, vitamin A, vitamin B1, vitamin B2, vitamin B3, vitamin B6, vitamin B12, vitamin C, vitamin E, or zinc.[13]

● **In multiple-study analysis: decreased risk of retinal vein occlusion in those with higher blood levels of folate** An analysis that looked at 4 studies of nearly 300 people with vein occlusions compared to nearly 300 control people found that those who had vein occlusions had lower levels of folate in their blood. The same study did not find any difference in blood levels of vitamin B12 between the two groups.[50]

● **In a small study: decreased risk of optic nerve dysfunction in those with**

higher blood levels of folate

A study of 26 people with nutritional amblyopia (a disorder of poor nutrition and optic nerve dysfunction) found that those with nutritional amblyopia had lower levels of folate in their blood than the control groups. Interestingly, vitamin B12 levels were not found to be reduced, even though vitamin B12 is known to be associated with similar optic nerve dysfunction.[52]

● Several studies found a benefit: past use of folate associated with decreased risk of cataract

A large study of nearly 3,000 people age 49 to 97 found that past use of folate reduced the risk of having cataracts by 40 to 60% depending on the type of cataract. Likewise, the past use of multivitamins was associated with a decreased risk of having cataracts as well. The use

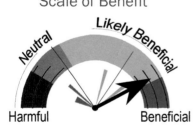

Folate for
Cataract
Scale of Benefit

of vitamin A in higher doses reduced the risk of having cataracts by 90%, the use of vitamin B1 in higher doses reduced the risk of having cataracts by 30 to 40% depending on the type of cataract, the use of vitamin B2 in higher doses reduced the risk of having cataracts by 30%, and the use of vitamin B3 in higher doses

reduced the risk of having cataracts by 30%. The study did not find any link (neither protective nor harmful) between the use of vitamin B6 or vitamin B12 and cataract.[51]

A study of nearly 500 people age 53 to 73 found that past intake of *higher* amounts of folate decreased the risk of having cataracts by about 10%, and past intake of *higher* amounts of vitamin B2 decreased the risk of having cataracts by over 60%. The study found that the past intake of *higher* amounts of vitamin C decreased the risk of having cataracts by nearly 70%. It also found that long-term intake of vitamin C for over 10 years decreased the risk of having cataracts by nearly 65%. Long-term intake of vitamin E for over 10 years decreased the risk of having cataracts by over 50%, even though the study found no link (neither protective nor harmful) between the past intake of *higher* amounts of vitamin E and the risk of having cataracts. The finding of no beneficial link with higher doses of vitamin E may be related to increased risks associated with the higher doses. Furthermore, the use of a multivitamin for over 10 years reduced the risk of having cataract by over 40%. However, the study found no link (neither protective nor harmful) between the intake of beta-carotene, carotenoids, lutein and zeaxanthin, or lycopene and the risk of having cataracts.[20]

An Italian study of over 900 people found that those who consumed higher dietary levels of folate and vitamin E had a lower risk of developing cataracts that required surgery. However, no link (neither protective nor harmful) was found between intake of higher levels of beta-carotene, methionine, vitamin A, or vitamin D and the risk of having cataracts.[22]

A study of 300 women age 56 to 71 from a group of over 120,000 people found that folate in higher doses reduced the risk of having cataracts by nearly 75%. The study also found that in non-smokers, the past use of beta-carotene in higher doses reduced the risk of having cataracts by over 70%. In fact, carotenoids, as a group, in higher doses reduced the risk of having cataracts by over 80%. In addition, past use of higher doses of vitamin C decreased the risk of having cataract by nearly 60% and the use of vitamin C for over 10 years decreased the risk by 60%. However, the study found no link (neither protective nor harmful) between the use of vitamin E or B2 and cataract.[23]

A study of over 2,000 people found that the past intake of folate, vitamin A, vitamin B1, vitamin B2, vitamin B3, vitamin B6, vitamin C, and vitamin E were each associated with a decreased risk of having a certain type of cataract (called nuclear sclerosis). However, each of these nutrients was also associated with an increased risk of having another type of cataract (called cortical cataract).[53] The researchers suggest that the finding of increased cortical cataracts reflects the possibility that the presence of nuclear sclerosis cataracts masked the finding of cortical cataracts and skewed the results. This study exemplifies how difficult it is at times to interpret results and make meaningful extrapolations.

Body Absorption, Metabolism, & Excretion

Folate is absorbed by the intestines and stored in the liver, and from there delivered through the bloodstream to all organs for constant use in cellular activities.

Folate is excreted mostly by being filtered out by the kidneys. Folate, however, is broken down as it is used by the body, and it is usually the breakdown of by-products of folate that are filtered out by the kidneys rather than folate itself. Folate also gets excreted by the liver back into the intestines. However, when the liver excretes it into the intestines, most of the folate is then recycled by being reabsorbed by the intestines and sent back to the liver for storage and distribution.

Deficiency

Folate deficiency is known to produce birth defects, particularly deficiency during the first trimester of pregnancy.

Folate deficiency results in anemia (insufficiency of the red blood cells that carry oxygen). Some of the symptoms of anemia include fatigue, shortness of breath, increased heart rate, mouth sores or ulcers, tongue soreness, pale skin, and brittle nails.

Folate deficiency can result in build-up of the toxic chemical, called homocysteine (see page 128), in the bloodstream. Elevated levels of homocysteine are associated with vascular disease including blood clots, heart disease, stroke, and vein occlusions in the retina, as well as Alzheimer's disease (see section on interactions with other nutrients).

Folate deficiency has also been associated, more rarely, with optic neuropathy (a disorder of the optic nerve that can cause blind spots and blurred vision). Folate deficient optic neuropathy is often associated with poor nutrition in alcoholism or with vitamin B12 deficiency.

Toxicity & Side Effects

Some of the side effects of folate include upset stomach, nausea, bloating, diarrhea, hair loss, skin rashes and itching, fatigue, excitability and hyperactivity, difficulty sleeping, and even impairment of judgment.

At extremely high doses, the gastrointestinal side effects can be quite severe as can be the neurological side effects. High doses of folate can also cause seizures in those who are predisposed to seizure activity. These types of toxicities often occur from ingesting high-dose folate supplements. Folate from dietary sources rarely causes toxicities.

Folate supplementation can mask the anemia of vitamin B12 deficiency. High doses of folate can correct anemia caused by vitamin B12 deficiency, without correcting the neurological disorders that are caused by vitamin B12 deficiency. Thus, high doses of folate can perpetuate the neurologic disorders caused by vitamin B12 deficiency.

Interactions with Other Nutrients

There are numerous interactions between folate and other nutrients. The important concept is that a balance should be achieved between intake of folate and other nutrients.

There are several nutrients (vitamin B12, vitamin B6, folate, selenium, SAMe, methionine, and N-acetyl-cysteine) that act in the same complex circular pathway and are all interrelated when it comes to: (1) the toxicity of homocysteine and decreasing its levels, and (2) the activities of SAMe as a donator of methyl groups (see sections on vitamin B12, vitamin B6, selenium, SAMe, methionine, and N-acetyl-cysteine).

Folate plays an important role in the process of converting the toxic chemical homocysteine into methionine. The particular enzyme that converts homocysteine back to methionine is, in fact, one of only two enzymes throughout our body that depend on vitamin B12 for their activity. SAMe participates in this cycle by donating methyl groups (see sections on vitamin B12 and SAMe).

Not only do vitamin B12 and folate work together in regulating homocysteine levels, vitamin B6 and zinc regulate homocysteine levels by helping convert homocysteine into glutathione, which, by doing so, ensures lower levels of toxic homocysteine. Selenium is required in this pathway as these glutathione enzymes are selenoproteins, composed of selenium with the protein. N-acetyl-cysteine may lower homocysteine levels as well by converting homocysteine into the protein building block cysteine, an amino acid.

Choline also interacts in this complex homocysteine pathway. Choline forms a chemical called betaine in the body, and betaine works to convert homocysteine to methionine, in order to decrease levels of homocysteine in the body.

In addition to their interactions together in the homocysteine pathway, the activities of vitamin B12 and folate are so interrelated that a deficiency of vitamin B12 results in a deficiency of folate within cells.

Vitamin B2 is required for the activation of folate and vitamin B6.

There is controversial data that suggest that folate absorption interacts with zinc absorption, such that low zinc levels cause low folate absorption while high folate levels cause low zinc absorption. The studies are not consistent on these findings however. A zinc-dependent enzyme is involved in folate absorption though, and, as such, the need to balance zinc and folate supplementation is vital.

Ideal Dosage

The minimum recommended daily allowance is 400 µg per day. In pregnant women, the minimum amount increases to 600 µg per day, and in lactating women, the minimum amount increases to 500 µg per day. In children age 14 to 18, the minimum recommended daily allowance is 400 µg per day.

Doses of 800 to 1,000 µg per day may be required to assist in reduction of homocysteine levels, so it may be best to obtain a daily dose of 800 to 1,000 µg per day. The upper limit of safe dosages of folate is 5,000 µg per day. However, most physicians recommend people ingest no more than 1,000 µg per day, since doses of 1,000 µg or more can mask a vitamin B12 deficiency and result in permanent neurological damage.

Sources (Where to Find It)

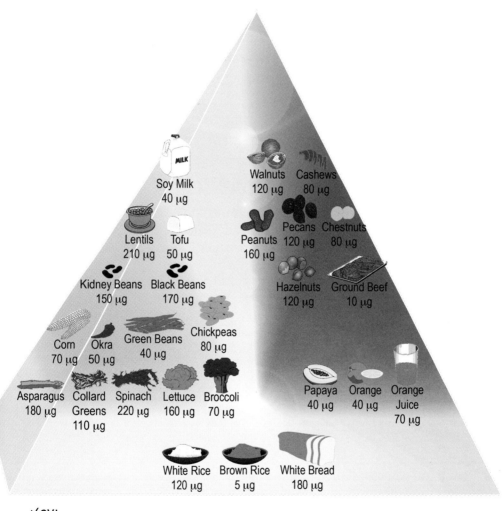

Soy Milk
40 µg

Walnuts
120 µg

Cashews
80 µg

Lentils
210 µg

Tofu
50 µg

Peanuts
160 µg

Pecans
120 µg

Chestnuts
80 µg

Kidney Beans
150 µg

Black Beans
170 µg

Hazelnuts
120 µg

Ground Beef
10 µg

Corn
70 µg

Okra
50 µg

Green Beans
40 µg

Chickpeas
80 µg

Asparagus
180 µg

Collard
Greens
110 µg

Spinach
220 µg

Lettuce
160 µg

Broccoli
70 µg

Papaya
40 µg

Orange
40 µg

Orange
Juice
70 µg

White Rice
120 µg

Brown Rice
5 µg

White Bread
180 µg

Pyramid Key:

Fats & Sweets

Dairy   Meats & Nuts

Vegetables   Fruits

Breads & Grains

Top sources of folate include nuts, beans especially lentils, asparagus, and greens such as spinach, lettuce, and collard greens. Oranges and papaya also contain moderately high amounts of folate. White bread and white rice are often enriched with high amounts of folate.

*See Guides on Pages 467-468.

GENISTEIN

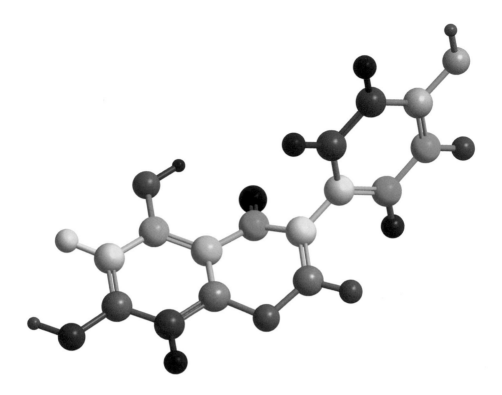

Category

Genistein is a bioflavonoid in the isoflavones subgroup (see section on bioflavonoids).

Cellular Location

Because genistein is not required for cellular function, it is not stored in any particular location.

Structure

Genistein is a moderately-sized compound consisting of three hexagonal rings. The rings are carbon-based with the central ring containing oxygen. The ring pattern is called isoflavone.

Mechanisms of Action

The isoflavone group of bioflavonoids, and genistein in particular, has strong estrogenic activity. Genistein is a plant estrogen, known as a phytoestrogen. In addition, genistein functions as an antioxidant.

Biological & Ocular Importance

● **Blocks cell growth factors**
In addition to its antioxidant functions as a bioflavonoid (see section on bioflavonoids), it is an anti-growth factor that works by blocking the action of tyrosine kinase, an enzyme that transfers phosphate groups to proteins to activate and de-activate them.

● **Helps starve cancer cells**
Isoflavones particularly genistein have estrogenic activity and can affect transcription factors (proteins that turn specific genes on or off). One such transcription factor that is blocked by genistein is known as CCAAT, and blocking it can help starve cancer cells of nutrients that allow them to grow.

● **Raises levels of the good type of cholesterol (HDL)**
Estrogen is important in raising the levels of high-density lipoproteins, also known as HDL or good cholesterol, and therefore prevents or reduces the risk of heart or blood vessel disease. HDL is also important in the transport of lutein and zeaxanthin to the retina, two essential carotenoids.

● **Protects against osteoporosis** Estrogenic activity is shown to help protect bones against osteoporosis.

● **Acts as an antioxidant and prevents cataract formation**
As an antioxidant, genistein is believed to play a role in preventing many types of eye diseases (see introduction). Furthermore, as a phytoestrogen, it also helps prevent cataract formation.

● **Blocks the growth of abnormal blood vessels in the eye** Also, genistein has been found to inhibit angiogenesis (the formation of abnormal new blood vessels). Angiogenesis is particularly harmful in the retina, cornea, and trabecular meshwork (filtration site of the eye) and can cause loss of vision. The problems that result are called choroidal neovascularization (seen in wet macular degeneration), or retinal neovascularization (seen in severe diabetic retinopathy or retinal disease), or corneal neovascularization (seen in corneal injury or disease), or iris neovascularization (seen in angle-closure glaucoma and inflammatory eye disease). Bioflavonoids, such as genistein, act to inhibit the expression of enzymes and cellular growth factors that stimulate new blood vessel growth, in order to prevent angiogenesis in the eye (see section on bioflavonoids).

● Relaxes eye filtration site to prevent glaucoma

Genistein is also believed to relax the trabecular meshwork. The trabecular meshwork is the site of filtration of fluid from the eye, a critical component in the fluid balance of the eye. Malfunction of this filtration site is a common mechanism of glaucoma.

Human Studies on Utility

There are no human studies on genistein use in eye disease reported in the scientifically-reviewed medical literature. Nevertheless, the fact that there are no reported clinical studies does not necessarily imply a benefit or lack of benefit. Looking at the mechanism of action, the use of genistein in moderation may be possibly of benefit in certain eye diseases.

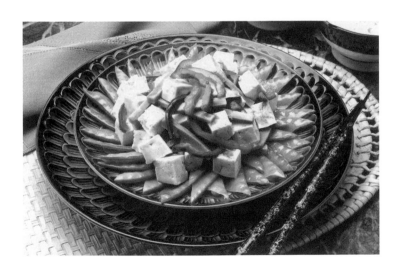

Body Absorption, Metabolism, & Excretion

Digestion of fruits, vegetables, herbs and other sources of bioflavonoids occurs in the stomach with the assistance of stomach acids that help break down the fruits, vegetables, and herbs to release the bioflavonoids. In the intestines, though, enzymes often further break down the bioflavonoids. Some bioflavonoids, particularly those bound to sugars, are absorbed in the small intestines, while most bioflavonoids pass to the large intestines where they are further broken down.

Overall, a small amount of the bioflavonoids are absorbed in the digestive tract and then into the bloodstream. The majority of bioflavonoids are not absorbed and remain in the digestive tract, where they are either broken down by enzymes or are excreted.

Of the bioflavonoids absorbed in the bloodstream, excretion occurs mostly through the kidneys.

Deficiency

There are no known disorders of bioflavonoid deficiency, as bioflavonoids are non-essential nutrients. Instead, any deficiency that ensues is often from a widespread nutritional deficiency.

Toxicity & Side Effects

There is data from animal studies that suggests that extremely high doses of genistein may be toxic to the retina, depending on where the genistein dose is given. While the mechanisms of this toxicity are unknown, a recurring theme in ocular nutrition is moderation. Too much of a good nutrient may end up being detrimental.

Interactions with Other Nutrients

There is limited knowledge of the interaction of genistein with other nutrients.

Ideal Dosage

Although some studies have suggested doses of 25 to 75 mg per day, there is no established ideal dosage because the bioflavonoids are non-essential. Furthermore, the body absorbs relatively little of the bioflavonoids in the digestive tract.

Sources (Where to Find It)

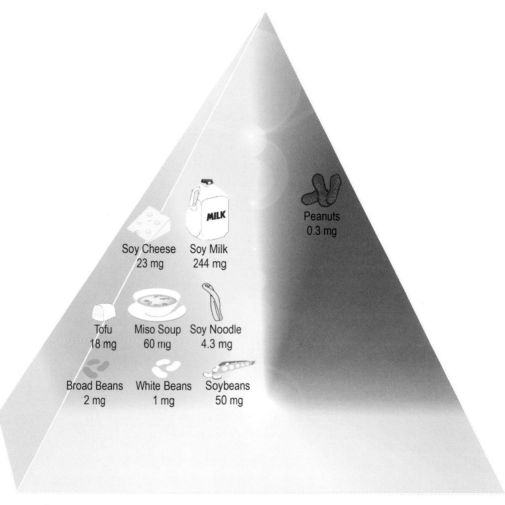

Soy Cheese
23 mg

Soy Milk
244 mg

Peanuts
0.3 mg

Tofu
18 mg

Miso Soup
60 mg

Soy Noodle
4.3 mg

Broad Beans
2 mg

White Beans
1 mg

Soybeans
50 mg

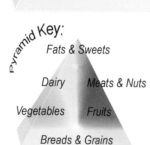

Pyramid Key:

Fats & Sweets

Dairy   Meats & Nuts

Vegetables   Fruits

Breads & Grains

The most abundant source of genistein is soybeans. A 4 ounce serving of soybeans often contains over 50 mg of genistein.

Genistein may also be obtained through a nutrient known as "genistein combined polysaccharide", which is genistein combined with complex sugars from mushrooms.

*See Guides on Pages 467-468.

GINKGO

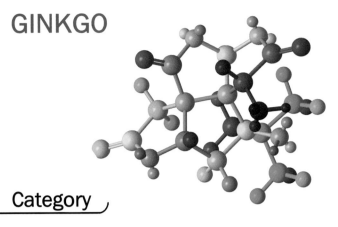

Category

The ginkgo tree, also known as the maidenhair tree, is a unique tree in its own class, order, family, and genus with only one species, the ginkgo biloba. The tree is believed to have been around for 250 million years, originating in the Permian period of the Paleozoic era. While people have been known to eat its seeds, which can be toxic in high concentrations because of the presence of cyanide, its leaves are known to have medicinal effects. These effects are believed to result from chemical compounds within the leaves that are called ginkgolides and bilobalides, which are isoprenoid or isoprene unit multi-ring carbon compounds. Steroids are derived from isoprenoid precursors. Other medicinal effects are believed to result from flavonoid glycosides, or bioflavonoids bound to sugar groups (see section on bioflavonoids). Ginkgo leaves contain numerous types of ginkgolides and bioflavonoids as well as other compounds including vitamin C.

Some of the bioflavonoids include procyanidin, prodelphinidin, quercetin, kaempferol, isorhamnetin, and myricetin. The ginkgolides and bilobalides are labeled with letters such as A, B, C, J, and M. A standardized extract of ginkgo is often referred to as EGb761. A non-standardized extract of ginkgo may also contain alkylphenols such as ginkgolic acids, ginkgol, and bilobol, which may have toxic or allergic effects.

Cellular Location

Because ginkgo is not required for cellular function, it is not stored in any particular location.

Structure

The ginkgolides and bilobalides found in ginkgo are moderately-sized compounds consisting of multiple pentagonal rings.

Mechanisms of Action

Ginkgo can act as an antioxidant. It also acts to inhibit activity of an enzyme called platelet-activating factor. There is some data to suggest that ginkgo also acts to regulate certain genes.

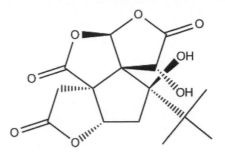

Biological & Ocular Importance

● **Acts as an antioxidant to protect the eye** Ginkgo acts as an antioxidant by scavenging or removing oxygen free radicals (toxic chemicals that result in oxidation), particularly peroxyl and superoxide radicals. It is a potent donator of electrons, and acts to prevent oxidation. It can also act as an antioxidant indirectly by stimulating glutathione activity. Many of the antioxidant effects of ginkgo are believed to result from its bioflavonoids (see section on bioflavonoids). A primary site of the antioxidant benefits of ginkgo appears to be in cell membranes.

The antioxidant properties of ginkgo make it useful in protecting against cataract, which has been shown in animal models. And it is the same antioxidant properties that are believed to protect photoreceptors in animal models of light damage.

Another mechanism of protection of retinal cells is by protecting the cells against oxidative damage. For example, animal models have shown that ginkgo can protect mitochondria (the energy-producing organelles in the body's cells) from oxidative damage, in cells such as Muller cells of the retina. These Muller cells are the support cells for the photoreceptors and signaling neurons and remove excess neurotransmitters, maintain appropriate electrolyte balances, provide fuel for metabolism, remove excess carbon dioxide and ammonia waste, and synthesize retinoic acid from retinol.

● **Potent blocker of the platelet-clotting enzyme**
The ginkgolide acts to inhibit the enzyme, platelet-activating factor. This enzyme is involved in inflammation and leakage of fluid from blood vessels as well as activation of platelets which are responsible for blood clotting. As such, the ginkgolide "type B" is one of nature's most potent blockers of this platelet clotting enzyme.

These anti-inflammatory actions extend to other mediators of inflammation. In experimental animal studies, ginkgo has been shown to block inflammation by blocking other molecular mediators of inflammation. Some of these blocked pathways involve nitric oxide and others involve arachadonic acid, an omega-6 fatty acid (see section on omega-3 and omega-6 fatty oils), which is a potent stimulator of the inflammation pathways.

The effects of decreasing inflammation make ginkgo a useful nutrient in the treatment of many inflammatory diseases, such as asthma.

● **Protects the retina through antioxidant and platelet-blocking activities** These antioxidant and anti-platelet activities protect the retina. In animal models, ginkgo provides protection against many retinal and retinal-vascular disorders, such as diabetic retinopathy and retinopathy of prematurity. There is similar thought that ginkgo may be beneficial in protecting neural cells that degenerate in glaucoma, again by its ability to provide protection to neurons of the retina while also promoting good blood flow.

● **Relaxes muscle cells around blood vessels to improve blood flow and protect the retina** Through its antioxidant functions and through its inhibition of the platelet-activating factor, ginkgo improves the flow of blood through vessels. This function is believed to be beneficial in vascular and heart disease, and particularly in a disorder called claudication,

whereby leg pain develops from clogging of leg arteries. Ginkgo can also relax the smooth muscle cells of blood vessels to improve blood flow. The mechanism is not fully known and is believed to be related to a non-bioflavonoid and non-ginkgolide component in ginkgo. As such, ginkgo also provides protection to neurons of the brain, or retina, during injury, stroke, or disease

● **Protects the retina by blocking signaling in cells** Through these same mechanisms, anti-oxidant, inhibition of platelet-activating factor, and relaxation of smooth muscle cells of blood vessels, ginkgo is believed to provide protection to the neural cells of the retina and the brain. Other mechanisms of protecting neural cells of the retina and brain involve blocking molecular signaling in cells involved neuronal injury. Some of these mechanisms involve nitric oxide, phospholipase, and calcium-initiated signaling. These neuroprotective mechanisms are believed to provide benefit in numerous diseases of the brain as well as retinal diseases and glaucoma.

● **Assists in wound healing** There is also some evidence that ginkgo may even help in wound healing, such as after laser corneal surgery for refractive procedures, such as lasik. The exact process is unknown but is believed to involve combinations of the mechanisms described above.

● **Regulates genes, prevents cancer**   There is some data to suggest that ginkgo also acts to regulate genes. Combined with its antioxidant activities, this may be a mechanism for prevention of cancer.

● **Enhances memory, decreases vertigo, diminishes depression, improves Alzheimer's**   Ginkgo is believed to play an important role as a memory enhancer and for treatment of vertigo. It may also be useful in the treatment of depression. There are some experimental studies in animals and clinical trials in humans showing such benefits. In fact, a study in the Journal of the American Medical Association reported the benefits of ginkgo on the cognitive impairments in Alzheimer's disease. This and other studies strongly demonstrate the benefits of ginkgo in Alzheimer's disease.

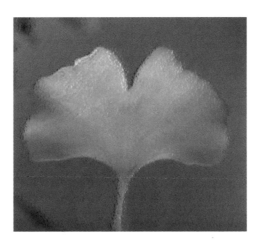

Human Studies on Utility

Currently, there are only a handful of human studies on ginkgo use in eye disease reported in the scientifically-reviewed medical literature. These studies are summarized below. Of note, the studies involve only small numbers of people, so the benefits found may be found by chance, and it is difficult to assess the broad applicability of the findings.

● **Three small studies show use of ginkgo in macular degeneration improves visual acuity or retinal sensitivity over time**   Ginkgo was shown to be effective as an antioxidant in increased photoreceptor functioning in diabetic retinopathy. A recent 2002 study in Germany of daily use of ginkgo for the treatment of 99 people with dry macular degeneration found an improvement in visual acuity over a 6 month period in people taking ginkgo, at doses of 240 mg per day as well as at doses of 60 mg per day. Those taking the higher dose had greater improvement.[54]

A study in France of 10 people with macular degeneration found improvement in visual acuity in those people who took Ginkgo at a dose of 160 mg per day compared to placebo.[55]

A small study of 24 elderly people found an improvement in their retinal sensitivity to light stimulus on a visual field test in people when taking ginkgo.[56] The authors believed that retinal-vascular improvements accounted for these results.

Although these 3 studies are not definitive due to small size and fluctuations in the measured responses, these studies provide important clues to believe that there is possibly a benefit to the use of ginkgo for retinal disease. It is indeed remarkable that improvement in vision was found in patients with macular degeneration, in which improvement is typically uncommon.

● Two small studies show use of ginkgo in diabetic retinopathy improves blood flow or color vision over time

Ginkgo was shown to be effective in improving photoreceptor functioning in diabetic retinopathy. A 2004 study found that blood flow in the capillaries of the retina improved by nearly 15% in 25 diabetic people with retinopathy, after taking 240 mg of ginkgo per day for 3 months.[57]

Another study of 29 diabetic people found that some people had improvements in their color vision after taking ginkgo for 6 months.[58]

● One small study shows use of ginkgo in healthy eyes improves blood flow over time

A 1999 study of 11 young healthy people found that taking 120 mg of ginkgo daily for 2 days results in improved blood flow to the eye.[59]

● One small study shows use of ginkgo in glaucoma improves visual fields

A 2003 study of 27 people with glaucoma, who did not have high eye pressures but had defects in their peripheral visual fields from glaucoma, found that visual fields actually improved during an 8 week time period taking ginkgo (120 mg per day). Unfortunately though, when the ginkgo was stopped, the defects in the visual field returned.[60]

There is some thought that the ginkgo was beneficial to ocular blood flow, which resulted improvements in the visual fields. However, because the benefit was transient, a more likely explanation is that ginkgo helped brain function, such as improving ability to think or concentrate. This cognitive benefit may be a result of improved blood flow in the brain. Similarly, the changes in the macular degeneration studies above also may be a result of cognitive benefits.

Body Absorption, Metabolism, & Excretion

Digestion of ginkgo occurs in the stomach with the assistance of stomach acids that help break down the ginkgo to release the ginkgolides, bilobalides, and other bioflavonoids. In the intestines, the ginkgolides and bilobalides are rapidly absorbed in high amounts. Over 80% of the ginkgolides and bilobalides ingested are often absorbed. In contrast, the bioflavonoids in the ginkgo leaf are poorly absorbed.

Excretion of ginkgolides and bilobalides occurs mostly through the kidneys.

Deficiency

There are no known disorders of ginkgo deficiency, as ginkgo is a non-essential nutrient.

Toxicity & Side Effects

Ginkgo may cause upset stomach, nausea, vomiting, and diarrhea. Muscle weakness has been reported as a side-effect of high doses of ginkgo.

Ginkgo should be avoided during pregnancy.

Furthermore, because of its effects on small blood vessels, ginkgo increases the risk of bleeding, and should be avoided in people taking anti-coagulants such as aspirin or coumadin or who have blood clotting disorders. Bleeding complications in the eye and the brain have been reported in people on ginkgo with or without anti-coagulants, such as aspirin. Some of the serious consequences of bleeding have included seizures. Blood evaluations, including a blood clotting evaluation, should be performed before starting ginkgo. The risk of bleeding complications in those who are taking ginkgo may be exacerbated if combined with omega-3 oils or high doses of vitamin E. Ginkgo should be used only with caution in those who are susceptible to bleeding and should be avoided prior to any surgery.

Ginkgo should not be combined with anti-depressant drugs, such as monoamine oxidase inhibitors, since one of ginkgo's activities is to inhibit monoamine oxidase. Combining ginkgo with certain anti-depressant drugs may result in overdose.

When not extracted from its leaves properly, ginkgo can cause an allergic reaction in the skin similar to poison ivy. This effect may be caused by alkylphenols such as ginkgolic acids, ginkgol, and bilobol, found in non-standardized extracts of ginkgo. These alkylphenols may also cause toxicity by damaging DNA. It may be best to avoid ginkgo obtained from non-standardized extraction.

Interactions with Other Nutrients

The risk of bleeding complications in those taking ginkgo may be exacerbated if combined with high dose omega-3 oils or high doses of vitamin E.

Ginkgo can act as an antioxidant indirectly by stimulating glutathione activity (see section on glutathione).

Ideal Dosage

A possible recommended daily dosage is up to 60 mg to 240 mg per day, in divided doses. Some physicians recommend doses of 30 mg per day, which may be the best recommended level. It is likely best not to exceed 250 mg per day.

Sources (Where to Find It)

Ginkgo is extracted from the ginkgo tree.

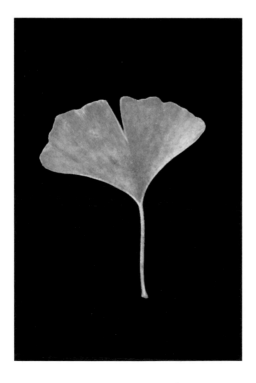

GLUTATHIONE

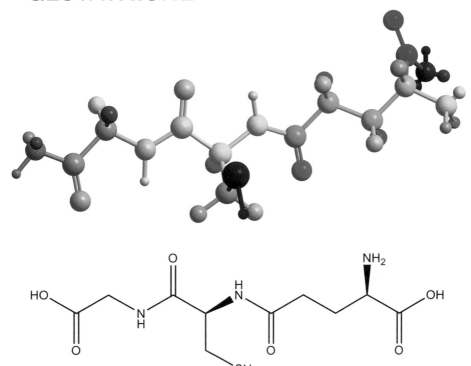

Category

Glutathione is a "tripeptide," composed of three amino acids (building blocks of proteins). The three amino acids in glutathione are: cysteine, glutamic acid, and glycine. Cysteine contains sulfur, and thus sulfur is required to produce glutathione.

Cellular Location

Glutathione-S-transferase comprises 10% of the volume of the soluble proteins in the liver! That is a lot! It is also highly concentrated in the lens of our eyes.

Since proteins cannot be stored by the human body, unused proteins are metabolized and excreted.

Structure

Glutathione consists of a chain of three amino acids linked together. One of the amino acids contains sulfur.

Mechanisms of Action

Glutathione has several important functions in our body's cells. Glutathione is involved in regulating the cell's manufacturing of DNA and proteins, in sending signals between cells, in regulating immune system responses, in controlling proliferation (an increase in the number of cells), and, quite importantly, in functioning as an antioxidant that protects against oxidants such as reactive oxygen species (toxic chemicals that result in oxidation).

Biological & Ocular Importance

● **Acts as a powerful antioxidant**   Glutathione acts as an antioxidant by donating electrons. For example, it "reduces" disulfide bonds of cell proteins that have become oxidized. With the help of an enzyme, glutathione peroxidase, it removes free peroxides from inside cells, which prevents oxidative damage to DNA (DNA hydroperoxidation) and to cell membranes (lipid peroxidation).

By acting as an antioxidant, it assists vitamin E in its antioxidant activities (saving cell membranes from oxidative damage). Vitamin E performs the first steps of preventing lipid peroxidation by converting strong and dangerous oxidants, hydroperoxyl radicals, into weaker but still harmful hydroperoxides. Thioredoxin, another antioxidant protein, and glutathione perform the second steps of safely removing the hydroperoxides, without which these hydroperoxides would turn back on lipids and cause damage (see sections on selenium and vitamin E).

Other glutathione-dependent

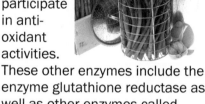

enzymes also participate in anti-oxidant activities. These other enzymes include the enzyme glutathione reductase as well as other enzymes called dehydrogenases.

There are actually four varieties of glutathione peroxidase that have been identified. Glutathione peroxidase is called a selenoprotein because it includes 4 selenium-containing amino acids and requires selenium to be produced (see page 152). There are at least four selenium-containing glutathione peroxidase enzymes that have been identified, including classical cellular glutathione peroxidase and phospholipid hydroperoxide glutathione peroxidase. Because these glutathione peroxidases remove free peroxides, such as hydrogen peroxide, from cells, they are very potent antioxidants and play an essential role in eye tissues from the cornea and lens to the retina and optic nerve.

When glutathione acts to remove free peroxides or oxidized protein disulfide bonds, it becomes oxidized itself, and becomes ineffective. The enzyme glutathione reductase converts the oxidized form of glutathione back to its "monomeric" form so that it can act in its antioxidant capacity.

Glutathione as an antioxidant that can also neutralize reactive nitrogen species called peroxynitrites and convert them to safe s-nitrosoglutathione.

Glutathione-S-transferase is an enzyme that functions in the same manner as glutathione peroxidase to help glutathione remove free peroxides within cells, except that it acts on peroxides other than hydrogen peroxide. Furthermore, glutathione-S-transferase is not a selenoprotein and does not require selenium to be produced. Also, it may be the predominant enzyme assisting glutathione when selenium levels are low.

● Recycles vitamin C

Glutathione is also involved in recycling of vitamin C. Vitamin C functions as an antioxidant by reducing reactive oxygen species. It donates electrons and, in doing so, it oxidizes itself and converts into dehydroascorbic acid or into ascorbyl free radical. These forms cannot act as antioxidants and must be recycled back to vitamin C with the help of glutathione, the glutathione-dependent enzymes such as dehydroascorbate reductase, or the selenium-containing enzyme

called thioredoxin reductase (see section on selenium).

● Protects the retina from oxidative damage

Light exposure is high in the retina, and the highest amount of oxygen consumption of any tissue in the body occurs in the retina. Therefore, the retina is particularly susceptible to oxidative damage. Glutathione plays a major role in protecting the retinal pigment epithelium (the layer of cells behind the retina that serve to nourish the retina and remove the excess debris from the retina) from oxidative damage. Similarly, high glutathione levels within Muller cells of the retina help protect photoreceptors and signaling neurons of the retina from oxidative damage. These Muller cells are the support cells for the photoreceptors and signaling neurons and remove excess neurotransmitters, maintain appropriate electrolyte balances, provide fuel for metabolism, remove excess carbon dioxide and ammonia waste, and synthesize retinoic acid from retinol (see section on vitamin A). Thus, as an antioxidant, glutathione plays an important role in the health of the retina, as related to retinal diseases as well as the retinal neurons and their axons (or nerve fibers) that are affected in glaucoma.

● Protects against glaucoma

Oxidation is believed to be involved in some of the cell death in glaucoma, and glutathione

149

plays a central role in protecting against such oxidation. Excess oxidative stress during glaucoma is believed to result in depletion of glutathione in retinal cells, such as the nourishing Muller cells of the retina, while depletion of the antioxidant glutathione causes further oxidative stress, resulting in a vicious cycle of cell injury during glaucoma.

Furthermore, glutathione protects the trabecular meshwork against oxidative damage. The trabecular meshwork is the site of filtration of fluid from the eye, a critical component in the fluid balance of the eye. Malfunction of this filtration site is a common mechanism of glaucoma.

● **Protects the lens from cataract formation** Similarly, light exposure is very high in the lens, and glutathione may protect against cataract formation. In fact, among the first discoveries of glutathione peroxidase was that of Dr. Antoinette Pirie in 1965: glutathione peroxidase's presence in the lens. In the past decade, another form of glutathione peroxidase has been found in the ciliary body (the muscular tissue behind the iris that makes the aqueous fluid). This aqueous fluid is located behind the cornea and bathes the natural lens, and has glutathione peroxidase, among other enzymes and vitamins, which gives it its high antioxidant capacity.

Levels of glutathione within the lens are the highest of any tissue in the body! As an antioxidant, glutathione is so important in the lens that every day the lens remakes half of its store of glutathione. With age, though, these levels decrease, and a decrease is associated with increased cataracts. Glutathione protects against cataract formation through its antioxidant functions as well as through its role in preventing protein cross-linkage, which results in decreased clarity of the lens. Glutathione also maintains sulfhydryl groups on proteins that are important for the lens cell activities, such as transport of cations.

● **Protects the cornea from oxidative damage** In addition, because light exposure to the cornea is high, glutathione helps protect the cornea from oxidative damage. This protection occurs at both the front surface of the cornea as well as the back surface of the cornea, which is responsible for maintaining the adequate lubrication of the inner layers of the cornea. This role for glutathione in maintaining hydration or lubrication of the inner layers of cornea, particularly under oxidative stress, may be beneficial in protecting against corneal disorders where swelling of the cornea occurs, such as in Fuch's corneal dystrophy. The cornea also plays an important role in defending the eye against infections, and glutathione helps in degrading infectious agents.

Human Studies on Utility

Currently, there are only two human studies on glutathione use in eye disease reported in the scientifically-reviewed medical literature. Nevertheless, the fact that there are only two reported clinical studies, both of which suggest no benefit, does not necessarily imply a benefit or lack of benefit. Looking at the mechanism of action, the use of glutathione in moderation may be possibly of benefit in many eye diseases.

Studies have shown that circulating blood levels of glutathione are lower in people with diabetes as well as in people with macular degeneration. Therefore, among many other potential groups, these are two groups of people who could especially benefit from glutathione supplementation.

● **In one small study: no benefits from the use of glutathione with other antioxidants on the future risk of macular degeneration over time**   A small study of 71 people with macular degeneration found no benefit to the macular degeneration or to vision in those who took a daily antioxidant combination, for over 1½ years, that consisted of glutathione (5 mg), beta-carotene (20,000 IU), vitamin B2 (25 mg), vitamin C (750 mg), vitamin E (200 IU), chromium (100 µg), selenium (50 µg), zinc (12.5 mg), taurine (100 mg), N-acetyl cysteine (100 mg), and selected bioflavonoids, compared to placebo.[17] It is impossible, however, to ascertain the individual effect of glutathione from this type of study.

● **In one study: no link between blood levels of glutathione and cataract**
A study of over 1,000 people found no link (neither protective nor harmful) between higher levels of glutathione, beta-carotene, or vitamin A in the blood and the risk of having cataracts. However, the study did find that higher levels of vitamin C in the blood decreased the risk of one type of cataract by nearly 50%. Of concern, the study found that higher levels of vitamin E in the blood increased the risk by nearly twice of having cataracts (this finding may be related to increased risks associated with higher doses of vitamin E)![25]

Body Absorption, Metabolism, & Excretion

Glutathione is digested by the stomach with the help of stomach acids. Digestive enzymes from the pancreas further break down glutathione, which is then absorbed into the bloodstream through the intestines. Little is known of glutathione metabolism, but it is believed that it is broken down into amino acids in the intestines prior to being absorbed.

As proteins are broken down, ammonia is formed. Since ammonia is extremely toxic to cells, it must be converted into a nitrogen-containing chemical known as urea. When ammonia builds up in excess, it can cause poor coordination, difficulties with balance, tremors, seizures, difficulty breathing, swelling of the brain, and can eventually lead to a coma. A normally functioning liver works to remove excess ammonia by creating urea, which is then filtered into the urine by the kidneys.

Deficiency

Since the body can make its own glutathione, deficiency is rare.

Toxicity & Side Effects

Excess glutathione, like other proteins, is often broken down and converted into sugars or fats, and used for energy, or stored as fat in the body's fat stores. Excess proteins and amino acids can stress the kidneys, stress the bloodstream, and cause dehydration. Furthermore, proteins and excess amino acids can cause the kidneys to lose calcium, which results in weakened bones. As with any protein, excessive glutathione in someone with liver disease or with kidney disease may result in build-up of ammonia or urea in the body, resulting in severe illness (see above).

In diabetics, excess amino acids can result in an increased sugar load on the body, or increased fat deposits in the body!

Interactions with Other Nutrients

There are numerous interactions between glutathione and other nutrients, though the important concept is that a balance should be achieved between intake of glutathione and other nutrients.

Selenium, along with vitamin B2 and vitamin E, is required for production of glutathione peroxidase, an enzyme involved in the functioning of antioxidant glutathione. Actually, glutathione peroxidase is called a selenoprotein as it includes 4 selenium-containing amino acids. Selenite, selenomethionine, and selenocysteine can be used as dietary supplements in order for cells to produce glutathione peroxidase. Organic selenium and selenomethionine are preferred sources of selenium for raising selenium and glutathione peroxidase levels, unlike the inorganic forms selenate and selenite.

Glutathione acts with vitamin E, vitamin C, bioflavonoids, and alpha-lipoic acid to form a highly protective antioxidant team. Vitamin C and alpha-lipoic acid protect glutathione from being used up by donating electrons to the oxidized form of glutathione so that it can be reduced to usable glutathione that can act again as an antioxidant (see sections on vitamin C, alpha-lipoic acid, and glutathione).

Glutathione can be made through a pathway that involves alpha-lipoic acid, vitamin B3, and cysteine. The conversion of lipoic acid into dihydrolipoic acid often occurs by the co-enzyme (or enzyme helper) nicotinamide adenine dinucleotide, NAD, or nicotinamide adenine dinucleotide phosphate, NADP (see section on vitamin B3). In this process, the oxidized sulfur amino acid cystine is converted to the biologically useful sulfur amino acid cysteine. Cysteine can then be recycled into the cell and used to form glutathione (see section on N-acetyl-cysteine).

Vitamin B2 is required to make glutathione reductase, which consists of flavin rings.

Increased levels of other sulfur-containing nutrients, such as cysteine, taurine, alpha-lipoic acid, and methylsulfonylmethane, also result in increased level of glutathione, a sulfur-containing tripeptide.

Ginkgo can indirectly act as an antioxidant by stimulating glutathione activity (see section on gingko).

Experimental studies have shown that the antioxidant enzyme, glutathione-S-transferase, can bind to hypericin (the active ingredient of Saint John's Wort) and block the phototoxic effects of hypericin, along with blocking the beneficial effects of hypericin (see section on Saint John's Wort).

The synthetic form of vitamin K, called menadione, may interfere with the functioning of glutathione. Thus, it may be better to avoid this synthetic vitamin K.

Ideal Dosage

The liver produces about 13,000 mg of glutathione each day. It is produced with the help of sulfur as well as selenium (see interaction with other nutrients). A typical diet contains up to 125 mg of glutathione per day, far short of the 13,000 mg produced by the liver. Therefore, providing the building blocks for the liver to produce glutathione, a sulfur-containing tripeptide, is essential. These building blocks include nutrients, such as alpha-lipoic acid, cysteine, selenium, taurine, vitamin B2, vitamin B3, and vitamin E.

Therefore, glutathione supplementation in pills is often ineffective and believed to be useless. Nevertheless, supplemental oral doses up to 600 mg of glutathione per day have been reported to be safe.

Sources (Where to Find It)

Fruits & Vegetables:

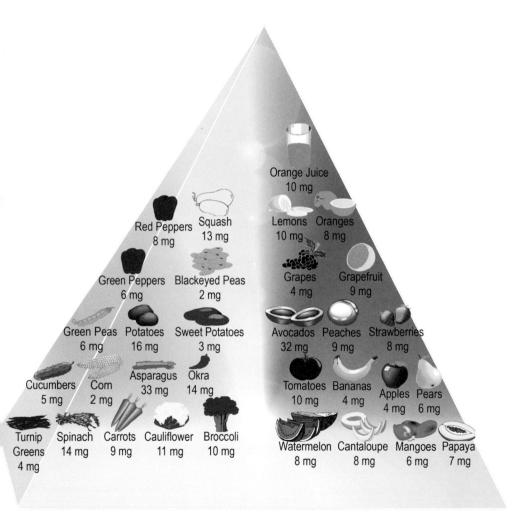

Orange Juice 10 mg

Red Peppers 8 mg
Squash 13 mg
Lemons 10 mg
Oranges 8 mg

Green Peppers 6 mg
Blackeyed Peas 2 mg
Grapes 4 mg
Grapefruit 9 mg

Green Peas 6 mg
Potatoes 16 mg
Sweet Potatoes 3 mg
Avocados 32 mg
Peaches 9 mg
Strawberries 8 mg

Cucumbers 5 mg
Corn 2 mg
Asparagus 33 mg
Okra 14 mg
Tomatoes 10 mg
Bananas 4 mg
Apples 4 mg
Pears 6 mg

Turnip Greens 4 mg
Spinach 14 mg
Carrots 9 mg
Cauliflower 11 mg
Broccoli 10 mg
Watermelon 8 mg
Cantaloupe 8 mg
Mangoes 6 mg
Papaya 7 mg

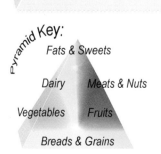

Pyramid Key:

Fats & Sweets

Dairy   Meats & Nuts

Vegetables   Fruits

Breads & Grains

*See Guides on Pages 467-468.

Dairy, Meats, & Grains:

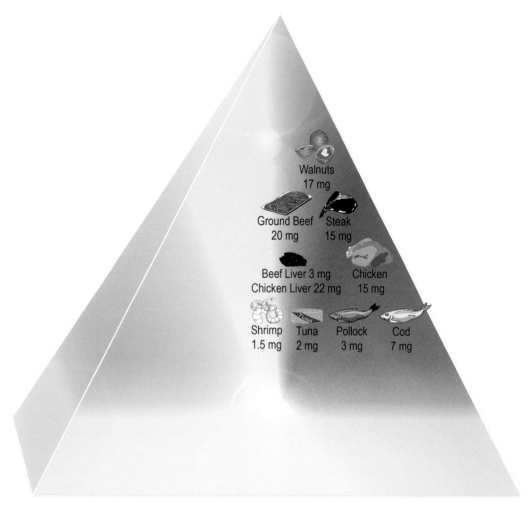

Walnuts
17 mg

Ground Beef   Steak
20 mg   15 mg

Beef Liver 3 mg   Chicken
Chicken Liver 22 mg   15 mg

Shrimp   Tuna   Pollock   Cod
1.5 mg   2 mg   3 mg   7 mg

Top sources of glutathione are steak, ground beef, chicken, and chicken liver. Walnuts are also high in glutathione. Asparagus is an all-star with 33 mg per 4 ounce serving. Other vegetables high in glutathione include spinach, okra, and potatoes.

However, it is evident that the amount of glutathione in food sources is low compared to the 13,000 mg of glutathione produced by the liver each day.

HYALURONIC ACID

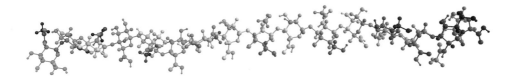

Category

Hyaluronic acid is often called hyaluronan. It is an alternating polymer of two sugars: glucosamine and glucuronic acid. In fact, it often contains thousands or tens of thousands of repeats of glucosamine and glucuronic acid!

Cellular Location

Hyaluronic acid was first discovered in 1934 in cow eyes. It is a major component of the vitreous gel and is also found in high concentrations in joints and in soft tissue below the skin.

Structure

Hyaluronic acid is composed of two sugars, called glucosamine and glucuronic acid, that alternate in a long and repeating chain that can keep going on in length.

Mechanisms of Action

Hyaluronic acid is a powerful water-holding compound. In fact, one and a half ounces of hyaluronic acid can hold over one cup of water!

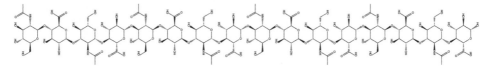

Biological & Ocular Importance

● Important for joints & skin

Connective tissue is a matrix of cells, proteins, and other molecular components that helps support and bind together other tissues such as skin and muscle. Cartilage is a specialized form of connective tissue that is flexible and found commonly in joints. Hyaluronic acid is important for the health of the joints and skin because of its role in the connective tissue matrix and cartilage. In fact, it is believed to be important in preventing arthritis as well as preventing the aging wrinkles in skin.

● Forms the vitreous gel

The major component of the vitreous gel is water, which is supported by hyaluronic acid and collagen (see section on vitamin C). In fact, the vitreous is 99% water supported in this collagen and hyaluronic acid meshwork. Vitreous floaters, which appear as cobwebs or spiders or spots floating in one's vision, occur when the vitreous begins to shrink. The vitreous shrinks at different ages for different people, often ranging from age 20 to age 70, though more commonly in the elderly. A decrease in hyaluronic acid is associated with premature shrinking of the vitreous. The shrinking of the vitreous is associated with tears in the retina, as well as detachments of the retina. Hyaluronidase is an enzyme that breaks down hyaluronic acid and increases the liquefaction of the vitreous gel. Excess vitamin B2, excess copper or iron release into the vitreous, along with ultraviolet light, may also result in early or accelerated liquefaction of the vitreous gel by increasing hyaluronidase.

● Forms support tissue in the retina

Hyaluronic acid supports the connective tissue matrix that surrounds the cells of the retina. Interestingly, estrogen levels help increase levels of hyaluronic acid. Low estrogen levels have been associated with the formation of macular holes, or holes within the retina in the macula. The macula is the center of the retina, where images are focused and vision is at its sharpest. Macular holes occur when there is pulling against the macula, presumably from the vitreous or a membrane on the surface of the retina. Some researchers have hypothesized that hyaluronic acid may play a role in the formation of macular holes by weakening the structure of the retina and/or altering the dynamics of the vitreous gel.

● **Supports the eye's filtration site & the optic nerve junction** Hyaluronic acid supports the trabecular meshwork (the filtration site of the eye) by preventing it from collapsing. Allowing enough fluid to exit the eye is essential to prevent pressure build-up in the eye, decreasing the risk of glaucoma, since malfunction of this filtration site is a common mechanism of glaucoma. In fact, a decrease in hyaluronic acid has been found in the trabecular meshwork in people affected by glaucoma.

Similarly, a decrease in hyaluronic acid has also been found around the optic nerve in people with glaucoma because hyaluronic acid supports the optic nerve at its junction with the retina as well.

● **Plays a role in the healing of the cornea & conjunctiva** Similarly, hyaluronic acid supports the connective tissue around the cornea and plays an important role in corneal and conjunctival healing after surgery, injury, or inflammation.

Human Studies on Utility

Hyaluronic acid is commonly used in several different forms to protect parts of the eye during surgery. Aside from this use, there are no reported human studies on hyaluronic acid use in eye disease in the scientifically-reviewed medical literature.

Nevertheless, the fact that there are no reported clinical studies does not necessarily imply a benefit or lack of benefit. Looking at the mechanism of action, hyaluronic acid may be possibly of benefit in certain eye diseases.

Body Absorption, Metabolism, & Excretion

There is little scientific literature on the absorption, metabolism, and excretion of hyaluronic acid. It is believed that hyaluronic acid is absorbed very poorly in the digestive system due to its high molecular weight (large size) and because of the fact that it does not dissolve well in solutions that contain fats, which is a preferred manner of absorption. Furthermore, it is likely that any absorbed hyaluronic acid may be broken down by enzymes.

On the other hand, the building blocks of hyaluronic acid (glucosamine and glucuronic acid) are easily absorbed into the bloodstream through the digestive tract. Glucosamine is believed to be rapidly absorbed by the intestines, though only about one-fifth or less of the ingested dose is actually absorbed. Glucuronic acid is known to be easily absorbed in high concentrations; in fact, many synthetic medicines are linked to glucuronic acid so that they can be absorbed more easily.

Deficiency

Hyaluronic acid deficiency is uncommon because the body makes its own hyaluronic acid using 3 different enzymes found within cells.

Toxicity & Side Effects

A skin rash has been reported in some users of hyaluronic acid. Actually, smaller chains of hyaluronic acid have been known to stimulate inflammation. Also, high synthesis of hyaluronic acid by cells is believed to be associated with certain types of cancer.

Interactions with Other Nutrients

Manganese plays an important role in the enzyme that makes glycosaminoglycans, an important component of hyaluronic acid.

As boron is essential in balancing estrogen levels, it plays an important role in maintaining appropriate levels of hyaluronic acid.

Bioflavonoids and phytic acid can help stabilize levels of hyaluronic acid.

Ideal Dosage

A possible recommended daily dosage of hyaluronic acid is 100 to 150 mg. However, no ideal dosage or recommended dosage range has been established.

Sources (Where to Find It)

Hyaluronic acid can be derived from rooster combs, the vitreous in cow eyes, or umbilical cords from cows. It is often made by bacteria that are engineered to produce hyaluronic acid.

Hyaluronic acid in the diet is likely poorly absorbed in the digestive system, though the building blocks of hyaluronic acid are readily absorbed (see page 159).

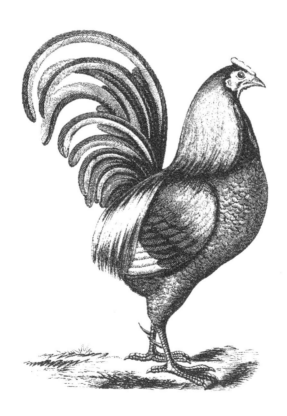

HYPERFORIN
(SEE SAINT JOHN'S WORT)

HYPERICIN
(SEE SAINT JOHN'S WORT)

INOSITOL HEXAPHOSPHATE (SEE
PHYTIC ACID)

INOSITOL TRIPHOSPHATE
(SEE PHYTIC ACID)

IRON

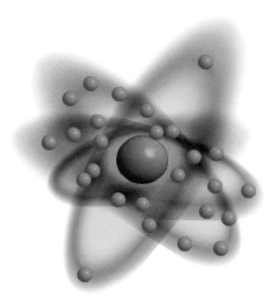

Category

Iron is an essential mineral.

Cellular Location

About two-thirds of the iron in our bodies is found within red blood cells. Iron is stored in the liver, spleen, and the bone marrow.

Structure

Iron is a metallic element. Its symbol on the periodic table of elements is Fe, and its atomic number is 26. It is found between manganese and cobalt on the periodic table.

Mechanisms of Action

Iron is the central metal required for red blood cells to carry oxygen. Iron is also essential in hundreds of proteins and enzymes.

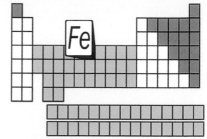

Biological & Ocular Importance

● **Essential for transporting oxygen through the body**
The highest amount of oxygen consumption of any tissue in the body occurs in the retina and iron is essential in carrying this oxygen in red blood cells throughout the body for tissue consumption.

● **Helps in energy production & in making DNA**   Iron also helps the mitochondria (the energy-producing organelles in the body's cells) in producing energy. In addition, iron plays a role in the production of DNA.

● **Plays a role in antioxidant enzymes but also creates oxidants**   Iron plays a role in enzymes that remove oxidants, such as hydrogen peroxide. It also plays a role in enzymes that create oxidants to kill off bacteria!

● **Excess causes oxidation and is associated with macular degeneration**
Excess iron leads to oxidation. Proteins such as ferritin, lactoferrin, and transferrin are produced by the liver and bind iron so that it can be stored and

transferred, in order to prevent oxidation. In the eye, the pigment protein melanin, which is found in the retina and in the iris, also binds iron so that it does not act as an oxidant. Decreasing levels of melanin in the retina as one ages are associated with increased oxidation and diseases such as macular degeneration. Similarly, increased levels of iron have been found in the retinas of people with both wet and dry types of macular degeneration.

Small areas of localized bleeding in the retina, which can occur in some forms of wet macular degeneration, lead to pockets of excess iron in the retina, as red blood cells degenerate and release their iron. These pockets of excess iron then result in localized areas of oxidative damage. The retina is particularly susceptible to oxidative damage, especially the photoreceptor discs (see introduction).

● **Excess in the vitreous causes break down of the gel and floater formation**
Similarly, bleeding in the vitreous can lead to iron release within the

vitreous, resulting in syneresis or breakdown of the vitreous gel. Vitreous floaters, which appear as cobwebs, spiders, or spots floating in one's vision, occur when the vitreous begins to shrink. Decrease in collagen is associated with earlier shrinking of the vitreous (see sections on vitamin C and copper).

Excess iron or copper release into the vitreous, excess vitamin B2, as well as ultraviolet light may result in early or accelerated liquefaction of the vitreous gel by increasing hyaluronidase. Hyaluronidase is an enzyme that breaks down hyaluronic acid, the major water-holding matrix compound in the vitreous gel, and increases the liquefaction of the vitreous gel (see section on hyaluronic acid).

Human Studies on Utility

Currently, there are only four human studies on iron use in eye disease reported in the scientifically-reviewed medical literature. These clinical trials involve large numbers of people. They look at the risk of macular degeneration and cataract. However, there is no definitive answer from these studies. Overall, looking at the studies, combined with understanding the mechanism of action of iron, there is suggestion that there may be good reason to use iron in moderation for decreasing the risk of cataract. The studies are as follows.

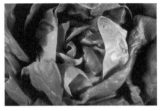

vitamin A, and vitamin C. However, a diet high in vitamin E decreased the risk of having macular degeneration by 20%. A diet high in multiple nutrients (beta-carotene, vitamin C, vitamin E, and zinc together) decreased the risk of having macular degeneration by about ½![18]

● **In one large study: no benefits in past use of iron found on risk of cataract** A study of nearly 1,800 people found no link (neither protective nor harmful) between iron and the risk

● **In one study: no benefits from the use of iron by itself on the future risk of macular degeneration over time** A study of nearly 4,000 people, looking forward over an average of 8 years, found no link (neither protective nor harmful) between macular degeneration and a diet high in iron, zinc, beta-carotene, lutein and zeaxanthin, lycopene,

Iron for
Cataract
Scale of Benefit

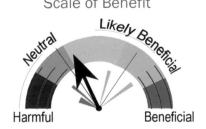

of having cataract. The study also found that the past intake of vitamin A, vitamin B1, vitamin B2, vitamin B3, vitamin C, and vitamin E was associated with a decreased risk of having certain types of cataract. This decrease in risk ranged between 40 to 55%. Also, the study found that use of any multivitamin was associated with a 30% decrease in the overall risk of having cataracts.[61]

● **Another large study found a benefit: past use of iron associated with decreased risk of cataract**   A study of nearly 3,000 people found that the past intake of iron, vitamin A, vitamin B1, vitamin B2, vitamin B3, and zinc decreased the risk of having certain types of cataract by 30 to 50%.[62] It is interesting to note that in this study (and the one below), iron was associated with a decrease in risk of having cataract, and not an increased risk, as some physicians have predicted. Furthermore, it is surprising that no link (neither protective nor harmful) was found between vitamin C use and cataract, despite other studies showing a benefit.

● **Decreased risk of cataract in those with higher blood levels of iron**   A study of nearly 1,800 people found that increased blood levels of either iron or vitamin E were associated with an over 50% decrease in the risk of having certain types of cataracts.[63]

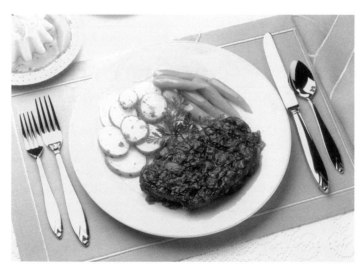

Body Absorption, Metabolism, & Excretion

Iron is absorbed mostly in the small intestines and transported in the bloodstream by carrier proteins.

Most of the iron excretion occurs in the intestines, as a result of the loss of the bile salts produced by the liver as well as through loss of exfoliated intestinal cells and degenerated red blood cells.

Most of the degenerated red blood cells are processed by the body in order to recycle the iron.

Deficiency

Despite the fact that iron is the most abundant metal on planet Earth, iron deficiency is the most common type of nutrient deficiency! It is estimated that up to 10% of adolescent girls and women in the US have iron deficiency, mainly because women lose high quantities of iron during menstruation.

Vegetarians are particularly vulnerable to iron deficiency since much of the daily iron consumption comes from meats. In addition, soy proteins can inhibit the absorption of iron.

Iron deficiency can result in anemia (insufficiency of the red blood cells that carry oxygen). Some of the symptoms of anemia include fatigue, shortness of breath, increased heart rate, mouth sores or ulcers, tongue soreness, pale skin, and brittle nails.

Iron deficiency is also known to produce thinning of the sclera.

Toxicity & Side Effects

Excess free iron can act as an oxidant and, therefore, can be toxic to cells.

Iron supplements can cause upset stomach, nausea, vomiting, diarrhea or constipation. Moreover, iron can discolor the stool as well as stain teeth.

An acute ingestion of extremely high doses of iron can result in death, and is a serious common cause of childhood poisoning. In a 20 pound child, 4 g of iron can be fatal, whereas in an adult the fatal dose is often 15 g or more.

Interactions with Other Nutrients

There are numerous interactions between iron and other nutrients. The important concept is that a balance should be achieved between intake of iron and other nutrients.

Over-the-counter and prescription supplements of iron can lead to decreased absorption of zinc, and thus decreased zinc levels. However, this decrease is not known to occur when supplementing iron levels through natural dietary sources.

When taken with iron, calcium can decrease the ability of the body to absorb iron.

Iron, as well as copper, zinc, and magnesium, may inhibit the absorption of vitamin B2.

Vitamin C increases intake of iron. Therefore, people taking vitamin C should be careful about the amount of iron they ingest.

Some nutrients are metal chelators (agents that bind the metals to remove them from action). Such nutrient chelators include alpha-lipoic acid, bioflavonoids such as quercetin, and phytic acid (see section on phytic acid). Phytic acid can be important in preventing oxidative damage because it can chelate (bind and remove) metals like iron and copper to prevent them from acting as oxidants. However, phytic acid can also block the absorption of iron, which results in iron deficiency.

Copper functions in iron oxidation and transport enzymes. Low copper levels are associated with low availability of iron for use by the body. However, a balance is needed between iron and copper. In fact, high iron levels can interfere with copper intake and decrease copper levels.

Iron, vitamin B3, vitamin B6, and vitamin C play roles in the pathway leading to the formation of carnitine, in which SAMe donates methyl groups to methionine, an amino acid (building blocks of proteins), in order to form lysine, which can then be made into carnitine.

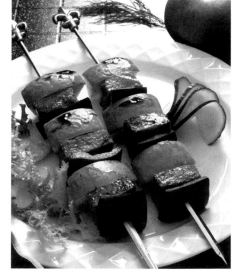

Iron, along with vitamin B2 and vitamin B6, plays a role in making vitamin B3 derivatives from an amino acid called tryptophan, when vitamin B3 is low (see section on vitamin B3).

Ideal Dosage

The ideal dose for iron differs depending on age. For boys age 11 to 18, the recommended dose is 12 mg per day, whereas for teenage menstruating girls, the recommended dose increases to 15 mg per day. For adult women, the recommended dose is 15 mg per day as well. For adult men and post-menopausal women, the recommended dose is lower, at 10 mg per day. During pregnancy, the recommended dose is 30 mg per day, and for lactating women, the recommended dose is 15 mg per day. These dosages are for elemental iron.

A 100 mg dose of ferrous gluconate provides only 12 mg of elemental iron, whereas a 100 mg dose of ferrous ascorbate provides 14 mg of elemental iron. Also, a 100 mg dose of carbonyl iron provides 20 mg of elemental iron, and a 100 mg dose of ferrous fumarate or of ferrous sulphate provides about 32 mg of elemental iron.

Spreading the full amount into smaller doses over the course of the day is preferable to a single, larger dose.

Sources (Where to Find It)

Fruits & Vegetables:

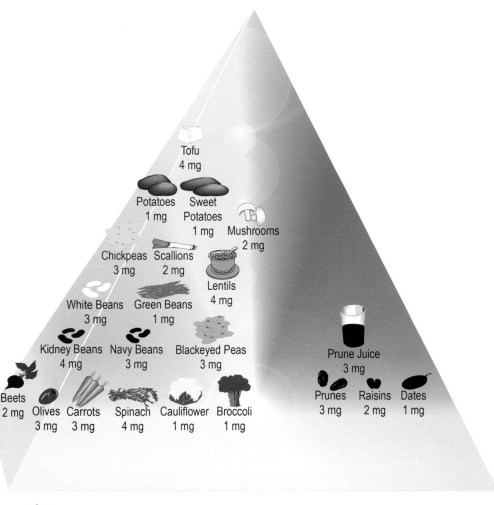

Tofu
4 mg

Potatoes
1 mg

Sweet
Potatoes
1 mg

Mushrooms
2 mg

Chickpeas
3 mg

Scallions
2 mg

Lentils
4 mg

White Beans
3 mg

Green Beans
1 mg

Kidney Beans
4 mg

Navy Beans
3 mg

Blackeyed Peas
3 mg

Prune Juice
3 mg

Beets
2 mg

Olives
3 mg

Carrots
3 mg

Spinach
4 mg

Cauliflower
1 mg

Broccoli
1 mg

Prunes
3 mg

Raisins
2 mg

Dates
1 mg

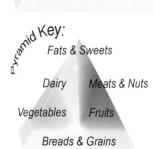

Pyramid Key:

Fats & Sweets

Dairy   Meats & Nuts

Vegetables   Fruits

Breads & Grains

*See Guides on Pages 467-468.

Dairy, Meats, & Grains:

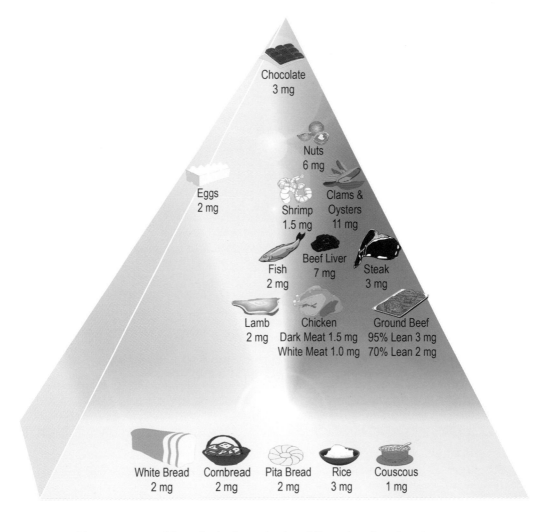

Chocolate
3 mg

Nuts
6 mg

Eggs
2 mg

Shrimp
1.5 mg

Clams &
Oysters
11 mg

Fish
2 mg

Beef Liver
7 mg

Steak
3 mg

Lamb
2 mg

Chicken
Dark Meat 1.5 mg
White Meat 1.0 mg

Ground Beef
95% Lean 3 mg
70% Lean 2 mg

White Bread
2 mg

Cornbread
2 mg

Pita Bread
2 mg

Rice
3 mg

Couscous
1 mg

Top sources of iron include nuts, beef liver, beef, spinach, beans, and tofu. Clams and oysters contain particularly high amounts of iron. In fact, a 4 ounce serving of clams and oysters in addition to a diet with other iron-rich foods may result in excess iron.

LIPOIC ACID
(SEE ALPHA-LIPOIC ACID)

LUTEIN

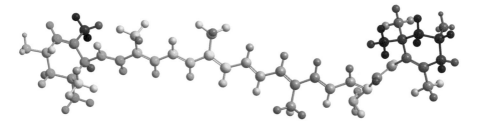

Category

Carotenoids are organic pigments that occur naturally in plants, but cannot be made by animals (see section on carotenoids).

The yellow carotenoids are lutein and zeaxanthin, both also known as xanthophylls. They are structurally nearly identical, differing only in the position of a double bond in one of their hydroxyl groups.

Cellular Location

The highest concentration of the xanthophylls, lutein and zeaxanthin, are found within the retina, predominantly in the macula (the central portion of the retina), where their concentration is 100 times that of the peripheral retina. Lutein is found throughout all areas of the retina from the peripheral retina to the central retina, while zeaxanthin is concentrated within the macula, and predominantly within the fovea (the center of the macula where images are focused).

The xanthophylls, lutein and zeaxanthin, are also concentrated in the nerve fiber layer that serves as the connection between the photoreceptors and the processing neurons of the retina, and within the outer segments of photoreceptor cells, where the photoreceptor discs are located. There are numerous reports that increased dietary consumption of lutein and zeaxanthin increase blood levels of lutein and zeaxanthin, and that increased blood levels of lutein and zeaxanthin are associated with increased levels of lutein and zeaxanthin in the macula. As a matter of fact, researchers as early as 1941 have shown that the amount of lutein and zeaxanthin in the macula is related to the amount in the diet.

Interestingly, lutein and zeaxanthin are also found to become concentrated in the lens, following a diet with higher levels of the nutrients. This finding suggests a protective role for lutein and zeaxanthin in the lens, likely as antioxidants. In past studies, other carotenoids have not been observed in the lens.

Structure

The xanthophylls lutein and zeaxanthin are polar because they have hydroxyl groups on both ends, unlike other carotenoids. This structure makes them particularly effective as retinal pigments since this polarity can enable them to lay in the photoreceptor discs with their ends sticking out, which enables them to function more effectively in their antioxidant role.

Lutein is composed of two rings connected by a long chain. The long chain contains many double bonds that give zeaxanthin its characteristic yellow color. Additionally, its structure causes it to be insoluble in water, so it prefers to be in the presence of oils and fats.

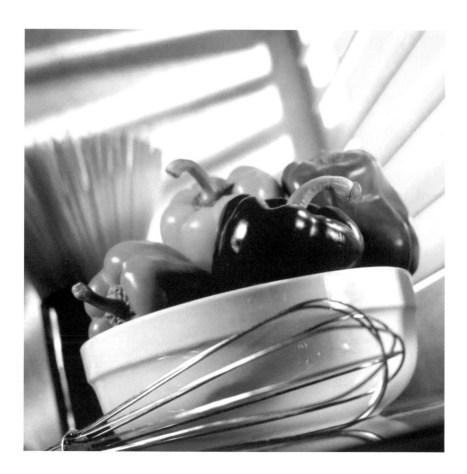

Mechanisms of Action

The carotenoids can function as antioxidants as well as light filters.

Biological & Ocular Importance

● **Acts as a powerful antioxidant**   The carotenoids have a long chain of carbons with alternating single and double bonds. In fact, the high number of double bonds is what makes these carotenoids able to function as antioxidants. They are able to donate electrons to free radicals (toxic chemicals that result in oxidation), which prevents the free radicals themselves from accepting electrons and damaging cell components. Lycopene is known as the most potent antioxidant of the carotenoids.

Light exposure is high in the retina, and the highest amount of oxygen consumption of any tissue in the body occurs in the retina. The retina's cells are therefore particularly susceptible to oxidative damage.

● **Acts as a light filter for the retina**   Furthermore, the long chain on the carotenoids gives these pigments their color, by absorbing light of various wavelengths. This absorption of light is biologically important since the yellow pigments lutein and zeaxanthin absorb blue light and ultraviolet light (forms of high-energy light). This absorption helps protect the macula from high-energy light exposure and oxidative damage. In fact, some studies show that lutein and zeaxanthin in the macula absorb anywhere from 40 to 90% of the high-energy blue light! In addition to being concentrated in the photoreceptor outer segments, lutein and zeaxanthin are concentrated in the nerve fiber layer that serves as the connection between the photoreceptors and the processing neurons of the retina. This nerve fiber layer sits on top of the photoreceptors in the macula and, because of the lutein and zeaxanthin, it acts to filter the light that passes through on its way to the photoreceptors.

There is also evidence to suggest that the absorption of blue light assists in improving the quality of the image we see. Lutein and zeaxanthin in the retina act by blocking excess light, improving the eye's contrast sensitivity, or the ability of the eye to distinguish different shades of contrast in dim light and in very bright light. Lutein and zeaxanthin pigments in the macula can absorb the shorter-wavelength blue light, reducing what is called "chromatic aberrations." This chromatic aberration would result in a blurred blue edge to the object that we see in the center of our vision. Alternative theories suggest that the macular pigments help prevent glare in bright daylight conditions.

● **Plays a role in a cell to cell communication protein**   In addition to their antioxidant and light-absorbing capabilities, carotenoids help upregulate expression of the gene to make connexin proteins and they stabilize connexin proteins as they are being made. These connexin proteins are important in cell to cell communication, and the loss of this communication is thought to play a role in the development of cancer.

● **Helps lower cholesterol** Carotenoids share similar synthesis pathways as cholesterol and may help lower cholesterol levels by interfering in this pathway or by inhibiting cholesterol-forming enzymes such as HMGCoA in this pathway. Also, carotenoids are believed to prevent the lipid oxidation in blood vessels that leads to atherosclerosis (blood vessel cholesterol clots and plaques that can result in heart disease and stroke, as well as artery or vein clots in the retina or optic nerve strokes).

● **Strengthens the immune defense system**   In addition, the carotenoids and notably vitamin A also play an essential role in immune protection. While vitamin A and the carotenoids assist in maintaining a healthy immune system, there is considerable controversy and unknown mechanism of how they function in this role. A deficiency in carotenoids and vitamin A can impair function of certain types of white blood cells, called neutrophils. The deficiency can also impair the ability of other types of white blood cells, known as macrophages, from ingesting and killing bacteria, while simultaneously causing an increased amount of inflammation, or the presence of excess white blood cells. It can also impair the response of other types of white blood cells, called T-cells.

Human Studies on Utility

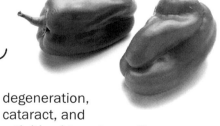

Currently, there are numerous human studies on lutein use in eye disease reported in the scientifically-reviewed medical literature. These studies involve the eye disease macular degeneration, cataract, and retinitis pigmentosa. These studies are described below.

- **Older studies suggested benefit of lutein for the retina and for retinitis pigmentosa**

In the 1940's to 1960's, several German researchers looked at the benefits of commercially-available xanthophylls. Some studies of healthy people found that taking the xanthophylls for several months improved their night vision. Other researchers found that night vision improved in people with a night-blindness retinal disease, called retinitis pigmentosa. On the other hand, some of the researchers found no benefits. One study found that there was no change in the electrical activity of the retinal cells after use of the xanthophylls. These studies were mostly small studies, often without control groups, making them quite difficult to interpret; however, they did provide a suggestion of the benefits of xanthophylls.[64]

- **In two recent studies: one found no benefit of the use of lutein in the future risk of retinitis pigmentosa over time, and another found a benefit in visual acuity improvement** A 2001 study of 23 people with retinitis pigmentosa or Usher's syndrome (retinitis pigmentosa with hearing loss) found that lutein supplementation (20 mg per day) had no benefit to visual acuity over 6 months, though it did increase the density of the lutein pigment in the central retina.[65]

> Looking at the mechanisms of action, there is good reason to use lutein in moderation for macular degeneration and cataract.

An earlier 2000 study of 13 people with retinitis pigmentosa found that taking lutein (40 mg daily for 9 weeks, followed by 20 mg daily for a total of 26 weeks) along with docosahexaenoic acid (500 mg daily), vitamin B complex, and digestive enzymes results in an improvement in visual acuities. In fact, visual acuity improved by nearly one line, on average, and in one person, improved by two-and-one-half lines. This study is remarkable in that it is the only scientifically validated study that has demonstrated an improvement in visual acuity for any type of therapy involving retinitis pigmentosa.[66] The concerns of the study are the limited number of people enrolled and that the visual acuity testing was performed by the subjects themselves in their own homes over the internet.

Summary of Studies for Macular Degeneration:

Over a dozen clinical trials have been performed looking at the role of lutein in both preventing and treating macular degeneration. These clinical trials are of many different types, some of which are very well-designed and well-performed studies.

As a whole, the clinical studies provide no definitive answer as to whether lutein is beneficial. Many of the studies found no benefit to lutein for macular degeneration. However, there is some suggestion that is may be beneficial, as 7 out of the 17 studies found a benefit.

Lutein for
Macular Degeneration
Scale of Benefit

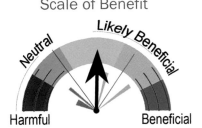

A Looking at the mechanisms of action, there is good reason to use lutein in moderation for macular degeneration.

The studies can be summarized as follows: one study found that those with macular degeneration had less lutein in their retinas. Three studies found a benefit in the past use of lutein in decreasing the risk of macular degeneration, while, one study found no benefit in the past use of lutein in decreasing the risk of macular degeneration. Interestingly, one study found that the past use of lutein actually increased the risk of macular degeneration, but this increased risk was in those who used lutein with high amounts of linoleic acid (see section on omega-6 oils). This finding supports the need for a well-balanced diet. Eating beneficial nutrients along with the bad may still cause harm. Several studies have shown no link (neither protective nor harmful) between

levels of lutein in the blood and macular degeneration, though two studies found that higher levels of lutein in the blood are associated with a decrease in the risk of macular degeneration. In following people over time, three large well-performed studies found that those who took lutein did not have any benefit in preventing macular degeneration compared to those who did not take lutein, while two small studies found that lutein in macular degeneration improves visual acuity over time.

● In one study: decreased lutein in the retina associated with macular degeneration
A study of over 100 autopsy cases found that those eyes with macular degeneration had lower levels of lutein and zeaxanthin in their retinas as compared to eyes without macular degeneration.[67]

● In one study: no benefits in past use of lutein found on risk of macular degeneration
A study of over 3,500 people age 49 and over found no link (neither protective nor harmful) between the risk of developing macular degeneration over a 5 year period and people who took the following nutrients, alone or in combination, in the past: lutein and zeaxanthin, beta-carotene, lycopene, vitamin A, or zinc. Surprisingly, however, the study found, that those who took vitamin C supplements combined with a diet high in vitamin C had a 2-fold increase in their risk of developing macular degeneration.[2] This finding is quite surprising, as

one would expect vitamin C to protect against macular degeneration, as opposed to increasing the risk of macular degeneration. However, the finding highlights the problems associated with these types of studies: namely, that the findings may occur coincidentally and other true findings may be missed. It is sometimes difficult to explain the findings or apply them to real life.

● One study found a harm: past use of lutein (with high amounts of linoleic acid) associated with *increased* risk of macular degeneration

A study of 2,000 people found that a diet high in lutein and zeaxanthin possibly decreased the risk of having dry or wet macular degeneration. However, when combined with a diet high in linoleic acid (a precursor of omega-6 fatty oils), the study found the risk of having dry or wet macular degeneration actually by increased by 2- to 5-fold![68] This finding of an increased risk with lutein and zeaxanthin is contrary to what one expects, but in the context of a diet high in linoleic acid, it supports the theory that a well-balanced diet is essential in protecting one's eyes. High amounts of linoleic acid by itself may be harmful (see section on omega-6 oils).

● Though the one study above found harm, several studies found a benefit: past use of lutein associated with decreased risk of macular degeneration

A large study of over 8,000 people age 40 and over found no link (neither protective nor harmful) between the risk of having macular degeneration (dry or wet) and a diet high in lutein and zeaxanthin. However, when the study population was divided, the study found that younger people age 40 to 59 who consumed diets high in lutein and zeaxanthin in the past had a 90% decrease in the risk of having *early* macular degeneration. Also, the study found that older people age 60 to 79 who consumed diets high in lutein and zeaxanthin in the past had a 90% decrease in the risk of having *advanced or severe* macular degeneration.[69]

A study of over 1,000 people age 55 to 80 found that those who consumed a diet high in lutein and zeaxanthin had a nearly 60% decrease in the risk of having wet macular degeneration compared to those who did not consume a diet high in lutein and zeaxanthin. Similarly, dietary beta-carotene decreased the risk by 40%, while dietary vitamin A and dietary carotenoids each decreased the risk by over 40%. The authors found no link (neither protective nor harmful) between macular degeneration and a diet high in vitamin C or E.[5]

A study of nearly 150 people age 60 and over found that those people who consumed higher amounts of lutein in their diets had over an 80% decrease in the risk of having wet macular degeneration.[70]

● In several studies: no link between blood levels of lutein and macular degeneration

A study of over 900 people age 60

to 80 found that the blood levels of lutein and of zeaxanthin were no different among people divided into 3 groups: with early macular degeneration, with advanced or severe macular degeneration, and without any macular degeneration.[71]

A study of over 300 people from a group of nearly 5,000 people found no difference in the blood levels of lutein and zeaxanthin, beta-carotene, or lycopene between those with or without macular degeneration. They also found that those who had macular degeneration had lower blood levels of vitamin E compared to those without macular degeneration. Interestingly, they also found that fewer people with macular degeneration use vitamin C than people without macular degeneration.[7]

Another study of nearly 100 people found no difference in the blood levels of lutein and zeaxanthin, carotenoids, beta-carotene, lycopene, vitamin A, vitamin C, zinc, or selenium between those with or without macular degeneration (looking at both early and severe or advanced macular degeneration). However, the study found that those who had severe or advanced macular degeneration had lower blood levels of vitamin E compared to those without macular degeneration. They found no differences in the blood levels of vitamin E between those with or without early macular degeneration.[6]

A study of 130 people also found no difference in the blood levels of lutein, beta-carotene, lycopene, vitamin A, or vitamin E

between those with or without macular degeneration.[9]

● **Though the four studies above found no link, two studies found a benefit: decreased risk of macular degeneration in those with higher blood levels of lutein**

A study of nearly 400 people age 66 to 75 found no link (neither protective nor harmful) between higher blood levels of lutein and macular degeneration. The study did find that those with higher blood levels of zeaxanthin had a 50% decrease in the risk of having macular degeneration (dry or wet). Interestingly, the study also found no link between macular degeneration and higher blood levels of zeaxanthin and lutein together.[72]

A study of over 1,000 people age 55 to 80 found that having higher blood levels of carotenoids decreased the risk of having wet macular degeneration by 60% compared to those who had lower blood levels of carotenoids.[11] Looking at specific carotenoids, the study found that having higher blood levels of lutein and zeaxanthin decreased the risk of having macular degeneration by 70%. Higher blood levels of beta-carotene also decreased the risk by 70% and higher blood levels of lycopene decreased the risk by 60%. Also, higher blood levels of a combination of three or more of four nutrients (carotenoids, vitamin C, vitamin E, and selenium) decreased the risk by 70%. The study found no link (neither protective nor harmful) between higher blood levels of vitamin C, vitamin E, or selenium by themselves and macular degeneration.[12]

● In large studies: no benefits from the use of lutein on the future risk of macular degeneration over time
A study of over 75,000 people (nurses and health professionals) followed over time for up to 18 years found no link (neither protective nor harmful) between the risk of developing macular degeneration (wet or dry) and a diet high in any of the following nutrients: lutein and zeaxanthin, carotenoids, beta-carotene, lycopene, vitamin A, vitamin C, or vitamin E. The study did find that those who consumed more than 3 servings of fruit each day were $1/3$ less likely to develop *wet* macular degeneration over time compared to those who consumed less than 1½ servings of fruit each day. No link (neither protective nor harmful) was found when looking at increased fruit consumption for dry macular degeneration, nor when looking at increased vegetable consumption for dry or wet macular degeneration.[15]

Looking over a 5-year period, a study of 2,000 people from a group of nearly 5,000, found no link (neither protective nor harmful) between macular degeneration and a diet high in lutein and zeaxanthin, beta-carotene, carotenoids, vitamin C, vitamin E, or zinc.[14]

A study of nearly 4,000 people, looking forward over an average of 8 years, found no link (neither protective nor harmful) between macular degeneration and a diet

high in lutein and zeaxanthin, beta-carotene, lycopene, vitamin A, vitamin C, iron, or zinc. However, a diet high in vitamin E decreased the risk of having macular degeneration by 20%. A diet high in multiple nutrients (beta-carotene, vitamin C, vitamin E, and zinc together) decreased the risk of having macular degeneration by about ½![18]

● Though the several studies above found no link, two small studies found a benefit: use of lutein in macular degeneration improves visual acuity over time
A study in 1999 of 14 people with macular degeneration found an actual improvement in visual acuity and other measures of visual functioning after one year of a lutein-rich diet.[73] It is unknown whether this finding represents a true improvement or simply a placebo effect, as there were no control groups in the study.

A recent 2004 study of 90 people with dry macular degeneration found that supplementation with lutein (12 mg per day), with or without additional antioxidants, resulted in a modest improvement in visual acuity (of about 1 line on a doctor's eye chart) over a period of 12 months.[74]

Summary of Studies for Cataract:
Over a half dozen clinical trials have been performed looking at the role of lutein in both preventing and treating cataract. These clinical trials are of many different

179

types, some of which are very well-designed and well-performed studies.

As a whole, the studies provide no definitive answer that lutein is beneficial. However, 5 of the 8 studies found a benefit. Looking at the mechanisms of action, there may be good reason to use lutein in moderation for cataract.

The studies can be summarized as follows: two

Lutein for
Cataract
Scale of Benefit

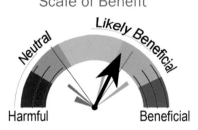

studies found no benefits from the past use of lutein on the risk of having cataract, while three larger studies that did find a benefit in the past use of lutein in decreasing the risk of cataract. One study found no link (neither protective nor harmful) between blood levels of lutein and the risk of having cataract while another study found that higher levels of lutein in the blood are associated with a decrease in the risk of cataract. There was one small study that had been reviewed by the scientific community that followed people taking lutein over time. This study found that vision improved in those who took lutein over a period of two years. However, the study was inconclusive as to whether the

improvement in visual acuity was related to the cataracts or the retina.

● **In two studies: no benefits in past use of lutein found on risk of cataract**   A study of nearly 500 people age 53 to 73 found no link (neither protective nor harmful) between the intake of lutein and zeaxanthin, beta-carotene, carotenoids, or lycopene and the risk of having cataracts. However, the study did show that the past intake of *higher* amounts of vitamin C decreased the risk of having cataracts by nearly 70%. It also found that long-term intake of vitamin C for over 10 years decreased the risk of having cataracts by nearly 65%. Similarly, past intake of *higher* amounts of vitamin B2 decreased the risk of having cataracts by over 60%, and past intake of *higher* amounts of folate decreased the risk by about 10%. It also found that long-term intake of vitamin E for over 10 years decreased the risk of having cataracts by over 50%, even though the study found no link (neither protective nor harmful) between the past intake of *higher* amounts of vitamin E and the risk of having cataracts. The finding of no beneficial link with higher doses of vitamin E may be related to increased risks associated with the higher doses. Furthermore, the use of a multivitamin for over 10 years reduced the risk of having cataract by over 40%.[20]

Another study of 400 people age 50 to 86 found no link (neither protective nor harmful) between the past use of lutein, beta-carotene, lycopene, vitamin A, or vitamin E and the risk of having cataract.[21]

● **Though the two studies above found no link, three large study found a benefit: past use of lutein associated with decreased risk of cataract** A 12-year study of over 75,000 nurses age 45 and over found that those who consumed the highest amounts of lutein and zeaxanthin in their diets had an over 20% reduction in the development of cataracts that required surgery.[75]

A similar 8-year study of over 35,000 male health professionals age 45 and over found that those who consumed the highest amounts of lutein and zeaxanthin in their diets had a nearly 20% reduction in the development of cataracts that required surgery.[76]

A study of over 1,300 people age 43 to 84 found that higher intake of lutein and zeaxanthin was associated with a decrease in the risk of having cataract by about a ½. No link (neither protective nor harmful) was found between cataract and the past use of vitamin C or of vitamin E over 10 years.[77]

● **In one study: no link between blood levels of lutein and cataract** A study of 400 people found no link (neither protective nor harmful) between higher blood levels of lutein, beta-carotene, or lycopene and the risk of having cataracts. However, the study found that higher blood levels of vitamin E decreased the risk of having cataracts by 60%.[26]

The study also looked at gender differences in this same group of people and found that some nutrients, such as lycopene, are more beneficial in women and other nutrients, such as vitamin A, are more beneficial in men. These results, however, are much more difficult to interpret.[27]

● **Though the one study above found no link, one study found a benefit: decreased risk of cataract in those with higher blood levels of lutein** A study of nearly 400 people age 66 to 75 found that higher levels of lutein in the blood decreased the risk of having one type of cataract but not another. Similarly, higher levels of beta-carotene and alpha-carotene in the blood decreased risk of having one type of cataract, whereas higher levels of lycopene in the blood decreased risk of having another type of cataract. However, the study found no link (neither protective nor harmful) between higher levels of vitamin C or vitamin E or zeaxanthin and the risk of having any type of cataract.[28]

● **One small study found a benefit: use of lutein decreases the future risk of cataract over time** An interesting, but small, study of 15 people with cataracts found that vision actually modestly improved in the group that took about 7 mg of lutein each day over a period of 2 years, compared to placebo. The study also found that those who took about 14 IU of vitamin E each day did not do any better or worse than those who took placebo.[78] This study is remarkable in that it shows an improvement in vision in those people on lutein. However, the study was problematic because of its small size (only 15 people enrolled) and the fact that the some people dropped out to have cataract surgery. Furthermore, it is inconclusive in the study whether the improvement in visual acuity was related to the cataracts or the retina.

Body Absorption, Metabolism, & Excretion

Digestion of fruits and vegetables occurs in the stomach with the assistance of stomach acids that help break down the fruits and vegetables to release the lutein. Lutein is insoluble in water, and therefore needs to be dissolved in fat micelles (spherical soap-bubble-like conglomerates of fat) that can carry lutein into the bloodstream from the intestines. Accordingly, eating a small quantity of fat with lutein assists in the absorption of lutein and greatly increases the amount that is delivered to the bloodstream. Lutein is then transported to specific tissues with the assistance of fatty-proteins.

Excretion of lutein occurs mostly through the kidneys. Some excretion occurs through the digestive tract while excess lutein is often dumped back into the digestive tract through bile (a green fluid produced by the liver that is stored in the gallbladder to assist in digestion).

Deficiency

It has been shown that lutein and zeaxanthin levels are reduced in people with cystic fibrosis compared to healthy control people. Cystic fibrosis is an inherited lung disease and pancreas disease in which there is poor absorption of certain vitamin and nutrients, including lutein and zeaxanthin, as well as vitamins A, D, and E. However, a study that found the decreased lutein and zeaxanthin levels did not show any difference in visual functioning in people with cystic fibrosis.

Toxicity & Side Effects

Excess lutein and zeaxanthin can result in a yellow-bronze discoloration of the skin, called carotenodermia or xanthosis cutis. It is harmless and can be reversed upon cessation of the supplementation.

Interactions with Other Nutrients

Fat in one's diet is an essential component of good carotenoid nutrition. It is required for absorption of lutein and zeaxanthin by the digestive system. However, in people with excess fat stores in their bodies, lutein and zeaxanthin can accumulate in body fat rather than be sent to the eyes when needed.

Furthermore, HDL (good type of cholesterol) is required for transportation of lutein and zeaxanthin to the retinas. In people with less of HDL, there is less lutein and zeaxanthin in their retinas. In fact, this finding may be one of the reasons why women undergoing menopause have a higher risk of macular degeneration since their HDL levels decrease during menopause.

Ideal Dosage

The recommended dose of lutein is 6 to 12 mg each day. Interestingly, zeaxanthin can be made from lutein within cells of the retina.

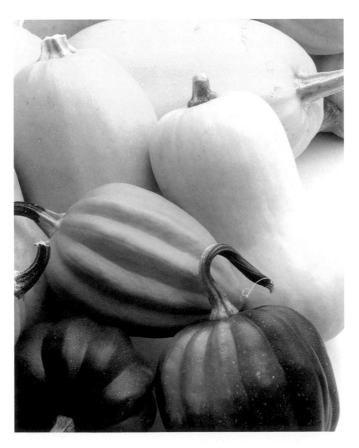

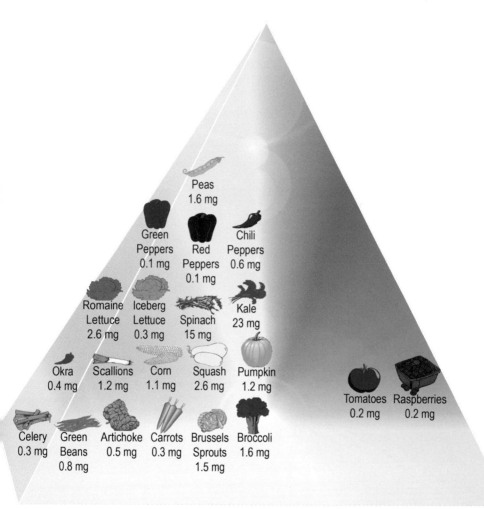

Peas
1.6 mg

Green Peppers
0.1 mg

Red Peppers
0.1 mg

Chili Peppers
0.6 mg

Romaine Lettuce
2.6 mg

Iceberg Lettuce
0.3 mg

Spinach
15 mg

Kale
23 mg

Okra
0.4 mg

Scallions
1.2 mg

Corn
1.1 mg

Squash
2.6 mg

Pumpkin
1.2 mg

Tomatoes
0.2 mg

Raspberries
0.2 mg

Celery
0.3 mg

Green Beans
0.8 mg

Artichoke
0.5 mg

Carrots
0.3 mg

Brussels Sprouts
1.5 mg

Broccoli
1.6 mg

Pyramid Key:

Fats & Sweets

Dairy

Meats & Nuts

Vegetables

Fruits

Breads & Grains

Sources above are for lutein and zeaxanthin together. The top sources are spinach and kale. Other high sources include squash, romaine lettuce, peas, broccoli, and Brussels sprouts.

*See Guides on Pages 467-468.

LYCOPENE

Category

Carotenoids are organic pigments that occur naturally in plants, but cannot be made by animals (see section on carotenoids).
Lycopene is a red carotenoid in the carotene family.

Cellular Location

Unlike the carotenoids, lutein and zeaxanthin, lycopene is not concentrated in the retina, and is not found in the lens or aqueous fluid that bathes the lens and occupies the front of the eye. It is most concentrated in the bloodstream, liver, lungs, colon, and skin.

Structure

Lycopene is a long compound composed of 8 units, called isoprenes in a chain. The presence of many double bonds in the long chain gives lycopene its characteristic red color. Additionally, its structure causes it to be insoluble in water, so it prefers to be in the presence of oils and fats.

Mechanisms of Action

Lycopene acts as an antioxidant by donating electrons to prevent oxidation.

Biological & Ocular Importance

● **Powerful antioxidant to preserve other antioxidants and prevent eye disease**
Lycopene is a very potent antioxidant and one of the most potent antioxidants against the harmful singlet oxygen. In fact, it is more powerful as an antioxidant against singlet oxygen than any other known carotenoid, such as lutein or zeaxanthin.

As an antioxidant, it is believed to be beneficial to retinal diseases, such as macular degeneration and childhood hereditary photoreceptor diseases, in which oxidative damage plays a role in the disease. It may also be beneficial in diseases, such as glaucoma or optic nerve diseases, in which oxidative damage plays a role as well. Furthermore, it may also help prevent cataract formation or corneal disease, again by preventing or decreasing oxidative damage.

Animal studies have shown that dietary lycopene can stop the formation and progression of cataracts that are caused by oxidative damage. Lycopene functions in these cases as an antioxidant itself and, by doing so, also preserves the concentrations and actions of other antioxidants found in the lens.

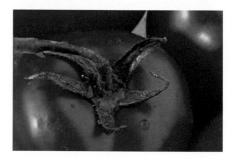

Human Studies on Utility

Currently, there are numerous human studies on lutein use in eye disease reported in the scientifically-reviewed medical literature. These studies involve the eye disease macular degeneration, cataract, and retinitis pigmentosa. These studies are described below.

Summary of Studies for Macular Degeneration:
Over a half dozen clinical trials have been performed looking at the role of lycopene in both preventing and treating macular degeneration. These clinical trials are of various types, some of which are very well-designed

and well-performed studies.

As a whole, the clinical studies provide no definitive answer as to whether lycopene is beneficial, and, in fact, the majority of studies found no benefit to lycopene for macular degeneration. However, there some suggestion that it may be beneficial, as 2 out of the 7 studies found a benefit. Looking at the mechanisms of action, there may be good reason to use lycopene in moderation for macular degeneration.

The studies can be summarized as follows: one

Lycopene for Macular Degeneration Scale of Benefit

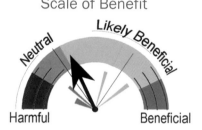

study found no benefit in the past use of lycopene on the risk of macular degeneration. Three studies have shown no link (neither protective nor harmful) between levels of lycopene in the blood and macular degeneration, while two studies found that higher blood levels of lycopene are associated with a decrease in the risk of macular degeneration. In following people over time, two large, well-performed studies found that those who took lycopene did not have any benefit in preventing macular degeneration compared to those who did not take lycopene.

● **In one study: no benefits in past use of lycopene found on risk of macular degeneration**   A study of over 3,500 people age 49 and over found no link (neither protective nor harmful) between the risk of developing macular degeneration over a 5 year period and people who took the following nutrients, alone or in combination, in the past: lycopene, lutein and zeaxanthin, beta-carotene, vitamin A, or zinc. Surprisingly, however, the study found, that those who took vitamin C supplements combined with a diet high in vitamin C had a 2-fold increase in their risk of developing macular degeneration.[2] This finding is quite surprising, as one would expect vitamin C to protect against macular degeneration, as opposed to increasing the risk of macular degeneration. However, the finding highlights the problems associated with these types of studies: namely, that the findings may occur coincidentally and other true findings may be missed. It is sometimes difficult to explain the findings or apply them to real life.

● **In several studies: no link between blood levels of lycopene and macular degeneration**   A study of over 300 people from a group of nearly 5,000 people found no difference in the blood levels of lycopene, beta-carotene, or lutein and zeaxanthin between those with or without macular degeneration. They also found that those who had macular degeneration had lower blood levels of vitamin E compared to those without macular degeneration. Interestingly, they also found that fewer people with macular degeneration use vitamin C than people without macular degeneration.[7]

Another study of nearly 100 people found no difference in the blood levels of lycopene, carotenoids, beta-carotene, lutein and zeaxanthin, vitamin A, vitamin C, zinc, or selenium between those with or without macular degeneration (looking at both early and severe or advanced macular degeneration). However, the study found that those who had severe or advanced macular degeneration had lower blood levels of vitamin E compared to those without macular degeneration. They found no differences in the blood levels of vitamin E between those with or without early macular degeneration.[6]

A study of 130 people also found no difference in the blood levels of lycopene, beta-carotene, lutein, vitamin A, or vitamin E between those with or without macular degeneration.[9]

● **Though the three studies above found no link, two studies found a benefit: decreased risk of macular degeneration in those with higher blood levels of lycopene** A study of 55 people found that lycopene levels in the blood are lower in people with macular degeneration than those without.[79] Because lycopene does not directly concentrate in the retina to act as an antioxidant, the researchers hypothesize that lycopene acts as an antioxidant in our bloodstream and, by doing so, preserves lutein and zeaxanthin from being used up as antioxidants. This preservation of lutein and zeaxanthin then allows them to be available for use in the retina.

A study of over 1,000 people age 55 to 80 found that having higher blood levels of carotenoids decreased the risk of having wet macular degeneration by 60% compared to those who had lower blood levels of carotenoids.[11] Looking at specific carotenoids, the study found that having higher blood levels of lycopene decreased the risk of having macular degeneration by 60%. Higher blood levels of lutein and zeaxanthin decreased the risk by 70% and higher blood levels of beta-carotene also decreased the risk by 70%. Furthermore, higher blood levels of a combination of three or more of four nutrients (carotenoids, vitamin C, vitamin E, and selenium) decreased the risk by 70%. The study found no link (neither protective nor harmful) between higher blood levels of vitamin C, vitamin E, or selenium by themselves and macular degeneration.[12]

● **In large studies: no benefits from the use of lycopene on the future risk of macular degeneration over time** A study of over 75,000 people (nurses and health professionals) followed over time for up to 18 years found no link (neither protective nor harmful) between the risk of developing macular degeneration (wet or dry) and a diet high in any of the following nutrients: lycopene, carotenoids, lutein and zeaxanthin, beta-carotene, vitamin A, vitamin C, or vitamin E. The study did find that those who consumed more than 3 servings of fruit each day were 1/3 less likely to develop *wet* macular degeneration over time compared to those who consumed less than 1½ servings of fruit each day. No link (neither protective nor harmful) was found when looking at increased fruit consumption for dry macular degeneration, nor when looking at increased vegetable consumption for dry or wet macular degeneration.[15]

A study of nearly 4,000 people, looking forward over an average of 8 years, found no link (neither protective nor harmful) between macular degeneration and a diet high in lycopene, beta-carotene, lutein and zeaxanthin, vitamin A, vitamin C, iron, or zinc. However, a diet high in vitamin E decreased the risk of having macular degeneration by 20%. A diet high in multiple nutrients (beta-carotene, vitamin C, vitamin E, and zinc together) decreased the risk of having macular degeneration by about ½![18]

 Summary of Studies for Cataract: Currently, four clinical trials have been performed looking at the role of lycopene in both preventing and treating cataract. These clinical trials are of various types, some of which are very well-designed and well-performed studies.

As a whole, the clinical studies provide no definitive answer as to whether lycopene is beneficial, and, in fact, the majority of studies found no benefit to lycopene for cataract. However, there some suggestion that it may be beneficial, as 1 out of the 4 studies found a benefit.

Lycopene for
Cataract
Scale of Benefit

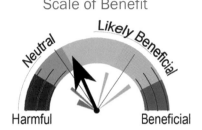

A Looking at the mechanisms of action, there may be good reason to use lycopene in moderation for cataract.

The studies can be summarized as follows: two studies found no benefits from the past use of lycopene on the risk of cataract. One study found no link (neither protective nor harmful) between blood levels of lycopene and the risk of cataract, while another study found a decreased risk of macular degeneration in those with higher blood levels of lycopene. There are no studies that have been reviewed by the scientific community that followed people taking lycopene over time.

● **In two studies: no benefits in past use of lycopene found on risk of cataract** A study of nearly 500 people age 53 to 73 found no link (neither protective nor harmful) between the intake of lycopene, lutein and zeaxanthin, beta-carotene, or carotenoids and the risk of having cataracts. However, the study did show that the past intake of *higher* amounts of vitamin C decreased the risk of having cataracts by nearly 70%. It also found that long-term intake of vitamin C for over 10 years decreased the risk of having cataracts by nearly 65%. Similarly, past intake of *higher* amounts of vitamin B2 decreased the risk of having cataracts by over 60%, and past intake of *higher* amounts of folate decreased the risk by about 10%. It also found that long-term intake of vitamin E for over 10 years decreased the risk of having cataracts by over 50%, even though the study found no link (neither protective nor harmful) between the past intake of *higher* amounts of vitamin E and the risk of having cataracts. The finding of no beneficial link with higher doses of vitamin E may be related to increased risks associated with the higher doses. Furthermore, the use of a multivitamin for over 10 years reduced the risk of having cataract by over 40%.[20]

Another study of 400 people age 50 to 86 found no link (neither protective nor harmful) between the past use of lycopene, beta-carotene, lutein, vitamin A, or vitamin E and the risk of having cataract.[21]

● In one study: no link between blood levels of lycopene and cataract   A study of 400 people found no link

(neither protective nor harmful) between higher blood levels of lycopene, beta-carotene, or lutein and the risk of having cataracts. However, unlike the other study, this study found that higher blood levels of vitamin E decreased the risk of having cataracts by 60%.[26] The study also looked at gender differences in this same group of

> Looking at the mechanisms of action, there is good reason to use lycopene in moderation for macular degeneration and cataract.

people and found that some nutrients, such as lycopene, are more beneficial in women and other nutrients, such as vitamin A, are more beneficial in men. These results, however, are much more difficult to interpret.[27]

● In another study: decreased risk of cataract in those with higher blood levels of lycopene   A study of nearly 400 people age 66 to 75 found that higher levels of lycopene in the blood decreased the risk of having one type of cataract but not another. Similarly, higher levels of lutein in the blood decreased risk of having one type of cataract, whereas higher levels of beta-carotene and alpha-carotene in the blood decreased risk of having another type of cataract. However, the study found no link (neither protective nor harmful) between higher levels of vitamin C or vitamin E or zeaxanthin and the risk of having any type of cataract.[28]

Body Absorption, Metabolism, & Excretion

Digestion of fruits and vegetables occurs in the stomach with the assistance of stomach acids that help break down the fruits and vegetables to release the lycopene. Lycopene is not soluble in water, and so it needs to be dissolved in fat micelles (spherical soap-bubble-like conglomerates of fat) that can carry lycopene into the bloodstream from the intestines. Accordingly, eating a small quantity of fat with lycopene assists in the absorption of lycopene and greatly increases the amount that is delivered to the bloodstream. Lycopene is then transported to specific tissues with the assistance of fatty-proteins.

Excretion of lycopene occurs mostly through the kidneys. Some excretion occurs through the digestive tract and excess lycopene is often dumped back into the digestive tract through bile (a green fluid produced by the liver that is stored in the gallbladder to assist in digestion).

Deficiency

There are no known disorders of lycopene deficiency. Instead, the deficiency that ensues is from a widespread deficiency of carotenoids, which is often associated with other nutritional deficiencies.

Toxicity & Side Effects

Lycopene may cause an allergic reaction in those who are sensitive to tomatoes.

Interactions with Other Nutrients

There is limited knowledge of the interaction of lycopene with other nutrients.

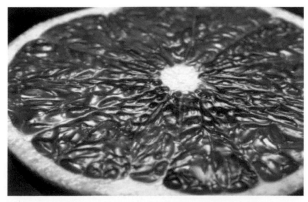

Ideal Dosage

The recommended dose of lycopene is about 4 to 8 mg each day; however, some researchers recommend doses as high as 15 mg per day.

Sources (Where to Find It)

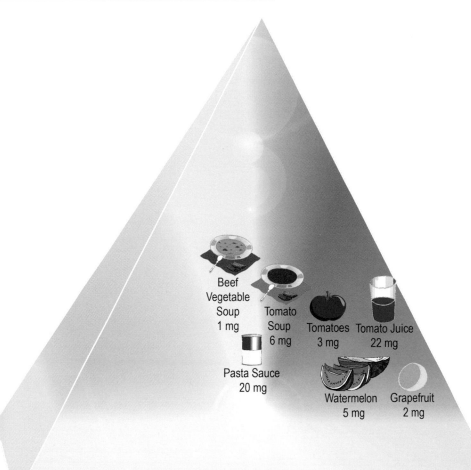

Beef Vegetable Soup
1 mg

Tomato Soup
6 mg

Tomatoes
3 mg

Tomato Juice
22 mg

Pasta Sauce
20 mg

Watermelon
5 mg

Grapefruit
2 mg

Pyramid Key:

Fats & Sweets

Dairy   Meats & Nuts

Vegetables   Fruits

Breads & Grains

The top sources for lycopene are tomatoes, watermelon, and pink grapefruit.

*See Guides on Pages 467-468.

LYSINE

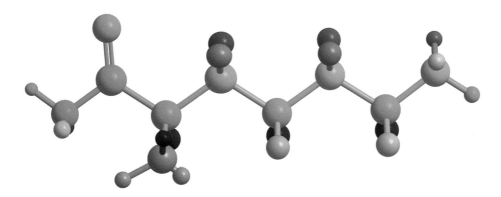

Category

Lysine is an essential amino acid (building block of proteins).

Cellular Location

Lysine is distributed through the bloodstream to various organs. Since proteins cannot be stored by the human body, unused proteins are metabolized and excreted.

Structure

Lysine is an amino acid with a relatively long chain, called an aminobutyl group.

Mechanisms of Action

Lysine is a building block of proteins and is a component of collagen.

Biological & Ocular Importance

● **Makes collagen which provides support for the cornea, vitreous, retina, eye filtration site, & optic nerve support site** Collagen is an important component of many parts of the eye, as well as other parts of the body, including bones. Collagen is formed with the help of vitamin C and copper, as well as lysine and proline (see section on vitamin C).

Collagen is the major protein of the cornea and its uniformity and pattern of arrangement is essential in maintaining the clarity of the cornea. Along with elastin, it forms the layers of Bruch's membrane, a support layer that separates the retinal pigment epithelium from the underlying choroidal blood vessels. In wet macular degeneration as well as in extremely high myopia (near-sightedness), cracks can develop in Bruch's membrane through which new blood vessels grow that can lead to bleeding and scarring as well as detachment and distortion of the retina.

Collagen maintains the trabecular meshwork, (the filtration site of the eye) by preventing it from collapsing. Allowing enough fluid to exit the eye is essential to prevent pressure build-up in the eye, decreasing the risk of glaucoma, since malfunction of this filtration site is a common mechanism of glaucoma.

Collagen also forms the lamina cribrosa, a structure that supports individual nerve fibers as they pass from the retina into the optic nerve. One mechanism of glaucoma is damage to these nerve fibers when the lamina cribrosa is unable to support them.

Collagen is also the major structural component of the vitreous. The vitreous gel is water supported by collagen and hyaluronic acid (see section on hyaluronic acid). In fact, the vitreous is 99% water supported in this collagen and hyaluronic acid meshwork. Vitreous floaters, which appear as cobwebs or spiders or spots floating in one's vision, occur when the vitreous begins to shrink. The vitreous shrinks at different ages for different people, often ranging from age 20 to age 70, though more commonly in the elderly. Decrease in collagen is associated with premature shrinking of the vitreous. Vitreous shrinking is associated with tears in the retina as well as detachments of the retina.

Collagen is also an important protein that forms skin, tendons, ligaments, and blood vessels as well. Capillaries are where the arteries thin to the point of supplying tissue with nutrients and oxygen from the blood supply, in exchange for waste materials and carbon dioxide that must be transported out in veins.

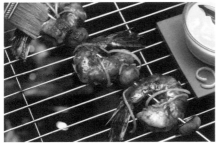

Capillary malfunction can result in tissue swelling, bleeding, and inappropriate control of tissue nutrition and oxygenation.

Finally, because collagen is also important in bone formation, lysine may play a role in preventing osteoporosis as well. Lysine may also assist in the absorption of calcium in the intestines.

● Blocks viruses & pink eye

Lysine is believed to interfere with replication of viruses, and, in animal models of the disease, it has been shown to decrease the severity of pink eye, or conjunctivitis, when it is caused by the herpes virus.

● Maintains fluid balance in cells

Lysine, as with other amino acids, plays an important role in osmoregulation (the maintenance of the fluid concentration of a cell through osmosis, whereby fluids move from areas of low protein and low ionic content to areas of high protein and high ionic content).

● Prevents damaging effects of high sugars on the eye

In addition, lysine may also act to prevent the formation of "advanced glycation end products" or AGEs, the toxic products that damage the retina, the lens, and other ocular structures (see introduction). Other amino acids, particularly taurine, act in these roles and may be beneficial in combination with lysine (see section on taurine).

Human Studies on Utility

There are no human studies on the use of lysine in eye disease reported in the scientifically-reviewed medical literature. Nevertheless, the fact that there are no reported clinical studies does not necessarily imply a benefit or lack of benefit. Looking at the mechanism of action, the use of lysine in moderation may be possibly of benefit in certain eye diseases.

Body Absorption, Metabolism, & Excretion

Lysine is digested by the stomach with the help of stomach acids. Digestive enzymes from the pancreas further break down proteins, which are then absorbed into the bloodstream through the intestines.

As proteins are broken down, ammonia is formed. Since ammonia is extremely toxic to cells, it must be converted into a nitrogen-containing chemical known as urea. When ammonia builds up in excess, it can cause poor coordination, difficulties with balance, tremors, seizures, difficulty breathing, swelling of the brain, and can eventually lead to a coma. A normally functioning liver works to remove excess ammonia by creating urea, which is then filtered into the urine by the kidneys.

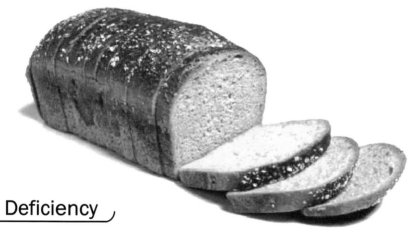

Deficiency

Lysine deficiency was made popular in a recent novel and movie in which dinosaurs were recreated in modern times from their DNA that was found; however, these dinosaurs were genetically engineered to have a lysine deficiency. When in captivity, they would be fed a diet with lysine, but if they escaped, they would not receive the lysine and would go into a coma and die within 12 hours. While this tale is pure fiction, it is important to note that lysine is an essential amino acid, and that the human body cannot produce lysine on its own.

Lysine deficiency may cause nausea, loss of appetite, dizziness, and fatigue. Weight loss and delayed growth may also occur. Neurologic and psychologic manifestations of lysine deficiency include anxiety, irritability, poor concentration, and lack of energy.

Toxicity & Side Effects

Excess lysine is believed to induce the breakdown of arginine (see section on arginine), and as a result, elevated levels of cholesterol have been reported.

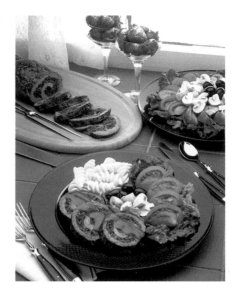

Excess lysine, like other amino acids, is often broken down and converted into sugars or fats, and used for energy, or stored as fat in the body's fat stores. Excess amino acids can stress the kidneys, stress the bloodstream, and cause dehydration. Furthermore, excess amino acids can cause the kidneys to lose calcium, resulting in weakened bones. As with any amino acid in excess, lysine in someone with liver disease or with kidney disease may result in build-up of ammonia or urea in the body, resulting in severe illness (see above).

In diabetics, excess amino acids can result in an increased sugar load on the body, or increased fat deposits in the body!

High amounts of lysine have been reported to cause gallstones.

Also, high doses are associated with upset stomach, nausea, vomiting, diarrhea, and abdominal cramping.

Interactions with Other Nutrients

Lysine assists in the absorption of calcium. Consequently, a deficiency of lysine may cause a deficiency of calcium, resulting in weak bones or osteoporosis.

Lysine is required in the pathway of making carnitine because lysine forms the backbone of carnitine. Therefore, lysine deficiency may result in carnitine deficiency, though the carnitine deficiency that ensues is often only a minimal deficiency.

Ideal Dosage

The recommended dose is 800 to 1,200 mg per day. In cases of viral infection, doses of up to 3,000 mg per day have been suggested.

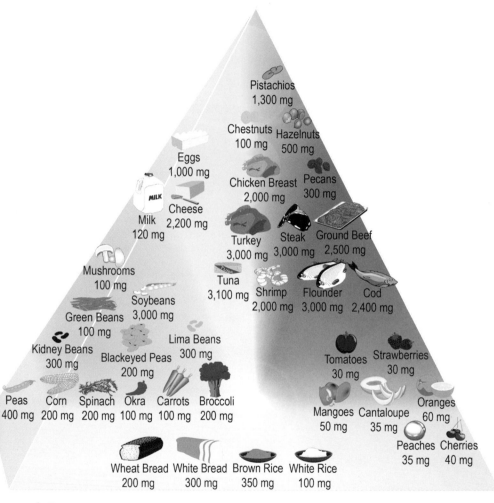

Pistachios
1,300 mg

Chestnuts Hazelnuts
100 mg   500 mg

Eggs
1,000 mg

Chicken Breast Pecans
2,000 mg   300 mg

Milk Cheese
120 mg 2,200 mg

Turkey   Steak   Ground Beef
3,000 mg 3,000 mg 2,500 mg

Mushrooms
100 mg

Tuna
3,100 mg Shrimp Flounder Cod
          2,000 mg 3,000 mg 2,400 mg

Soybeans
3,000 mg

Green Beans
100 mg

Kidney Beans   Lima Beans
300 mg   300 mg
     Blackeyed Peas
     200 mg

Tomatoes Strawberries
30 mg   30 mg

Peas   Corn   Spinach Okra   Carrots Broccoli
400 mg 200 mg 200 mg 100 mg 100 mg   200 mg

Mangoes Cantaloupe Oranges
50 mg   35 mg   60 mg

Peaches Cherries
35 mg   40 mg

Wheat Bread White Bread Brown Rice White Rice
200 mg   300 mg   350 mg   100 mg

Pyramid Key:

Fats & Sweets

Dairy   Meats & Nuts

Vegetables   Fruits

Breads & Grains

Top sources of lysine include meats (beef, turkey, chicken, and seafood) and dairy products (eggs and cheese). Soybeans contain very high amounts of lysine. Some nuts such as pistachios are also rich in lysine.

MAGNESIUM

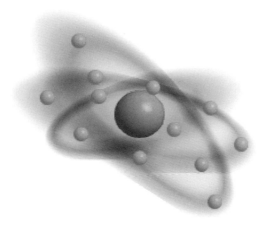

Category

Magnesium is an essential element.

Cellular Location

About one-half to two-thirds of the body's magnesium is located in the bones. Another ¼ of the body's magnesium is located in muscle, while the remainder is distributed throughout various organs in the body.

Structure

Magnesium is a metallic element. Its symbol on the periodic table of elements is Mg, and its atomic number is 12. It is found next to sodium, above from calcium, and diagonally adjacent to potassium on the periodic table.

Mechanisms of Action

Magnesium plays a role in several hundred different enzymes.

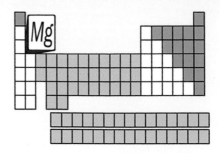

Biological & Ocular Importance

● **Essential for building proteins & creating energy**
Magnesium is important in several hundred enzymes as well as in the synthesis of proteins. In fact, magnesium activates almost all the enzyme reactions that involve the creation of ATP (the universal energy chemical of all living cells), from sugars and fats in our diet. In fact, 90% of all ATP in our cells is bound to magnesium!

Magnesium is involved in the process of vitamin B1 forming thiamine pyrophosphate, an important enzyme involved in metabolism and energy production. An essential function of vitamin B1 is to form the enzyme thiamine pyrophosphate (see section on vitamin B1).

Magnesium plays an important role in many enzymes involved in energy metabolism, synthesis of proteins, and glucose transportation across membranes of cells. As such, magnesium supplementation has been shown to help decrease blood glucose levels and insulin sensitivity in diabetes in some studies, but not in others.

● **Helps regulate blood flow through vessels**   Magnesium is essential in regulating the release of nitric oxide from the insides of cells. When nitric oxide is released, it helps maintain the proper dilation of blood vessels and helps prevent the development of hypertension (high blood pressure). Nitric oxide is also believed to be important in maintaining blood flow in the retina in diseases such as diabetic retinopathy and glaucoma. Furthermore, nitric oxide helps prevent infections in our bodies, particularly in our throats, sinuses, and lungs. Along with other agents, nitric oxide also helps block the bone-eating osteoclasts that are involved in the development of osteoporosis. When nitric oxide resides inside the cell for too long, it can form peroxynitrites, or chemicals that cause oxidation, or damage to the cells.

Magnesium is also involved in helping enzymes that regulate proper dilation of blood vessels by promoting those that dilate the blood vessels and decreasing the activity of those that constrict blood vessels.   As such, magnesium can also help regulate and reduce blood pressure.

● **Assists in muscle relaxation**   Magnesium helps regulate and decrease the release of acetylcholine (a nerve signaling agent) from nerve ends. Decreasing the acetylcholine prevents unnecessary muscle contractions. Magnesium deficiency can be associated with uncontrollable muscle contractions.

Because of its role in muscle relaxation, magnesium can help treat disorders of muscle spasm around the eyes, such as blepharospam, a disease of excess spasms or contractions of the eye lids. It has also been suggested that magnesium can play a similar role in treating other disorders in which muscle spasm around the eye plays a role, such as ocular migraines. Magnesium also helps to relax muscle fibers by counteracting the contraction of muscle fibers by calcium. As a muscle relaxant, magnesium can also lessen arterial spasms that result from arterial muscle contractions. Fewer spasms can be of benefit to the optic nerve and tissues around the eye.

Magnesium may also help reduce muscle pains and premenstrual cramps. It has been shown to relieve chronic fatigue as well.

● **Regulates neurotransmitter release &**

prevents cell injury
Glutamate is a natural signaling chemical in neural cells that enables signals to transfer from one cell to another. It is the main signal producer in the circuitry of the eye. There is experimental evidence that magnesium can help regulate the release of glutamate from rod and cone photoreceptors, other retinal circuit neurons, and the retinal ganglion cells that form and send axons that comprise the optic nerve. Of note, excess glutamate is toxic to surrounding cells. When a cell dies, for example in glaucoma, it can release excess glutamate, resulting in toxic injury and death of surrounding cells. Magnesium can help regulate glutamate release and prevent toxicity.

Magnesium also has been found to help reduce the frequency of migraines. Also, it is believed that magnesium can help block "photosensitive migraines," or migraines that form upon "photo-stress" or stimulation with bright lights.

● **Assists in stabilizing cell membranes & preventing cell injury**   Magnesium also helps stabilize cell membranes, which can help maintain proper heart rhythms.

Magnesium also stabilizes membrane mineral channels and helps regulate calcium influx into cells because excessive calcium influx into cells can lead to degeneration and death of cells. Excess calcium can also over-stimulate neural cells such as the cells of the retina and optic nerve, through a process called excitotoxicity. Magnesium helps regulate the calcium levels.

● **Plays a role in enzymes of the retina** Magnesium plays an important role in many enzymes of the retina. In some animal models, magnesium deficiency is also associated with disease of the retinal pigment epithelium that can mimic some inflammatory diseases of the retinal pigment epithelium, such as acute posterior multifocal placoid pigment epitheliopathy.

● **Helps the lens maintain its clarity** There is evidence that magnesium is essential to an important enzyme of the lens, which helps the lens maintain its clarity. In fact, animal studies have shown that magnesium deficiency is associated with cataract formation.

● **Prevents corneal infections & dry eye** In the cornea, magnesium may help ward off infections as well as prevent dryness. One method that magnesium may help prevent infection is by enhancing production of enzymes that attack bacteria.

● **Prevents thinning of the cornea** There is also evidence that magnesium may play a role in the development of the corneal disorder, keratoconus, where the cornea thins out over time and starts to bulge forward abnormally because of its thinness. Magnesium deficiency has been associated with multiple findings in the cornea: thinness, degeneration of the cells, and degeneration of the collagen fibers, and abnormal production of proteins. Keratoconus involves these aforementioned processes and may involve magnesium deficiency as part of the how the disorder develops.

● **Forms other antioxidant enzymes** Other enzymes in which magnesium plays a role are antioxidant enzymes. Antioxidant enzymes are believed to be beneficial to retinal diseases, such as macular degeneration and childhood hereditary photoreceptor diseases, in which oxidative damage plays a role in the disease. Also, they may be beneficial in diseases such as glaucoma or optic nerve diseases in which oxidative damage plays a role. They may also help prevent cataract formation or corneal disease, again by preventing or decreasing oxidative damage.

● **Helps remove metals from the body** Magnesium helps in the removal of metals from the body. When magnesium levels are low, heavy metals, including lead and cadmium and other metals such as iron and aluminum, are more easily retained in the body. The damaging effects of these metals are known to inflict many organs, including the brain.

Human Studies on Utility

Currently, there are only three human studies on magnesium use in eye disease reported in the scientifically-reviewed medical literature. Nevertheless, the fact that there are only three reported clinical studies does not necessarily imply a benefit or lack of benefit. Looking at the mechanism of action, the use of magnesium in moderation may be possibly of benefit in many eye diseases.

● **Studies show link with diabetic retinal disease and low levels of magnesium in the blood**   There are several studies that have shown that decreased levels of magnesium in the blood are associated with both higher levels of retinopathy in diabetics or progression of retinopathy in diabetics.

● **One study shows no link between blood levels of magnesium and cataract**   A study of 165 people found no link (neither beneficial nor harmful) between cataracts and magnesium, zinc, copper, vitamin

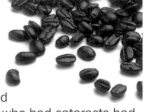

A, and vitamin E levels in the blood. However, the study found that those who had cataracts had lower levels of carotenoids and vitamin D in their blood compared to those who did not have cataracts. On the other hand, the study found that those who had cataracts had higher levels of selenium in their blood.[41]

● **One small study shows no benefits to the visual fields with the short-term use of magnesium in those with glaucoma**   A 1995 study of 10 people with glaucoma found no link (neither beneficial nor harmful) between visual field worsening or improvement and supplementation with 121.5 mg of magnesium each day for 4 months. However, the authors did suggest the role of magnesium in acting as a natural "calcium-channel blocker" to help improve ocular blood flow.[80]

Body Absorption, Metabolism, & Excretion

Magnesium absorption is quite a demanding task. It requires both vitamin D and a protein hormone called parathyroid hormone. Interestingly, when parathyroid hormone is extremely low, it requires magnesium in order to release the parathyroid hormone. This scenario is certainly a catch-22, as magnesium absorption requires parathyroid hormone and parathyroid hormone cannot be released if magnesium is too low. In addition, low levels of vitamin

B6 can prevent the absorption of magnesium. Similarly, high levels of saturated fats, the "bad oils," can block the absorption of magnesium. As such, only about $^1/_3$ to $^1/_2$ of the intake of magnesium is absorbed into the bloodstream.

The kidneys filter magnesium and play a central role in maintaining the appropriate magnesium levels in the bloodstream by either decreasing filtration when concentrations are low or by increasing filtration when concentrations are high. The filtered magnesium is excreted in the urine.

Deficiency

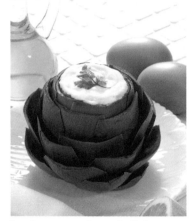

Magnesium deficiency may be caused by dietary deficiency or by metabolic abnormalities. Muscle twitches, muscle spasms, tremors, nausea, and vomiting are possible manifestations of a deficiency in magnesium. Hypertension (high blood pressure) is also a common result of magnesium deficiency.

Magnesium deficiency has been associated with osteoporosis and with diabetes. It has also been associated with atherosclerosis (blood vessel cholesterol clots and plaques that can result in heart disease and stroke, as well as artery or vein clots in the retina or optic nerve strokes) as well as with heart disease and abnormal heart rhythms.

Magnesium may play a role in maintaining appropriate blood vessel dilation and antioxidant activities in retinopathy of prematurity (a blinding retinal disease in new born infants who are born premature and exposed to oxygen in their incubator). There is some evidence to suggest that some forms of retinopathy of prematurity may be related to magnesium deficiency in the setting of oxygen use in the incubator.

Toxicity & Side Effects

Excess magnesium results in relaxation of muscle fibers that can result in, for example, loose stools. Abdominal cramping can occur with or without the diarrhea. In mild excess, magnesium can cause diarrhea, nausea, vomiting, and cramps.

Severely excess magnesium can also cause drowsiness and confusion. It can also cause severely low blood pressure as well as a slowed heart, heart block, and heart attacks. Difficulty breathing can also occur as can death from lung malfunction.

Interactions with Other Nutrients

There are numerous interactions between magnesium and other nutrients. The important concept is that a balance should be achieved between intake of magnesium and other nutrients.

In order to have proper magnesium absorption, the body requires vitamin D and vitamin B6 (see above).

When selenium levels are low, magnesium is more easily eliminated through the kidneys, a process that results in high levels of iron in the body.

High doses of zinc can result in blocked magnesium absorption.

Magnesium, copper, zinc, and iron may inhibit the absorption of vitamin B2.

When magnesium levels are low, vitamin B1 cannot form thiamine pyrophosphate, an important enzyme involved in metabolism and energy production. An essential function of vitamin B1 is to form the enzyme thiamine pyrophosphate (see section on vitamin B1). In fact, in states of low magnesium, instead of forming thiamine pyrophosphate, calcium pyrophosphate is formed, which can cause painful crystal formation in the body. In addition to the metabolism and energy problems, low levels of thiamine pyrophosphate are associated with gastrointestinal infections as well as brain disturbances such as hallucinations, confusion, disorientation, and even encephalopathy, a disorder of brain function involving confusion or even coma. Even in the presence of normal vitamin B1 levels in the body, magnesium deficiency can cause low levels of thiamine pyrophosphate, which looks just like vitamin B1 deficiency without deficiency of vitamin B1.

Ideal Dosage

The recommended daily dose of magnesium is about 300 to 400 mg. For boys age 14 to 18, the recommended dose is 410 mg per day, for men age 19 to 30, it is 400 mg per day, and for men over age 30, it is 420 mg per day. For girls age 14 to 18, the recommended dose is 360 mg per day, and for women age 19 to 30, it is 310 mg per day, and for women over age 30, it is 320 mg per day. For pregnant women, the dose is increased to 350 to 400 mg per day.

However, many diets consist of excess calcium, creating an imbalance between calcium and magnesium. In fact this excess ends up being over 2-to-1 and at times as high as 3-to-1 in favor of calcium. Some researchers suggest that the most appropriate ratio is 1-to-1, or at the very least under the 2-to-1 ratio in favor of calcium. Therefore, the recommended allowance of magnesium must be increased to 400 mg daily to achieve this balance. However, care must be taken to delicately balance magnesium doses and avoid excess doses of magnesium.

Sources (Where to Find It)

Fruits & Vegetables:

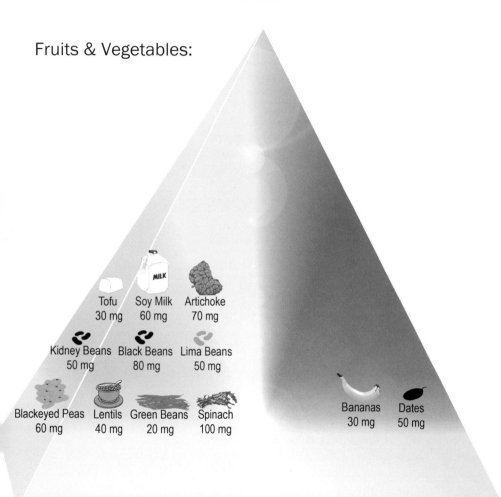

Tofu
30 mg

Soy Milk
60 mg

Artichoke
70 mg

Kidney Beans
50 mg

Black Beans
80 mg

Lima Beans
50 mg

Blackeyed Peas
60 mg

Lentils
40 mg

Green Beans
20 mg

Spinach
100 mg

Bananas
30 mg

Dates
50 mg

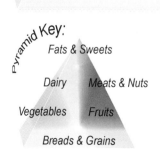

Pyramid Key:

Fats & Sweets

Dairy   Meats & Nuts

Vegetables   Fruits

Breads & Grains

*See Guides on Pages 467-468.

Dairy, Meats, & Grains:

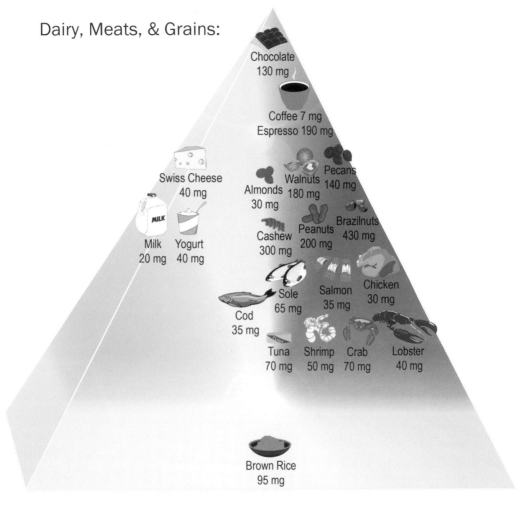

Chocolate 130 mg

Coffee 7 mg
Espresso 190 mg

Swiss Cheese 40 mg

Pecans

Walnuts 140 mg

Almonds 30 mg

Milk 20 mg   Yogurt 40 mg

Cashew 300 mg

Peanuts 200 mg

Brazilnuts 430 mg

Sole 65 mg   Salmon 35 mg   Chicken 30 mg

Cod 35 mg

Tuna 70 mg   Shrimp 50 mg   Crab 70 mg   Lobster 40 mg

Brown Rice 95 mg

Top sources of magnesium include nuts, espresso, and spinach. Other magnesium-rich sources include beans and fish.

MANGANESE

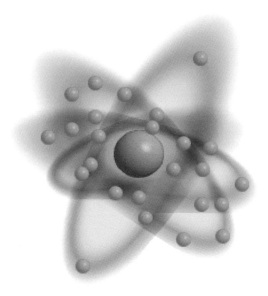

Category

Manganese is an essential element.

Cellular Location

Manganese is diffusely distributed throughout the body, though there are areas where it is more densely concentrated. The two most concentrated areas are in pigmented skin and behind the retina in the retinal pigment epithelium (the layer of cells behind the retina that serve to nourish the retina and remove the excess debris from the retina). Other areas were it is in high concentration include the liver, kidneys, pancreas, and bones.

Structure

Manganese is a metallic element. Its symbol on the periodic table of elements is Mn, and its atomic number is 25. It is found between chromium and iron on the periodic table.

Mechanisms of Action

There are numerous enzymes that require manganese to function.

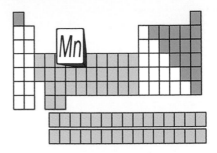

Biological & Ocular Importance

● Essential for a powerful antioxidant enzyme

Manganese plays a central role in the enzyme manganese superoxide dismutase, a powerful antioxidant enzyme that works in mitochondria (the energy-producing organelles in the body's cells). Oxidation is the process whereby chemical compounds lose electrons resulting in potentially toxic modifications to proteins, lipids, and DNA, that can eventually lead to degeneration and even death of cells.

Antioxidant enzymes are believed to be beneficial to retinal diseases, such as macular degeneration and childhood hereditary photoreceptor diseases, in which oxidative damage plays a role. They may be beneficial in diseases such as glaucoma or optic nerve diseases in which oxidative damage plays a role. They may also help prevent cataract formation or corneal disease, again by preventing or decreasing oxidative damage.

● Plays a role in making hyaluronic acid

Manganese plays an important role in the enzyme that makes glycosaminoglycans, an important component of hyaluronic acid (see section on hyaluronic acid). As such, it may play a role in preventing diseases ranging from glaucoma to osteoporosis.

● Assists in glucose utilization   Manganese is also believed to play a role in preventing diabetes, as evidenced by the fact that diabetics may have lower manganese levels and that manganese assists in glucose utilization.

● Required for many enzymes   Manganese is involved in enzymes that help create the coating of nerve fibers and the clotting factors.

Manganese is often recommended for treatment of muscle sprains or menstrual cramps from uterine muscle pain.

Human Studies on Utility

There are no human studies on the use of manganese in eye disease reported in the scientifically-reviewed medical literature. Nevertheless, the fact that there are no reported clinical studies does not necessarily imply a benefit or lack of benefit. Looking at the mechanism of action, the use of magnesium in moderation may be possibly of benefit in certain eye diseases.

Body Absorption, Metabolism, & Excretion

Manganese is absorbed in the intestines, though it is not always efficiently absorbed. Absorption ranges from 2 to 15%, depending on the amount of dietary chelators (nutrients that bind metals). For example, absorption of manganese is higher with leafy green vegetables than with fiber-rich meals or soy meals.

Manganese is excreted by being dumped back into the digestive tract through bile (a green fluid produced by the liver that is stored in the gallbladder to assist in digestion).

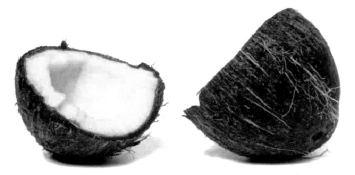

Deficiency

Manganese deficiency during adulthood can cause skin rashes and scaly skin, decreased growth of hair and nails, weight loss, abnormal glucose utilization mimicking diabetes, and full-fledged diabetes.

Toxicity & Side Effects

High levels of manganese can cause headaches, muscle cramps, nervousness, and increased sleepiness. In high doses, liver failure is known to occur. Also, damage to the reproductive system can occur as well as damage to the immune system, the pancreas, kidneys, and lungs.

In addition, a disease called "manganese madness" can occur. Manganese madness was originally described in miners in Chile where manganese dust fills the mines. Manganese madness consists of hallucinations associated with Parkinson's disease like symptoms such as tremors, slowed movements and slowed walking, decreased facial expressions, and rigid muscles, as it attacks the part of the brain that regulates movement and muscle tone.

Interactions with Other Nutrients

Manganese is required for an enzyme that makes proline from other amino acids (see section on proline).

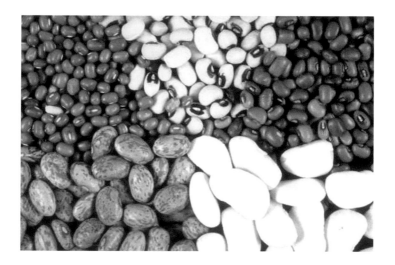

Ideal Dosage

The minimum dose of manganese recommended is 2 mg per day, in children ages 11 to 18 and in adults. Doses of 3 to 6 mg are often recommended by some scientists for its health benefits and doses up to 10 mg are considered safe. A dose of 3 to 5 mg per day may be the best recommended dose.

Sources (Where to Find It)

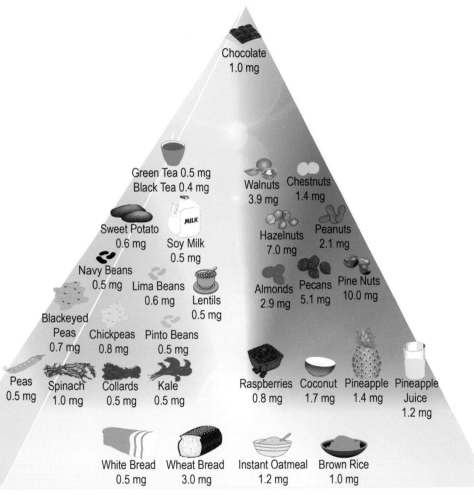

Chocolate
1.0 mg

Green Tea 0.5 mg
Black Tea 0.4 mg

Walnuts 3.9 mg   Chestnuts 1.4 mg

Sweet Potato 0.6 mg   Soy Milk 0.5 mg

Hazelnuts 7.0 mg   Peanuts 2.1 mg

Navy Beans 0.5 mg   Lima Beans 0.6 mg   Lentils 0.5 mg

Almonds 2.9 mg   Pecans 5.1 mg   Pine Nuts 10.0 mg

Blackeyed Peas 0.7 mg   Chickpeas 0.8 mg   Pinto Beans 0.5 mg

Peas 0.5 mg   Spinach 1.0 mg   Collards 0.5 mg   Kale 0.5 mg   Raspberries 0.8 mg   Coconut 1.7 mg   Pineapple 1.4 mg   Pineapple Juice 1.2 mg

White Bread 0.5 mg   Wheat Bread 3.0 mg   Instant Oatmeal 1.2 mg   Brown Rice 1.0 mg

Pyramid Key:

Fats & Sweets

Dairy   Meats & Nuts

Vegetables   Fruits

Breads & Grains

The top source of manganese is nuts, particularly pine nuts, hazelnuts, and pecans. Other manganese-rich foods are wheat bread, pineapple, and coconut.

    *See Guides on Pages 467-468.

MENADIONE
(SEE VITAMIN K)

MENAQUINONE
(SEE VITAMIN K)

METHIONINE

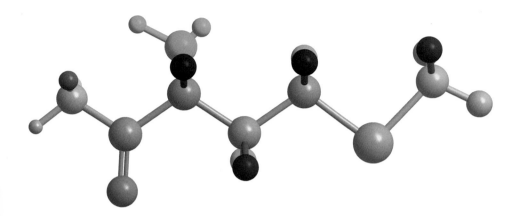

Category

Methionine is an essential amino acid (building block of proteins) that contains sulfur. Methionine is also known as 2-amino-4-methythiobutyric acid.

Cellular Location

Methionine is distributed through the bloodstream to various organs. Since proteins cannot be stored by the human body, unused proteins are metabolized and excreted.

Structure

Methionine is an acid that contains an amino group and also contains sulfur. Despite the fact that it is uncommon for a chemical reaction in the body to require three high-energy phosphate groups from ATP (the universal energy chemical of all living cells), methionine starts out by being transformed into the nutrient SAMe in a particularly high-energy reaction that requires three high-energy phosphate groups from ATP to be used in its production.

Mechanisms of Action

Methionine is a building block of proteins and plays a central role in other biochemical pathways involving amino acids.

Biological & Ocular Importance

● **Makes energy-boosting creatine**   Methionine is used to make creatine, an important energy producing molecule. Creatine is often used by athletes for improved performance and energy boosts. Creatine can also be made from the amino acids arginine and glycine.

● **Precursor to SAMe**
Methionine is also a precursor in the formation of SAMe (see section on SAMe).

● **Good & bad: acts as antioxidant but also precursor to toxic oxidant homocysteine**
Methionine itself can act as an antioxidant, though it is also a precursor to the toxic oxidant homocysteine (see below).

● **Precursor to cysteine which forms antioxidant glutathione**   Methionine is a precursor to the amino acid cysteine, which is a precursor to the antioxidant glutathione (see section on glutathione). Higher levels of methionine in the lens have been associated with a decreased risk of cataract formation.

● **Assists in removal of debris from behind retina**
One study has shown that chromium in the presence of methionine can assist in removal of lipofuscin from the body. Lipofuscin is a residue debris, which in the presence of light and oxygen results in the production of reactive oxygen species (toxic chemicals that result in oxidation). Excess lipofuscin can result in oxidative damage to the retina. Of course light exposure is high in the retina, and the highest amount of oxygen consumption of any tissue in the body occurs in the retina. Therefore, the retina is particularly susceptible to oxidative damage.

● **Helps form taurine**
Methionine can also assist in the formation of taurine (see section on taurine), an important amino acid for the eye and particularly the retina.

● **Other protective effects**
Methionine is also believed to prevent urinary tract infections. It may also protect the liver from potential damage from the pain-reliever acetaminophen.

Human Studies on Utility

Currently, there is only one human study on methionine use in eye disease reported in the scientifically-reviewed medical literature. Nevertheless, the fact that there is only one reported clinical study does not necessarily imply a benefit or lack of benefit. Looking at the mechanism of action, the use of methionine in moderation may be possibly of benefit in many eye diseases.

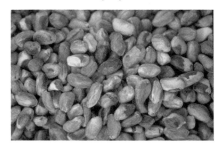

● **In one study: no benefits in past use of methionine found on risk of cataract** An Italian study of over 900 people also found no link (neither protective nor harmful) between intake of higher levels of methionine, beta-carotene, vitamin A, or vitamin D and the risk of having cataracts. However, this study found that those who consumed higher dietary levels of folate and vitamin E had a lower risk of developing cataracts that required surgery.[22]

Body Absorption, Metabolism, & Excretion

Methionine is digested by the stomach with the help of stomach acids. Digestive enzymes from the pancreas further break down proteins, which are absorbed into the bloodstream through the intestines.

As proteins are broken down, ammonia is formed. Since ammonia is extremely toxic to cells, it must be converted into a nitrogen-containing chemical known as urea. When ammonia builds up in excess, it can cause poor coordination, difficulties with balance, tremors, seizures, difficulty breathing, swelling of the brain, and can eventually lead to a coma. A normally functioning liver works to remove excess ammonia by creating urea, which is then filtered into the urine by the kidneys.

Deficiency

Some of the symptoms of methionine deficiency include nausea, vomiting, rashes, weakness, and liver disease characterized by fat accumulation within the liver.

Severe methionine deficiency is rare, as methionine can be reformed from homocysteine and from a chemical called glycine betaine.

Methionine deficiency can cause SAMe deficiency (see section on SAMe) as well as folate deficiency (see section on folate), as both are used to make more methionine from homocysteine.

Toxicity & Side Effects

Methionine in high levels can cause headaches, nausea, and vomiting.

High doses of methionine can result in increased production of homocysteine. Elevated levels of homocysteine are associated with Alzheimer's disease as well as vascular disease, including blood clots, heart disease, stroke, and vein occlusions in the retina (see interactions with other nutrients below). High doses of methionine can also decrease folate levels.

There is some suggestion that high doses of methionine can also cause an increased risk of cancers, particularly stomach cancer.

Excess methionine, like other amino acids, is often broken down and converted into sugars or fats, and used for energy, or stored as fat in the body's fat stores. Excess amino acids can stress the kidneys, stress the bloodstream, and cause dehydration. Furthermore, excess amino acids can cause the kidneys to lose calcium, resulting in weakened bones. As with any amino acid, methionine in excess in someone with liver disease or with kidney disease may result in build-up of ammonia or urea in the body, resulting in severe illness (see page 216).

In diabetics, excess amino acids can result in an increased sugar load on the body, or increased fat deposits in the body!

Interactions with Other Nutrients

There are several nutrients (methionine, vitamin B12, vitamin B6, folate, selenium, SAMe, and N-acetyl-cysteine) that act in the same complex circular pathway and are all interrelated when it comes to: (1) the toxicity of homocysteine and decreasing its levels, and (2) the activities of SAMe as a donator of methyl groups (see sections on folate, vitamin B12, vitamin B6, selenium, SAMe, and N-acetyl-cysteine).

These nutrients work to convert toxic homocysteine into methionine. However, high levels of methionine can result in increased production of homocysteine (see toxicity & side effects).

Folate plays an important role in the process of converting the toxic chemical homocysteine into methionine. The particular enzyme that converts homocysteine back to methionine is, in fact, one of only two enzymes throughout our body that depend on vitamin B12 for their activity. SAMe participates in this cycle by donating methyl groups (see section on vitamin B12 and SAMe).

Not only do vitamin B12 and folate work together in regulating homocysteine levels, vitamin B6 and zinc regulate homocysteine levels by helping convert homocysteine into glutathione, which ensures lower levels of toxic homocysteine. Selenium is required in this pathway as these glutathione enzymes are selenoproteins, composed of selenium with the protein. N-acetyl-cysteine may lower homocysteine levels as well, by converting homocysteine into the protein building block cysteine, an amino acid.

Choline also interacts in this complex homocysteine pathway. Choline forms a chemical, called betaine, in the body, and betaine works to convert homocysteine to methionine, in order to decrease levels of homocysteine in the body.

SAMe plays a role in providing methyl groups to methionine, which follows a pathway into carnitine.

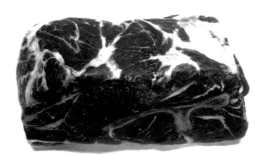

Ideal Dosage

No ideal dosage or recommended dosage range has been established; however, some physicians recommend doses of 500 to 1,000 mg per day.

Sources (Where to Find It)

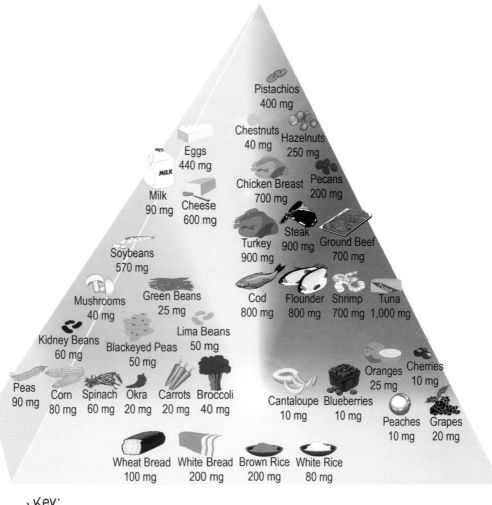

Pistachios
400 mg

Chestnuts
40 mg

Hazelnuts
250 mg

Eggs
440 mg

Chicken Breast
700 mg

Pecans
200 mg

Milk
90 mg

Cheese
600 mg

Turkey
900 mg

Steak
900 mg

Ground Beef
700 mg

Soybeans
570 mg

Mushrooms
40 mg

Green Beans
25 mg

Cod
800 mg

Flounder
800 mg

Shrimp
700 mg

Tuna
1,000 mg

Kidney Beans
60 mg

Blackeyed Peas
50 mg

Lima Beans
50 mg

Peas
90 mg

Corn
80 mg

Spinach
60 mg

Okra
20 mg

Carrots
20 mg

Broccoli
40 mg

Cantaloupe
10 mg

Blueberries
10 mg

Oranges
25 mg

Cherries
10 mg

Peaches
10 mg

Grapes
20 mg

Wheat Bread
100 mg

White Bread
200 mg

Brown Rice
200 mg

White Rice
80 mg

Pyramid Key:

Fats & Sweets

Dairy

Meats & Nuts

Vegetables

Fruits

Breads & Grains

Top sources of methionine include meats (beef, chicken, turkey, and seafood) and, to a lesser extent, dairy products (cheese and eggs) as well as nuts. Soybeans are also a rich source of methionine.

METHYLCOBALAMIN

Category

Methylcobalamin is an active form of vitamin B12 and the preferred form of vitamin B12 (see section on vitamin B12).

N-ACETYL-CYSTEINE
(NAC)

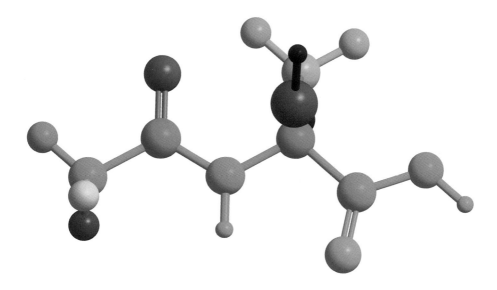

Category

N-acetyl-cysteine is a derivative of cysteine, an amino acid (building block of proteins). It is also known as N-acetyl-L-cysteine and N-acetylcysteine.

Cellular Location

Most of the N-acetyl-cysteine absorbed is sent to the liver and then rapidly broken down into cysteine, glutathione, taurine, and other proteins.

Structure

N-acetyl-cysteine is a moderately-sized compound that contains sulfur and nitrogen with carbon and oxygen.

Mechanisms of Action

N-acetyl-cysteine acts as an antioxidant and helps regenerate liver stores of glutathione.

Biological & Ocular Importance

● **Replenishes antioxidant glutathione levels**   Because N-acetyl-cysteine is broken down into the antioxidant glutathione, it helps replenish glutathione levels in the body. N-acetyl-cysteine is a rapid way to replenish glutathione levels in the body and provide antioxidant support (see section on glutathione).

In the process of converting the antioxidant lipoic acid into the antioxidant dihydrolipoic acid (see section on alpha-lipoic acid), the oxidized sulfur amino acid cysteine is converted to the biologically useful sulfur amino acid cysteine, which can then be recycled into the cell and used to form glutathione (see section on glutathione).

● **Treats pain-reliever overdose**   N-acetyl-cysteine is used to treat overdose of the pain-reliever acetaminophen, which is toxic to the liver.

● **Breaks down mucus on the surface of the eye & in the lungs**   N-acetyl-cysteine is used as an inhalant to treat acute and chronic bronchitis to break up lung mucus. It is believed to donate electrons to double-sulfur bonds in mucus, to break up

those bonds, and then liquefy the mucus.

Because of its ability to break down mucus, N-acetyl-cysteine has been suggested as an agent to break down mucus in certain diseases of the surface of the eye, such as filamentary keratitis, or a corneal disease involving mucus filament build-up on the surface of the cornea. Filamentary keratitis can be associated with dry eye syndrome, corneal ulcers, certain types of swelling of the cornea, superior limbic keratitis (a corneal and conjunctival disorder that is often associated with thyroid disease), and certain types of corneal scars. In certain types of chemical burns of the surface of the eye, N-acetyl-cysteine may be used to prevent melting of the cornea.

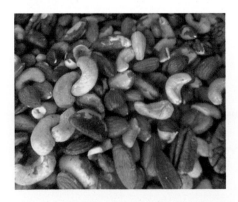

Human Studies on Utility

Currently, there is only one human study on N-acetyl-cysteine use in eye disease reported in the scientifically-reviewed medical literature. Nevertheless, the fact that there is only one reported clinical study does not necessarily imply a benefit or lack of benefit. Looking at the mechanism of action, the use of N-acetyl-cysteine in moderation may be possibly of benefit in many eye diseases.

● **In one small study: no benefits from the use of N-acetyl-cysteine with other antioxidants on the future risk of macular degeneration over time** A small study of 71 people with macular degeneration found no benefit to the macular degeneration or to vision in those who, for over 1½ years, took a daily antioxidant combination consisting of N-acetyl cysteine (100 mg), beta-carotene (20,000 IU), vitamin B2 (25 mg), vitamin C (750 mg), vitamin E (200 IU), chromium (100 µg), selenium (50 µg), zinc (12.5 mg), taurine (100 mg), glutathione (5 mg), and selected bioflavonoids, compared to placebo.[17] It is impossible, however, to ascertain the individual effect of N-acetyl-cysteine from this type of study.

Body Absorption, Metabolism, & Excretion

N-acetyl-cysteine is quickly absorbed in the intestines and transported to the liver. Stomach acids and digestive enzymes, however, may break down a portion of the N-acetyl-cysteine prior to being absorbed into the bloodstream. The N-acetyl-cysteine ingested can be quickly broken down and used to create cysteine, glutathione, taurine, and other proteins.

As proteins are broken down, ammonia is formed. Since ammonia is extremely toxic to cells, it must be converted into a nitrogen-containing chemical known as urea. When ammonia builds up in excess, it can cause poor coordination, difficulties with balance, tremors, seizures, difficulty breathing, swelling of the brain, and can eventually lead to a coma. A normally functioning liver works to remove excess ammonia by creating urea, which is then filtered into the urine by the kidneys.

Proteins and amino acids are filtered directly by the kidneys only to be recycled by the kidneys and sent back into the bloodstream. However, one amino acid, cystine (the oxidized form of cysteine) can cause stone formation in the kidneys (see below).

Deficiency

Since the body can make its own N-acetyl-cysteine, deficiency of N-acetyl-cysteine is rare. The body makes N-acetyl-cysteine from the amino acid cysteine.

Toxicity & Side Effects

Side effects of N-acetyl-cysteine include headaches, nausea, vomiting, diarrhea, skin rashes, and irritation of the conjunctiva mimicking pink eye. It may also cause stomach ulcers, as it may break down the protective mucosal barrier in the stomach wall. Severely low blood pressure and asthma attacks also have been reported.

One of N-acetyl-cysteine's breakdown products is cysteine, which can be oxidized into cystine. Kidney stone formation has been reported rarely as a result of cystine formation and build-up in the kidneys. As with any amino acid, excessive N-acetyl-cysteine in someone with liver disease or with kidney disease may result in build-up of ammonia or urea in the body, resulting in severe illness (see page 223).

Interactions with Other Nutrients

Cysteine and N-acetyl-cysteine are precursors of taurine (see section on taurine).

There are several nutrients (N-acetyl-cysteine, vitamin B12, vitamin B6, folate, selenium, SAMe, and methionine) that act in the same complex circular pathway and are all interrelated when it comes to: (1) the toxicity of homocysteine and decreasing its levels, and (2) the activities of SAMe as a donator of methyl groups (see sections on folate, vitamin B12, vitamin B6, selenium, SAMe, and methionine). Homocysteine is a toxic chemical that is associated with Alzheimer's disease as well as vascular disease, including blood clots, heart disease, stroke, and vein occlusions in the retina. N-acetyl-cysteine may lower homocysteine levels as well, by converting homocysteine into cysteine, an amino acid.

Ideal Dosage

Some researchers recommend doses of 500 mg to 1,500 mg per day. In these doses, kidney stones may form. Therefore, drinking 6 to 8 glasses of water daily is recommended alongside doses of 500 to 1,500 mg per day. Some physicians recommend doses of 500 mg to 750 mg, or less, per day in efforts to avoid kidney stones.

Sources (Where to Find It)

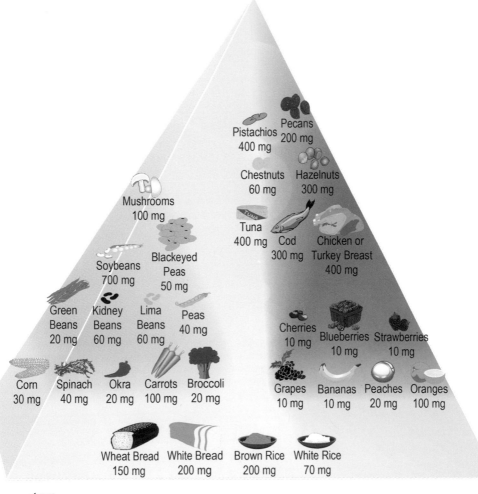

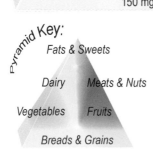

Pyramid Key:

Fats & Sweets

Dairy   *Meats & Nuts*

Vegetables   *Fruits*

Breads & Grains

Sources above are for cysteine. N-acetyl-cysteine is a derivative of cysteine. The body makes N-acetyl-cysteine from the amino acid cysteine. Top sources for cysteine are chicken, turkey, fish, nuts, and soybeans.

N-ACETYL-L-CYSTEINE
(SEE N-ACETYL-CYSTEINE)

NIACIN
(SEE VITAMIN B3)

OMEGA-3 OILS

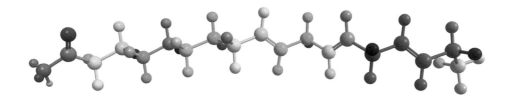

Category

Omega-3 oils are essential fatty oils, known as fatty acids.

Cellular Location

Most of the fatty acids are sent to the liver and to fat stores throughout the body and distributed to particular tissues of interest.

In its general form, fat is the second most abundant substance in the body, only second to water. Of note, all human brain cells, nerve cells, and retinal cells are made of more than 70% fat! Much of the fat is specialized fat, such as fatty acids. In fact, the highest concentrations of the fatty acid, DHA, anywhere in the body are in the outer segments of photoreceptors.

Structure

Omega-3 oils are long-chain fatty acids, with greater than 18 carbons forming their chain. They are unsaturated fatty acids with numerous double bonds. Omega-3 oils contain a double bond at the third carbon position, while omega-6 oils contain a double bond at the sixth carbon position.

Mechanisms of Action

Fatty acids play a central role in the formation of phospholipids. Phospholipids are large unique fatty compounds that serve the following functions: forming cell membranes, maintaining the structure of cell membranes, anchoring proteins in cell membranes, sending signals within cells, binding to transcription factors (proteins that turn specific genes on or off), and activating enzymes.

Biological & Ocular Importance

● **Form membranes of the retinal cells** The predominant phospholipids within the retina are phosphatidylcholine, phasphatidylethanolamine, and phosphatidylserise, of which the latter two predominantly contain the omega-3 oil docosahexaenoic acid (DHA) as their fatty acid. In addition to being the main fatty acids of the membranes of the neural (eg. photoreceptor) components of the retina, omega-3 and omega-6 oils are the main components of the cells that line the blood vessels of the retina.

DHA accounts for over half of all the fatty acids in the outer segments of rod photoreceptors. In fact, the highest concentrations of DHA anywhere in the body are in the outer segments of photoreceptors. DHA is also in high concentration in other retinal cells, such as the cells that line blood vessel and the Muller cells within the retina.

These Muller cells are the support cells for the photoreceptors and signaling neurons and also remove excess neurotransmitters, maintain appropriate electrolyte balances, provide fuel for metabolism, remove excess carbon dioxide and ammonia waste, and synthesize retinoic acid from retinol.

● **Important for proper development of the retina in infants** In infants, DHA is important in the proper development of the brain and retina, resulting in better visual acuity. A mother's breast milk has DHA, while cow's milk and many types of infant milk formulas do not.

● **Assist photoreceptor response to light by providing proper fluidic movement of compounds within**

photoreceptor membranes

Photoreceptors contain up to 1,000 discs arranged in layers to detect photons, or light particles. Within these discs are the light-sensing compounds, the chromophores, of the retina that are necessary for visual transduction (the process whereby a light signal is converted into a chemical signal that is sent through the retina and eventually to the brain). These photoreceptor discs contain exceedingly low levels of cholesterol and high levels of unsaturated fatty acids, particularly the omega-3s. In fact, anywhere from 50 to 90% of the lipid content of the disc membranes is unsaturated fatty acids.

This membrane composition is essential in providing the right microenvironment for visual transduction to occur, allowing for proper membrane component interactions and proper membrane fluidics (the movement of compounds within the membranes). The fluidity of the photoreceptor membranes allow for faster responses to light stimuli. There is also evidence that DHA in photoreceptor membranes directly affects the speed of response to light through its effects on the dynamics of the light processing pathway. For example, the formation of specialized membrane pigments (such as metarhodopsin) upon light stimulation, may be enhanced by the presence of DHA, which thereby speeds activation to the next step in the light processing pathway.

● **Play both antioxidant and pro-oxidant role**   However, whether or not omega-3 oils provide a substrate for oxidation or assist in decreasing the effects of oxidation remains controversial. Conflicting studies describe both a pro-oxidant role for these unsaturated fatty acids, as well as an antioxidant role.

What makes these fatty acids unsaturated is the presence of an increased proportion of double bonds. It is this same high number of double bonds, however, that makes these fatty acids prone to oxidation and oxidative damage. Oxidation is the process whereby chemical compounds lose electrons, resulting in potentially toxic modifications to proteins, lipids, and DNA that can eventually lead to degeneration and even death of cells. The presence of light and oxygen results in the production of reactive oxygen species (toxic chemicals that result in oxidation). Of course light exposure is high in the retina, and the highest amount of oxygen consumption of any tissue in the body occurs in the retina. Therefore, the photoreceptor discs are particularly susceptible to oxidative damage.

Omega-3 oils can act to decrease oxidative load on cells by making mitochondria (the energy-producing organelles in the body's cells) more efficient by improving the composition of the mitochondrial membrane. The mitochondria, the major energy-producing organelle found within cells of the body, are the major cellular source of oxidants. Almost all, 98%, of the oxygen that is metabolized in the body is handled by a single enzyme, cytochrome oxidase, within the mitochondria. By making mitochondria more efficient, energy production is improved and oxidative load is decreased.

DHA may also assist in removing and recycling the light-bleached pigments of the photoreceptors, since the bleached pigments and their byproducts are toxic and can cause oxidative damage if not properly removed and recycled.

Of note, excess light has been shown to decrease retinal concentrations of fatty acids such as DHA by releasing omega-3's bound to phospholipids in cell membranes.

● Participate in sending signals between retinal cells

There is a growing body of evidence that omega-3 and omega-6 oils participate in neurotransmission or sending of signals between neural cells of the retina. This participation may be direct or indirect by modulating and regulating neurotransmitters. However, the clinical and physiological implications of this process are unknown. The role of omega-3 and omega-6 oils may be beneficial, harmful, or neutral.

● Turn on & off genes involved in growth & metabolism

The omega-3 and omega-6 fatty acids also bind to transcription factors (proteins that turn specific genes on or off). Some of the transcription factors that are bound by omega-3 and omega-6 fatty acids are also involved in the growth and metabolism of cells. DHA also affects the growth of cells by acting to stimulate processes involved in photoreceptor growth. In animal models, survival of photoreceptors is prolonged by DHA.

● Block inflammation & growth of abnormal blood vessels

The omega-3 and omega-6 fatty acids are also involved in other signaling pathways. Derivatives of omega-3 and particularly omega-6 oils are involved in initiation of inflammation, blood clotting, constricting blood vessels, as well as angiogenesis (the formation of abnormal new blood vessels). However, they can also be balanced by other omega-3 and omega-6 oil derivatives that help prevent blood clotting, maintain vascular flow, respond to infections, and assist in physiologic functions during pregnancy. Because of this wide array of good and bad effects of omega-3 and omega-6 oils, what ends up being of particular importance is the balance between different types of omega-3 and omega-6 oil derivatives and the balance between the primary omega-3 and omega-6 oils themselves. In fact, in moderation, many of the seemingly harmful effects are quite beneficial: for example, blood clotting to prevent excess bleeding in injury, or a balanced inflammatory response to prevent infection.

The omega-3 fatty acids docosahexaenoic acid (DHA) and eicosapenaenoic acid (EPA) are both associated with the initiation of both inflammation and angiogenesis. Angiogenesis is particularly harmful in the retina, cornea, and trabecular meshwork (filtration site of the eye) and can cause loss of vision. The problems that result are called choroidal neovascularization (seen in wet macular degeneration), or retinal neovascularization (seen in severe diabetic retinopathy or retinal disease), or corneal neovascularization (seen in corneal injury or disease), or iris neovascularization (seen in angle-closure glaucoma and inflammatory eye disease). Inflammation is central to certain eye diseases, such as uveitis, and has been implicated in a broad range of other eye diseases, such as macular degeneration and diabetic retinopathy.

This information may suggest that one should avoid omega-3 fatty acids. On the contrary, their benefit is found in competing with and blocking of arachadonic acid, an omega-6 fatty acid (see section on omega-3 fatty acids). Aracadonic acid is a potent stimulator of the inflammation and angiogenesis pathways, much more so than DHA or EPA. Therefore, DHA and EPA are highly beneficial in decreasing the inflammatory and angiogenic effects of arachadonic acid.

Evidence suggests that omega-3 oils and particularly EPA may also directly inhibit certain factors along the angiogenesis pathway to block or decrease angiogenesis. There is a lot to be learned about these pathways and the omega-3 oils may both stimulate and inhibit angiogenesis depending on the circumstance. Overall, though, the omega-3 oils appear to be beneficial in inhibiting angiogenesis, primarily through competing with and blocking of arachadonic acid and its pathways.

● **Beneficial to numerous inflammatory conditions**
There is good evidence that omega-3 oils can aid in inflammatory diseases of the eye and throughout the body, such as rheumatoid arthritis. In addition,

231

there is suggestion that omega-3 oils can help out in other inflammatory conditions, such as Crohn's disease or ulcerative colitis, which are inflammatory gastrointestinal disorders. Omega-3 oils also seem to help out in certain types of cancer that involve inflammation as a predisposing risk factor. Benefits to a variety of other inflammatory conditions, ranging from asthma to lupus to psoriasis, have been suggested as well.

● **Improve blood flow**   In addition, omega-3 oils also participate in regulating blood flow in vessels by serving as precursors to eicosanoid compounds that improve blood flow through their actions on blood vessels and pericytes (the cells that nourish blood vessels). This process is important in many ophthalmic diseases, such as diabetes, in which compromised blood flow results in disease.

● **Prevent heart disease, blood vessel disease, & stroke**   Overall, though, omega-3 oils have been found to be extremely beneficial in moderate doses by decreasing heart and blood vessel disease, by decreasing blood pressure particularly in cases of hypertension (high blood pressure), by decreasing inflammation and atherosclerosis (blood vessel cholesterol clots and plaques that can result in heart disease and stroke, as well

as artery or vein clots in the retina or optic nerve strokes), and by decreasing blood clotting in general. Interestingly, these effects were first noted in Eskimos who ate high quantities of fish.

Because DHA also maintains the membrane fluidity of red blood cells, there is also evidence that it reduces the thickness or viscosity of the blood and improves blood flow. As such, there is clinical evidence that some people with glaucoma caused by microvascular blood flow abnormalities, may have low DHA levels.

Because of the beneficial cardiovascular effect, there is suggestion that omega-3 oils are beneficial in preventing strokes.

● **Decrease blood pressure & certain types of cholesterol but may cause bleeding & other complications**   Omega-3 oils at dangerously high levels have been shown to decrease blood pressure, as well as decrease fats such as triglycerides in the bloodstream. While it is good to decrease levels of these triglycerides or fats in the bloodstream, the problem is that omega-3 oils can actually increase levels of LDL cholesterol. Furthermore, the other problem is that high doses of greater than 3 or 4 g per day are associated with a high risk of bleeding and bleeding complications, which can be life-threatening (see below, under toxicity).

Human Studies on Utility

Currently, there are numerous human studies on omega-3 oils in eye disease reported in the scientifically-reviewed medical literature. These studies involve several eye diseases, including dry eyes, cataract, glaucoma, and diabetes, as well as macular degeneration, retinitis pigmentosa, and visual development in infants. The studies are described below.

Looking at the mechanisms of action, there is good reason to use omega-3 oils in moderation for dry eyes, macular degeneration, retinitis pigmentosa, and visual development in infancy.

● One large study found past use of omega-3 oils decreased risk of dry eyes

A study of over 30,000 women age 45 to 84, found that a diet higher levels of omega-6 oils compared to omega-3 oils had a 2½ times higher risk of having dry eyes.

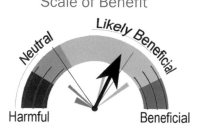

Omega-3 Oils for
Dry Eyes
Scale of Benefit

Eating higher amounts of dietary omega-3 oils decreased the risk of dry eyes. Eating more servings of tuna, as opposed to other types of fish or seafood, also decreased the risk of dry eyes.[81]

● A small study found use of omega-3 oils decreases the future risk of dry eyes

A study of 40 people found that dietary supplements of omega-3 and omega-6 oils for 2 months decreased corneal dryness and symptoms of dry eyes, compared to placebo.[82]

● One large study found past use of higher amounts omega-3 oils associated with decreased risk of cataract, while another study found no benefit

An Australian study of 2,900 people over the age of 49 found that a diet high in omega-3 and omega-6 oils (12 g or 17 g per day) were 30% less likely to develop one type of cataract (called cortical cataract) compared with a diet low in omega-3 and omega-6 oils (7 g or less per day).[83]

An Icelandic study of over 1,000 people over the age of 49 found no link (neither protective nor harmful) between cataract and increased quantities of fish or cod liver oil.[84]

A Japanese study of 14 people with cataracts found that DHA (540 mg for 3 months) improved their visual acuity. However, the study did not measure the cataracts, so no information is available as to whether or not the visual improvements represent improvements in the cataracts or another type of improvement in eye function and health or even a mental improvement, as these people were all nursing home residents participating in a dementia study. Furthermore, there was no control group to determine whether or not the improvement was a placebo effect.[85]

● **A small study found decreased risk of glaucoma in those with higher blood levels of DHA** A study of 18 people found that glaucoma is associated lower blood levels of DHA, eicosapenaenoic acid, and omega-3 oils. This study suggests that omega-3 oils are beneficial in glaucoma as well, through the protective mechanisms described above.[86]

● **A small study found omega-3 oils improved blood flow in diabetics** A study of 48 people with diabetic retinopathy found that the omega-3 eiconol from fish oil improved blood flow in diabetic retinopathy. The study though is unfortunately quite limited and much of the data not presented, making the study difficult to interpret.[87]

Summary of Studies for Macular Degeneration:
Nearly a dozen clinical trials have been performed looking at the role of omega-3 oils in both preventing and treating macular degeneration. These clinical trials are of many different types, some of which are very well-designed and well-performed studies.

As a whole, the clinical studies suggest that omega-3 oils may be beneficial in macular degeneration. Out of the 11 studies, 9 found a benefit. Furthermore, looking at the mechanisms of action, there may be good reason to use omega-3

Omega-3 Oils for
Macular Degeneration
Scale of Benefit

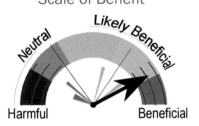

oils in moderation for macular degeneration.

The studies can be summarized as follows: several studies have found a benefit to the past use of omega-3 oils in decreasing the risk of macular degeneration. One study found the use of omega-3 oils improves vision over time in macular degeneration and decreases debris accumulation. However, one large study also found that the omega-3 oils DHA and EPA in moderately high doses with low doses of other omega-3 and omega-6 oils is quite beneficial in preventing retinal diseases such as macular degeneration. However, this study found that high doses of omega-3 in combination with high doses of omega-6 oils may actually be harmful to the retina. The take home message is that the benefits of high doses of omega-3 oils are counteracted by high doses of omega-6 oils.

● **One large study found conflicting evidence: past of use of DHA associated with a decreased risk of macular degeneration, but past use of omega-3 oil precursor associated with increased risk of macular degeneration** A 12 year study of over 70,000 people found that a diet low in DHA (50 mg per day) increased the risk of macular degeneration by about $1/3$ compared to a diet higher in DHA (500 mg per day). Similarly, 4 or more servings of fish per week decreased the risk by 35% compared to less than 4 servings per month! These findings provide strong support for the benefits of DHA and omega-3 oils. However, they must be tempered by the fact that a diet high in the omega-3 oil precursor alpha-linolenic acid (2 g per day) increased the risk of macular degeneration by about $1/3$ compared to a diet lower in alpha-linolenic acid ($1/2$ g per week).[88] One explanation is that a diet high in alpha-linolenic acid may also contain higher amounts of omega-6 oil precursor linoleic acid, which may result in toxic and deleterious effects, such as inflammation or angiogenesis, to the retina. The importance of this study is in the finding that DHA itself in moderately higher doses decreases the risk of macular degeneration.

● **Several studies found a benefit: past use of omega-3 oils associated with decreased risk of macular degeneration** A study of about 3,000 people age 49 and over found that higher consumption of fish in the past, such as 1 to 3 servings per month as compared to 1 per month, decreased the risk of developing severe macular degeneration by 75%. With even higher consumption of fish, the trend towards less macular degeneration was present, though the results were not statistically significant.[89]

A study of over 2,300 people from a population of nearly 5,000 found that a diet high in omega-3 oils decreased the risk of having early macular degeneration by nearly 60%. Similarly, a diet with at least 1 serving of fish per week or at least 3 servings of fish per week decreased the risk of having early macular degeneration by about 40% compared to a diet of 1 or less servings of fish per month. Also, a diet of at least 3 servings of fish per week decreased the risk of having late macular degeneration by 75% compared to a diet of 1 or less servings of fish per month.[90]

A smaller study of over 850 people found that a diet with higher amounts of the omega-3 fatty acids DHA and EPA (about 150 mg per day) and lower amounts of the omega-6 precursor linoleic acid (less than about 5 g per day) decreased the risk of having advanced macular degeneration by about 40%, compared to lower omega-3 (20 mg per day) and higher omega-6 precursor (5 g per day) oils. This study also found that consuming more than 2 servings of fish per week decreased the risk of having advanced macular degeneration by about 40%. A diet high in the omega-6 precursor linoleic acid (about 10 g per day) doubled the risk of having advanced macular degeneration, compared with a diet low in the omega-6 precursor (3½ g per day).[91]

A study of over 250 people over nearly 5 years found that in people whose intake of omega-6 precursor linoleic acid is less than 5 g per day, consumption of more than 2 servings of fish per week decreased the risk of having advanced macular degeneration by about 40%, compared with consumption of less than one serving of fish per week.[92]

Another study that was quite small, involving only 21 people, suggested similar findings.[93]

A study of 576 adults in rural Italy who consumed unprocessed fresh foods found that only 1.1% of these people developed macular degeneration, compared with the typical level of 3 to 4% of the population who develop macular degeneration. While this finding was attributed to an increased ratio of omega-3 oils to omega-6 oils in unprocessed fresh foods, it may be also attributed to increased presence or bioavailability of other nutrients.[94]

A recent study of nearly 700 twins found that those twins who consumed higher levels of omega-3 oils in the past had a 45% decrease in the risk of having macular degeneration compared to their twins who consumed less omega-3 oils. Those twins who consumed higher levels of omega-3 oils along with less omega-6 oil precursor linoleic acid had an over 75% decrease in the risk of having macular degeneration.[95]

Similarly, a study of nearly 8,000 people age 40 and over found a trend (that was not statistically significant) towards decreased risk of developing severe macular degeneration in those who consumed 5 or more servings of fish per month compared to those who consumed 1 or less serving,[96] while an earlier study found no link (neither protective nor harmful) between fish intake and severe macular degeneration.[97]

● **One study found a benefit: use of omega-3 oils improves vision over time in macular degeneration and decreases debris accumulation** A recent study in Italy looked at over 100 people with early macular degeneration. The study divided participants into two groups: one that took a cocktail of 3 supplements, consisting of 1060 mg of omega-3 oils, 200 mg of carnitine, and 20 mg of coenzyme Q10 daily for one year, and another that took placebo. The study found that those who took the supplement cocktail were less likely to develop worsening of their macular degeneration, as assessed by visual acuity and visual fields. In fact, on average, people who took the supplement cocktail showed an improvement in vision, compared to the average decline in vision in those who did not take the supplement cocktail! This finding is quite remarkable in that it is rare for macular degeneration to improve! Furthermore, the study found that the amount of drusen (damaging debris) that accumulates behind the retina in macular degeneration, actually decreased in people who took the supplement cocktail in comparison to those who did not. In those who took the supplement cocktail, the amount of drusen *decreased* by an average of 15% to 23%, while, in those who took the placebo, the amount of drusen *increased* by an average of 11% to 13%. This improvement in drusen is also unheard of![37] The same authors found similar results in their earlier pilot study involving 14 people taking a somewhat higher dose cocktail consisting of 1320 mg of omega-3 oils, 500 mg of carnitine, and 30 mg of coenzyme Q10.[38]

● One small study found no benefit in adding omega-3 oils during laser treatment for macular degeneration

A small study of 35 people with advanced wet macular degeneration found no benefit in adding omega oils and vitamin E to a treatment of photodynamic therapy (a laser-based treatment for wet macular degeneration). People were divided into two groups: both received the photodynamic therapy, but only one also received vitamin E and omega oils for 3 months after the photodynamic therapy.[98]

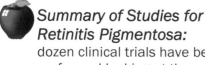 *Summary of Studies for Retinitis Pigmentosa:* A half dozen clinical trials have been performed looking at the role of omega-3 oils in treating retinitis pigmentosa. These clinical trials are of various types, some of which are very well-designed and well-performed studies.

As a whole, the clinical studies provide no definitive answer as to whether omega-3 oils are beneficial. However, overall, the studies suggest that there may be good reason to use omega-3 oils in moderation for retinitis pigmentosa.

Omega-3 Oils for
Retinitis Pigmentosa
Scale of Benefit

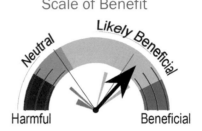

The studies can be summarized as follows. There are several small studies that looked at the use of omega-3 oils, particularly DHA, for retinitis pigmentosa. Of remark, one study found that the use of DHA slowed the appearance of the disease process in the retina over time. Another study found that in some groups of people, the use of DHA slowed the deterioration of visual fields over time. A third study found that people who took DHA with lutein and vitamin B complex had an improvement in their visual acuities.

● Several small studies found a benefit of omega-3 oils for retinitis pigmentosa

Two studies totaling over 300

people found that levels of DHA within red blood cells were anywhere from 14% to 40% lower in people with retinitis pigmentosa when compared with unaffected people.

A study of nearly 300 people found that circulating blood levels of omega-3 fatty acids, particularly DHA, were 10 to 15% lower in people with certain forms of retinitis pigmentosa. There was also suggestion that a gene involved in processing DHA may be affected in certain types of inherited macular dystrophies (degenerative diseases of the central retina).

A 4-year study of 44 people with retinitis pigmentosa found that the year-to-year worsening in the appearance of the retina was slowed down with DHA (400 mg per day) compared to taking corn and soy oil (400 mg per day). There was no difference between the two groups in terms of visual acuity, peripheral vision, or dark adaptation (ability to see in the dark). There was a trend (that was not statistically significant) that those who received DHA had less year-to-year worsening of rod and cone photoreceptor function (measured by the cell's electric activity). However, some of the people did not take their pills each day, and so the results may not represent the full benefit of the DHA. The study found that the DHA's benefit was in slowing rod photoreceptor loss in the younger group and in slowing cone photoreceptor loss in the older group. Characteristically in retinitis pigmentosa, rod photoreceptor loss occurs at an earlier age followed by cone photoreceptor loss.[100]

Another study of over 200 people found no link (neither protective nor harmful) between retinitis pigmentosa and DHA (1,200 mg per day for 4 years). In this study, everyone also received high doses of vitamin A (15,000 IU per day).[101] Looking in more detail, the study found that among those who were not on vitamin A before the study, taking DHA with vitamin A decreased the rate of decline of visual field sensitivity compared to taking only vitamin A. However, this benefit only lasted during the first two years. Among those who were already on vitamin A before the study, adding DHA did not make any difference in their disease progression. However, in people already on vitamin A before the study, higher amounts of fish (1 to 2 servings per week) and other dietary sources of omega-3 oils slowed the rate of decline of visual field sensitivity.[102]

An earlier 2000 study of 13 people with retinitis pigmentosa found that taking lutein (40 mg daily for 9 weeks, followed by 20 mg daily for a total of 26 weeks) along with docosahexaenoic acid (500 mg daily), vitamin B complex, and digestive enzymes results in an improvement in visual acuities. In fact, visual acuity improved by nearly one line, on average, and in one person, improved by two-and-one-half lines. This study is remarkable in that it is the only scientifically validated study that has demonstrated an improvement in visual acuity for any type of therapy involving retinitis pigmentosa.[66] The concerns of the study are the limited number of people enrolled and that the visual acuity testing was performed by the subjects themselves in their own homes over the internet.

Finally, a small study of 6 people with retinitis pigmentosa who were given DHA or EPA found no change after the treatment in the ability of the retinal cells to respond to light (measured by the cell's electric activity). However, this report looked at an extremely small number of people without any appropriate controls and outcome measures to determine any benefit of treatment.[99]

Summary of Studies for Visual Development in Infants:
Over a dozen clinical trials have been performed looking at the role of omega-3 oils in ensuring proper visual development in infants. These clinical trials are of various types, some of which are very well-designed and well-performed studies.

As a whole, the clinical studies suggest that omega-3 oils may be beneficial in ensuring proper visual development in infants. The majority of the studies found a benefit. Furthermore, looking at the mechanisms of action, there may be good reason to use omega-3 oils in moderation for ensuring proper visual development in infants.

The studies can be summarized as follows: several studies found that DHA supplementation, through DHA-fortified formula or breast-milk, during infancy was associated with improved visual development in healthy full-term

infants as well as in premature infants. A few studies found no

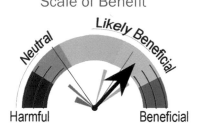

Omega-3 Oils for
Visual Development
in Infants
Scale of Benefit

Neutral — Likely Beneficial

Harmful   Beneficial

benefits or harms in DHA supplementation in healthy full-term infants. The importance and benefits of DHA go beyond supplementation of the infant to supplementation of the fetus during pregnancy. One study found that DHA during pregnancy associated with improved visual development in infants. These studies demonstrate the benefits of DHA, whether it comes from breast milk or DHA-fortified formula.

● **In several studies: DHA supplementation during infancy associated with improved visual development in healthy full-term infants** A study of 100 infants born full-term found that those who received formula supplemented with DHA or were breast-fed had better visual development (assessed by brain responses to fine visual stimuli) compared to those who received formula without DHA.[104]

A study of over 100 healthy infants born full-term found that those who received formula supplemented with DHA and arachadonic acid had better visual development (as assessed by brain responses to fine visual stimuli) compared to those who received formula without DHA.[105]

A study of 61 healthy infants found that those who were breast-fed until the age of 4 to 6 months and then received formula supplemented with DHA developed better visual health than those who received formula without DHA. Also, those who received the DHA had an increased ability of their retinas and brains to recognize finer objects and had an increased depth perception that was more finely tuned. In fact, in this study, those infants who were breast-fed until the age of 6 months, as compared to those who were breast-fed until the age of 4 months, did much better visually in these same tests.[106]

Similarly findings were found in another study of 83 full-term infants who were all breast-fed, but some received more DHA than others through differences in the mother's diet. Those babies that received higher amounts of DHA through the mother's breast-milk had better visual acuity and visual performance.[107] In fact, studies have shown that the breast-fed infants have higher levels of DHA in their blood when their lactating mothers eat diets with higher levels of DHA.[108]

● **Though the several studies above found benefits, a few studies found no benefits or harms in DHA supplementation in healthy full-term infants** Other studies in full-term infants have shown no link (neither beneficial nor harmful) between DHA (from breast-milk or DHA-supplemented formula) and visual acuity at 12 months or 39 months of age.[109 & 110] One study in full-term infants found no benefit of breast-milk compared to either formula with linoleic acid and alpha-linolenic acid or to formula with DHA. Of course, all groups contained omega-3 and omega-6 oils, so little or no difference is expected.[111]

Other studies found no difference in visual development in full-term infants who all received omega-3 precursors, but were fed different ratios of omega-3 to omega-6 precursors. Perhaps all the groups received enough DHA in their diets.[112 & 113]

● **In several studies: DHA supplementation during infancy associated with improved visual development in premature infants** A study of 470 *premature* infants found that those who were breast-fed had better visual acuity development at 6 months of age compared to those were received formula supplemented with DHA and arachadonic acid. Also, those who were fed formula supplemented with DHA and arachadonic acid had better visual acuity development at 6 months of age, compared to those who received formula without any additional omega-3 or omega-6 oils.[114]

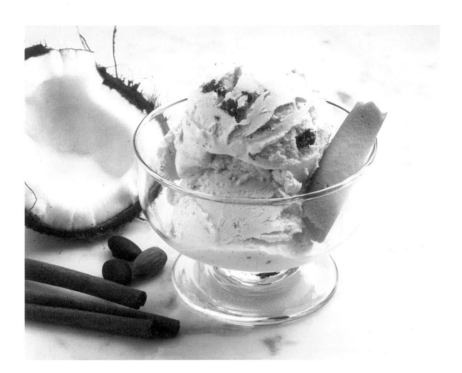

A study of 67 premature infants found better visual acuity at 4 months of age in those who were fed fish-oil supplemented formula compared to those who were fed non-fortified formula.[115]

Two studies of over 70 premature infants found better retinal sensitivity in the first few months after birth in those who received breast milk or DHA-fortified formula compared to non-fortified formula,[116] along with better visual development (assessed by brain responses to fine stimuli).[117]

In fact, a review that combined the results of 5 studies found that premature infants fed DHA-fortified formula had better visual development between the ages of 2 to 4 months when compared to being fed formula without DHA; however, at 6 to 12 months of age, there was no difference in visual development between the groups.[118]

● **In one study: DHA during pregnancy associated with improved visual development in infants** While the previous studies looked at DHA supplementation in infants, one study found benefits to the fetus during pregnancy. This study of 100 infants found that those born to pregnant women who took DHA during the pregnancy had better visual development than infants born to pregnant women who did not take DHA during pregnancy. The visual development was assessed by looking at both the electrical activity that the retina generates to dim light stimuli[119] and by brain responses to fine visual stimuli.[120]

Body Absorption, Metabolism, & Excretion

Omega-3 oils are absorbed in the intestines by being broken down into components by pancreas enzymes and bile (a green fluid produced by the liver that is stored in the gallbladder to assist in digestion). They are then absorbed into the intestinal cells, after which they are reformed and carried in fat and cholesterol transporters. These cholesterol transporters are called chylomicrons, which are composed of proteins and fats and require phospholipids. Rather than being directly absorbed into the bloodstream, these transporters are absorbed into the lymph circulation, and then taken into the bloodstream.

Most of the fatty acids are sent to the liver and to fat stores throughout the body and distributed to particular tissues of interest. Fat is primarily burned to provide energy to the body and fatty acids are a particularly rich source of energy. The excess fat is stored in the fat stores in the body.

Deficiency

Processed foods result in decreased omega-3s. Similarly, alcohol results in decreased omega-3 oil levels in the body.

Omega-3 oil deficiency has been associated with scaly skin and rashes, poor wound healing, and increased susceptibility to infections because of suppression of the immune system and inflammation.

Omega-3 oil deficiency has also been associated with rhodopsin deficiency in animals. Rhodopsin is the light-sensing protein used by retinal photoreceptors to detect light. Decrease in rhodopsin is associated with both night-blindness and decreased visual acuity. In fact, deficiency of the omega-3 oil DHA is associated with retinitis pigmentosa, a night-blinding retinal disease.

Toxicity & Side Effects

Common side effects of omega-3 oils include upset stomach, heartburn, abdominal bloating and cramps, diarrhea, and a fishy breath odor. Other side effects include skin rashes.

Allergic reactions to omega-3 oils and particularly fish oils have been reported in those who have a history of such allergies. Similarly, allergic reactions to nut-derived omega-3 oils have been reported in those who have a history of nut allergies.

There are also concerns that some fish and fish oils are contaminated with heavy metals, particularly mercury, and other environmental contaminants and toxins.

Another concern is that omega-3 oils may increase blood sugars in diabetes, so caution should be used when adding omega-3 oils to the diet of diabetics. Although the increase in the blood sugars is slight, a moderate dose of omega-3s is probably the best recommendation in diabetes.

Extremely high doses of omega-3 oils, in excess of 3 g per day, result in risk of bleeding due to the role of these fatty acids in blocking platelet actions. Furthermore, the risk of bleeding may be exacerbated in those taking ginkgo. Thus, omega-3 oils should be used only with caution in those who are susceptible to bleeding and also should be avoided prior to any surgery.

Interactions with Other Nutrients

Excess omega-3 will cause omega-6 deficiency while excess omega-6 will cause omega-3 deficiency. The discussions above regarding omega-6 oils make it clear that the ratio of omega-3 oils to omega-6 oils is important. The balance must be shifted towards omega-3 oils in order to provide a benefit to the health of the eye.

Long-term use of fish oils may result in a decrease in vitamin E levels in the body. However, many fish oil supplements include vitamin E, so care must be taken to avoid vitamin E excess with certain fish-oil supplements.

The risk of bleeding complications in those taking high doses of omega-3 oils may be exacerbated if combined with ginkgo or high doses of vitamin E.

Ideal Dosage

The average dose of omega-3 oils in the typical diet is 1.6 g per day, most of which is in the form of alpha-linolenic acid. The recommended dose of DHA and EPA together is 500 mg per day. While the total dose of omega-3 oils should not exceed 3 g per day (see toxicity), the recommended dose of omega-3 oils is around 2 to 2 ½ g per day.

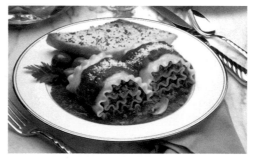

Sources (Where to Find It)

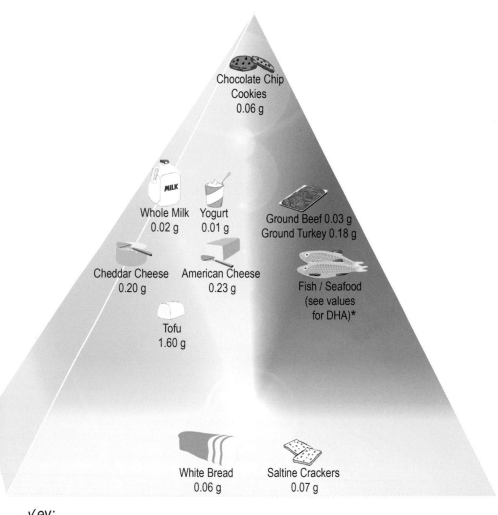

Chocolate Chip
Cookies
0.06 g

Whole Milk   Yogurt
0.02 g   0.01 g

Ground Beef 0.03 g
Ground Turkey 0.18 g

Cheddar Cheese   American Cheese
0.20 g   0.23 g

Fish / Seafood
(see values
for DHA)*

Tofu
1.60 g

White Bread   Saltine Crackers
0.06 g   0.07 g

Pyramid Key:

Fats & Sweets

Dairy   Meats & Nuts

Vegetables   Fruits

Breads & Grains

The top source of omega-3 oils is seafood (see section on DHA for food sources of DHA). Other sources of omega-3 oils include cheeses, tofu, and turkey. Other meats, grains, and sweets contain lower amounts of omega-3 oils.

*See Guides on Pages 467-468.

OMEGA-6 OILS

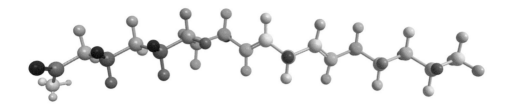

Category

Omega-6 oils are essential fatty acids.

Cellular Location

Most of the fatty acids are sent to the liver and to fat stores throughout the body and distributed to particular tissues of interest.

In its general form, fat is the second most abundant substance in the body, only second to water. Of note, all human brain cells, nerve cells, and retinal cells are made of more than 70% fat!

Structure

Omega-6 oils are long-chain fatty acids, with greater than 18 carbons forming their chain. They are unsaturated fatty acids, with numerous double bonds. Omega-6 oils contain a double bond at the sixth carbon position, while omega-3 oils contain a double bond at the third carbon position.

Mechanisms of Action

Fatty acids play a central role in the formation of phospholipids. Phospholipids are large unique fatty compounds that serve the following functions: forming cell membranes, maintaining the structure of cell membranes, anchoring proteins in cell membranes, sending signals within cells, binding to transcription factors (proteins that turn specific genes on or off), and activating enzymes.

Biological & Ocular Importance

● **Form membranes of the retinal cells**   The predominant phospholipids within the retina are phosphatidylcholine, phasphatidylethanolamine, and phosphatidylserise, of which the first predominantly contains the omega-6 oil arachadonic acid as its fatty acid. In addition to being the main fatty acids of the membranes of the neural (eg. photoreceptor) components of the retina, omega-3 and omega-6 oils are the main components of the cells that line the blood vessels of the retina.

Omega-6 oils can be used in place of omega-3s by retinal photoreceptors.

● **Helps maintain lubrication of the surface of the eye**
Omega-6 oils from primrose, borant, and black current seed provide the lubricant oil used to prevent tears from evaporating from the surface of the eye. The surface of the eye is coated by a thin layer of tear, called the tear film, which serves to lubricate and moisturize the eye surface. When this tear film evaporates, the cornea, which is particularly susceptible to dryness, begins to dry and the cells on its surface become damaged.

The tear film is composed of three layers. First, a mucin layer that is closest to the eye allows the tears to adhere more easily to the surface of the eye. This mucin component consists of glycoproteins (proteins conjugated with sugars). Second, an aqueous component consisting of water mixed with electrolytes or salts forms the bulk of the tear film and is the middle layer of the tear film. Third, a lipid component consisting of oils that stabilize the tear layer to prevent its evaporation. This lipid layer is the outermost layer of the tear film.

Omega-6 oils are involved in maintaining the lipid component of the tear film. These oils are secreted by oil-secreting glands of the eyelids. Similarly, vitamin A is required to ensure a proper tear film to lubricate the eye. The tear film is produced from nutrients and other components found in the bloodstream, and vitamin A is required for production of the mucins secreted from the eyelid glands for the natural tear layer.

● **Cause inflammation, blood clotting, blood vessels constriction, and formation of abnormal new blood vessels, but also prevent these harmful effects when balanced with omega-3 oils**

Derivatives of omega-3 and particularly omega-6 oils are involved in initiation of inflammation, blood clotting, constricting blood vessels, as well as angiogenesis (the formation of abnormal new blood vessels) (see under omega-3 oils). However, they can also be balanced by other omega-3 and omega-6 oil derivatives that help prevent blood clotting, maintain vascular flow, respond to infections, and assist in physiologic functions during pregnancy. Because of this wide array of useful and harmful effects of omega-3 and omega-6 oils, what ends up being of particular importance is the balance between different types of omega-3 and omega-6 oil derivatives and the balance between the primary omega-3 and omega-6 oils themselves. In fact, in moderation, many of the seemingly harmful effects are quite beneficial: for example, blood clotting to prevent excess bleeding in injury, or a balanced inflammatory response to prevent infection.

As such, omega-6 oils have been suggested for a wide variety of conditions, ranging from eczema to rheumatoid arthritis, to osteoporosis, to the neuropathy or nerve disease in diabetes. The important consideration is the balance between omega-6 and omega-3 oils. Omega-6 oils can serve as precursors for some omega-3 oils such as eicosapenaenoic acid (EPA), which acts to control inflammation.

Human Studies on Utility

See section on Omega-3 oils.

Body Absorption, Metabolism, & Excretion

Omega-6 oils are absorbed in the intestines by being broken down into components by pancreas enzymes and bile (a green fluid produced by the liver that is stored in the gallbladder to assist in digestion). They are then absorbed into the intestinal cells, after which they are reformed and carried in fat and cholesterol transporters. These cholesterol transporters are called chylomicrons, which are composed of proteins and fats and require phospholipids. Rather than being directly absorbed into the bloodstream, these transporters are absorbed into the lymph circulation, and then taken into the bloodstream.

Most of the fatty acids are sent to the liver and to fat stores throughout the body and distributed to particular tissues of interest. Fat is primarily burned to provide energy to the body and fatty acids are a particularly rich source of energy. The excess fat is stored in the fat stores in the body.

Deficiency

Omega-6 oil deficiency is rare in Western diets because of the high oil content in the types of foods typical to that diet. Interestingly, Mediterranean diets are often more balanced in their ratios of omega-6 to omega-3 oils.

Omega-6 oil deficiency has been associated with scaly skin and rashes, poor wound healing, and increased susceptibility to infections because of suppression of the immune system and inflammation. It has also been associated with dry eyes, hair loss, and changes in behavior.

Toxicity & Side Effects

One type of omega-6 fatty acid is arachadonic acid, which is associated with the initiation of both inflammation and angiogenesis (the formation of abnormal new blood vessels). Angiogenesis is particularly harmful in the retina, cornea, and trabecular meshwork (filtration site of the eye) and can cause loss of vision. The problems that result are called choroidal neovascularization (seen in wet macular degeneration), or retinal neovascularization (seen in severe diabetic retinopathy or retinal disease), or corneal neovascularization (seen in corneal injury or disease), or iris neovascularization (seen in angle-closure glaucoma and inflammatory eye disease). The omega-3 fatty acids docosahexaenoic acid (DHA) and eicosapenaenoic acid (EPA) both compete with arachadonic acid to decrease the inflammation and angiogenesis pathways that are triggered by arachadonic acid. It is important to note that while both DHA and EPA can decrease the effects of arachadonic acid, both DHA and EPA are known to stimulate inflammation and angiogenesis, though not to as extreme an extent as arachadonic acid (see section on omega-3 oils).

Interactions with Other Nutrients

Excess omega-6 will cause omega-3 deficiency while excess omega-3 will cause omega-6 deficiency. The discussions above regarding omega-6 oils make it clear that the ratio of omega-3 oils to omega-6 oils is important. The balance must be shifted towards omega-3 oils in order to provide a benefit to the health of the eye.

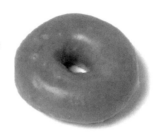

Ideal Dosage

The average dose of omega-6 oils in the typical diet is 12 to 16 g per day, most of which is in the form of linoleic acid. A balance between doses of omega-6 oils and doses of omega-3 oils must be achieved.

A typical ratio of omega-3 to omega-6 in the average Western diet is between about 1-to-6 and 1-to-20. The ratio of omega-3 to omega-6 in the Eskimo diet is about 1-to-2½. Although many scientists will recommend ratios of no more than 1-to-3, some researchers will recommend ratios of 1-to-2 or even 1-to-1. Ratios in favor of more omega-3 than omega-6 have been suggested as well; these ratios are 2-to-1 or 3-to-1.

The risk in a diet with a ratio of more omega-3 than omega-6 is that doses of omega-3 over 3 g per day are associated with a bleeding risk, and doses of less than 3 g per day of omega-3 will require omega-6 intake of less than 1½ g of omega-6, which is insufficient intake.

The recommended ratio of omega-3 to omega-6 is believed to be somewhere between 1-to-1 and 1-to-3. For example, an intake of 2½ g of omega-3 with about 6 or 7 g of omega-6 oils is well-balanced.

Sources (Where to Find It)

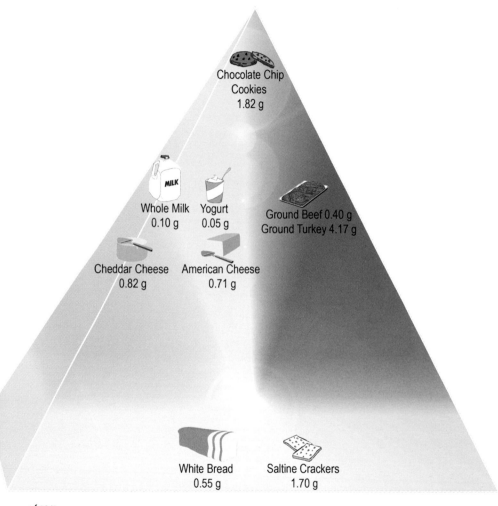

Chocolate Chip
Cookies
1.82 g

Whole Milk   Yogurt
0.10 g   0.05 g

Ground Beef 0.40 g
Ground Turkey 4.17 g

Cheddar Cheese   American Cheese
0.82 g   0.71 g

White Bread   Saltine Crackers
0.55 g   1.70 g

Pyramid Key:

Fats & Sweets

Dairy   Meats & Nuts

Vegetables   Fruits

Breads & Grains

The top sources of omega-6 oils are sweets and certain meats such as turkey. Other sources of omega-6 oils include cheeses, grains, and other meats.

*See Guides on Pages 467-468.

PHYLLOQUINONE
(SEE VITAMIN K)

PHYTIC ACID
(INOSITOL HEXAPHOSPHATE)

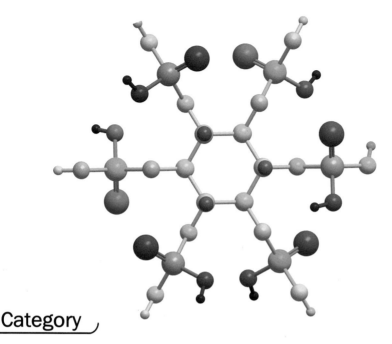

Category

Phytic acid is a nutrient found in grains and seeds.

Phytic acid is also called phytate and inositol hexaphosphate, and has the abbreviation, IP6. Other names include inositol hexakisphosphate, myo-inositol hexaphosphate and myo-inositol 1,2,3,4,5,6-hexakisphosphate.

It is a precursor to a cell-signaling compound, inositol triphosphate, which contains 3 phosphorus molecules. Inositol triphosphate is also known as IP3 or inositol 1,4,5-triphosphate. IP3 is composed of a central hexagonal ring of carbons surrounded by three phosphate groups.

Cellular Location

Phytic acid is distributed through the bloodstream diffusely throughout the body.

Structure

Phytic acid is composed of one inositol component with six phosphorus atoms that are bound to it. In essence, it is a hexagonal ring with six phosphorus groups surrounding it.

Mechanisms of Action

Phytic acid is a metal chelator, (an agent that binds the metals to remove them from action). It also acts as a precursor to a cell-signaling compound, inositol triphosphate.

Biological & Ocular Importance

● **Binds metals & prevents oxidation** Phytic acid binds and removes metals, such as copper, aluminum, cadmium, lead, mercury, and silver. In fact, plants use phytic acid to store phosphorus. Phytic acid does not bind electrolytic minerals such as potassium or sodium. Phytic acid is important in preventing oxidative damage because it can chelate (or bind to) metals like iron and copper to prevent them from acting as oxidants.

● **Binds metals & prevents enzyme function such as those that are associated with cancer** Phytic acid may prevent cell proliferation and, thus, may prevent cancers. This role may be due either to the binding of metals to block their ability to function in enzymes that are associated with proliferation (an increase in the number of cells) or to the regulation of cell signaling involved in cell proliferation. There is even some suggestion that phytic acid may inhibit platelet clotting.

● **Binding metals causes benefits but also harm, by causing deficiency of certain metals** However, phytic acid is a strong chelator of iron, which is essential for transport of oxygen in blood cells. Therefore, excess phytic acid results in iron deficiency, which results in anemia (insufficiency of the red blood cells that carry oxygen). Some of the symptoms of anemia include fatigue, shortness of breath, increased heart rate, mouth sores or ulcers, tongue soreness, pale skin, and brittle nails. Similarly, excess chelation of zinc in the intestine can lead to zinc deficiency. As with much of cellular function, balance of nutrients is critical.

● **Binds other minerals such as calcium** Phytic acid can also bind other minerals, such as calcium. Calcium deposits can build up behind the retina in Bruch's membrane, a supporting structure that separates the retinal pigment epithelium from the underlying choroid. Calcium accumulation in Bruch's membrane has been associated with macular degeneration.

253

• Precursor to a signaling molecule within cells

Phytic acid, or inositol hexaphosphate, contains 6 phosphorus molecules. It is a precursor to a cell-signaling compound, IP3, which contains 3 phosphorus molecules. Vitamin D assists in the conversion of phytic acid into IP3. IP3 often acts to signal the effects of chemical messengers that send signals to cells. When these messages are received by the cell, the molecule IP3 is activated and takes the message inside the cell to activate the specific chemical pathways requested by the original chemical messenger.

As a signaling molecule within cells, it often signals cells to release calcium stored within, which then mediates other important cellular activities.

• Precursor to IP3 that helps signal clean up of debris from the retina

IP3 functions as a cell-signaling compound that signals the retinal pigment epithelium (the layer of cells behind the retina that serve to nourish the retina and remove the excess debris from the retina) to increase its clean up of debris from photoreceptors. The retinal pigment epithelium serves to provide nutrition for the photoreceptors and to remove excess debris and waste from the photoreceptors. This debris and waste includes the discs of the photoreceptors, which are shed each day. In the presence of light and oxygen, excess debris results in the production of reactive oxygen species (toxic chemicals that result in oxidation), that can damage the retina. Of course light exposure is high in the retina, and the highest amount oxygen of consumption of any tissue in the body occurs in the retina. Therefore, the retina is particularly susceptible to oxidative damage, and IP3 assists in promoting the clean up of the debris that leads to oxidative damage.

Human Studies on Utility

There are no human studies on the use of phytic acid in treatment of eye disease reported in the scientifically-reviewed medical literature. Nevertheless, the fact that there are no reported clinical studies does not necessarily imply a benefit or lack of benefit. Looking at the mechanism of action, the use of phytic acid in moderation may be possibly of benefit in certain eye diseases.

Carbachol is a medication that through activation of cell messenger systems can increase levels of IP3. It has been shown to increase the removal (by the retinal pigment epithelium) of excess photoreceptor discs by from a level of 9% without carbachol to 34% with carbachol.

Body Absorption, Metabolism, & Excretion

Phytic acid is absorbed rapidly from the intestines into the bloodstream, though it is unclear how much of it is actually absorbed. There appears to be a limit to how much phytic acid can be absorbed at a given time; accordingly, the excess acid is excreted with the stool. Once absorbed though, phytic acid is filtered out and excreted by the kidneys.

Deficiency

Phytic acid can also be made from inositol in the body. Since it is non-essential, phytic acid dietary deficiency is not likely to cause any symptoms or illness. Instead, any deficiency that ensues is often from a widespread nutritional deficiency.

Toxicity & Side Effects

Because phytic acid is a metal chelator (an agent that binds the metals to remove them from action), it can chelate iron, which is essential for transport of oxygen in blood cells. Therefore, excess phytic acid results in iron deficiency, which results in anemia. As with much of cellular function, balance of nutrients is critical. Too much iron is toxic, while too little is harmful. Iron deficiency should be particularly avoided during pregnancy and in children.

While phytic acid has been proposed to treat bipolar disorder, it has also been shown to actually cause the manic component of bipolar disorder.

Because of the suggestion that phytic acid may inhibit platelet clotting, it should be used only with caution in those who are susceptible to bleeding and should also be avoided prior to any surgery. Moreover, the risk of bleeding may be exacerbated in those concurrently taking ginkgo or high doses of omega-3 oils.

Interactions with Other Nutrients

Nutrients such as alpha-lipoic acid, phytic acid, and bioflavonoids chelate (bind and remove) metals such as copper, aluminum, cadmium, lead, mercury, silver, zinc and iron. Therefore, excess of these nutrients can result in zinc deficiency or iron deficiency. Iron is essential for transport of oxygen in blood cells, and deficiency of iron results in anemia (see sections on zinc and iron).

High levels of calcium, especially when they are combined with phytic acid supplementation, can cause decreased zinc absorption in the intestines (see section on zinc).

Bioflavonoids and phytic acid can help stabilize levels of hyaluronic acid, a water-holding support compound of the eye (see section on hyaluronic acid).

IP3 is also involved in a cellular messaging pathway that is activated by vitamin E and helps improve blood flow through vessels. This mechanism is particular important in maintaining appropriate blood flow in the eye, especially in the retina in disorders such as diabetes or hypertension (high blood pressure).

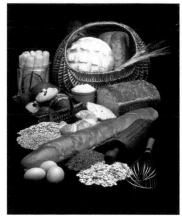

Ideal Dosage

A typical diet consists of 300 to 600 mg of phytic acid. However, phytic acid functions very poorly as a chelator in the body because it has already chelated minerals contained in the food ingested. Therefore, for phytic acid to be useful as a chelator in the body, it should be ingested separately from other foods, which can be achieved by taking it on an empty stomach with only water.

While there is no recommended minimum daily allowance, a recommended daily dose is about 1,500 to 2,000 mg, taken in conjunction with about 600 to 800 IU of vitamin D. It is important to note, however, that excess phytic acid should be avoided altogether during pregnancy and in children.

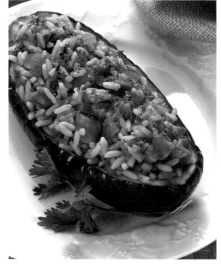

However, even in healthy non-pregnant adults, the risks of phytic acid toxicity can be minimized by taking breaks from the use of phytic acid. In other words, a six-week regimen of phytic acid should be followed by a six-week period free from the use of phytic acid.

Balance must be achieved between doses of phytic acid intake and mineral supplementation, particularly iron, selenium, and zinc, in order to avoid deficiencies of these minerals as well.

Sources (Where to Find It)

Sources of Phytic Acid (IP6):

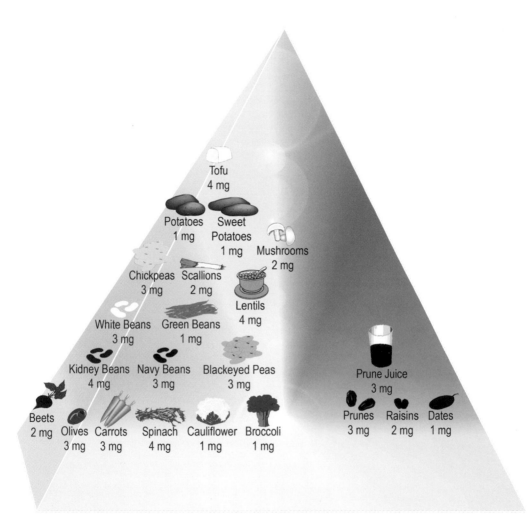

Tofu
4 mg

Potatoes   Sweet
1 mg   Potatoes
1 mg   Mushrooms
2 mg

Chickpeas Scallions
3 mg   2 mg

Lentils
4 mg

White Beans Green Beans
3 mg   1 mg

Kidney Beans Navy Beans Blackeyed Peas
4 mg   3 mg   3 mg

Prune Juice
3 mg

Beets
2 mg Olives Carrots Spinach Cauliflower Broccoli
3 mg   3 mg   4 mg   1 mg   1 mg

Prunes Raisins Dates
3 mg   2 mg   1 mg

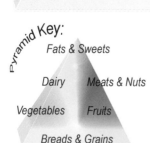

Pyramid Key:

Fats & Sweets

Dairy   Meats & Nuts

Vegetables   Fruits

Breads & Grains

The sources above are for phytic acid (IP6). The top sources of phytic acid are beans (particularly soybeans, lentils, and lima beans) and grains (such as wheat bread, wild rice, and pasta).

*See Guides on Pages 467-468.

Sources of IP3:

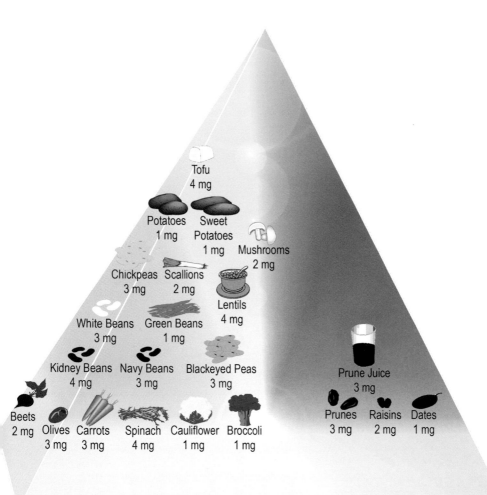

Tofu
4 mg

Potatoes
1 mg

Sweet Potatoes
1 mg

Mushrooms
2 mg

Chickpeas
3 mg

Scallions
2 mg

Lentils
4 mg

White Beans
3 mg

Green Beans
1 mg

Kidney Beans
4 mg

Navy Beans
3 mg

Blackeyed Peas
3 mg

Prune Juice
3 mg

Beets
2 mg

Olives
3 mg

Carrots
3 mg

Spinach
4 mg

Cauliflower
1 mg

Broccoli
1 mg

Prunes
3 mg

Raisins
2 mg

Dates
1 mg

Pyramid Key:

Fats & Sweets

Dairy   Meats & Nuts

Vegetables   Fruits

Breads & Grains

The sources above are for IP3. The top sources of IP3 are beans (particularly lentils, lima beans, and blackeyed peas).

PROLINE

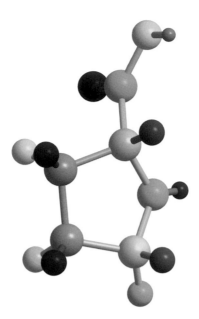

Category

Proline is often referred to as a non-essential amino acid (building block of proteins), though it is not truly an amino acid because it does not have an "amine" or "amino" group. It is still categorized with the amino acids, though, since it is still a building block of proteins.

Cellular Location

Proline is distributed through the bloodstream to various organs. Since proteins cannot be stored by the human body, unused proteins are metabolized and excreted.

The most abundant protein in the body is collagen. In fact ¼ to ½ of all the protein in the body is collagen. Collagen is the major structural support protein of skin, tendons, ligaments, and blood vessels and is the major protein that plays a support role in bones. It also plays an important role in the structure of many organs, including the eye. The amino acids proline and glycine form the most important parts of collagen, and the proline is what gives it its strength and its elasticity, which are two very important characteristics of the collagen needed for the eye.

Structure

Proline is an amino acid without an amine group. It is a relatively simple compound and is unique in its structural rigidity.

Mechanisms of Action

Proline is a building block of proteins.

Biological & Ocular Importance

● **Forms the connective protein collagen**   Proline is important in forming collagen. Collagen is an important component of many parts of the eye. It is the major protein of the cornea and its uniformity and pattern of arrangement is essential in maintaining the clarity of the cornea.

Collagen maintains the trabecular meshwork (the filtration site of the eye) by preventing it from collapsing. Allowing enough fluid to exit the eye is essential to prevent pressure build-up in the eye, decreasing the risk of glaucoma, since malfunction of this filtration site is a common mechanism of glaucoma.

Collagen also forms the lamina cribrosa, a structure that supports individual nerve fibers as they pass from the retina into the optic nerve. One mechanism of glaucoma is damage to these nerve fibers when the lamina cribrosa is unable to support them.

Collagen is also the major structural component of the vitreous. The vitreous gel is water supported by collagen and hyaluronic acid (see section on hyaluronic acid). In fact, the vitreous is 99% water supported in this collagen and hyaluronic acid meshwork. Vitreous floaters, which appear as cobwebs or spiders or spots floating in one's vision, occur when the vitreous begins to shrink. The vitreous shrinks at different ages for different people, often ranging from age 20 to age 70, though more commonly in the elderly. Decrease in collagen is associated with premature shrinking of the vitreous. Vitreous shrinking is associated with tears in the retina as well as detachments of the retina.

Collagen is also an important protein that forms skin, tendons, ligaments, and blood vessels as well. Capillaries are where the arteries thin to the point of supplying tissue with nutrients and oxygen from the blood supply, in exchange for waste materials and carbon dioxide that must be transported out in veins. Capillary malfunction can result in tissue swelling, bleeding, and inappropriate control of tissue nutrition and oxygenation.

● **Forms the connective protein elastin**   Proline also forms elastin, which is another protein that gives skin and connective tissue their elasticity. Elastin also plays an important role in providing elasticity to large blood vessels such as the aorta and organs, such as the lung.

Along with elastin, collagen forms the layers of Bruch's membrane, a support layer that separates the retinal pigment epithelium from the underlying choroidal blood vessels. In wet macular degeneration as well as in extremely high myopia (near-sightedness), cracks can develop in Bruch's membrane through which new blood vessels grow that can lead to bleeding and scarring as well as detachment and distortion of the retina.

● Important for the light sensing pigment rhodopsin

In addition, proline plays an important role in the structure of rhodopsin, particularly the region of rhodopsin that plays a role in transmitting signals. Rhodopsin is the light-sensing protein used by retinal photoreceptors to detect light.

Human Studies on Utility

Currently, there is only one human study on proline use in eye disease reported in the scientifically-reviewed medical literature. Nevertheless, the fact that there is only one reported clinical study does not necessarily imply a benefit or lack of benefit. Looking at the mechanism of action, the use of proline in moderation may be possibly of benefit in many eye diseases.

● No benefits from the use of proline for retinal disease

A 1985 study looked at proline supplementation for people with gyrate atrophy. Gyrate atrophy is a rare inherited disorder of cellular metabolism of ornithine (an amino acid that plays a role in the formation of arginine, another amino acid involved in building proteins). Ornithine also plays a significant role in the removal of excess nitrogen from cells through a process called the urea cycle. Deficiency of the enzyme involved in the cellular metabolism of ornithine results in excess build-up of ornithine and a disease called gyrate atrophy. Gyrate atrophy is a retinal disease resulting in night-

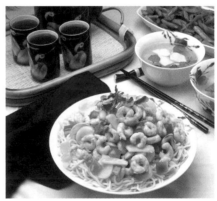

blindness and loss of peripheral (or side) vision.

The study looked at 4 people with gyrate atrophy who received proline supplements, and 2 who received vitamin B6 supplements. While the authors suggested possible benefits, there is no clear evidence of any benefit from proline supplementation and in fact the study found no increase in proline levels in the bloodstream.[121]

Body Absorption, Metabolism, & Excretion

Proline is digested by the stomach with the help of stomach acids. Digestive enzymes from the pancreas further break down proteins, which are then absorbed into the bloodstream through the intestines.

As proteins are broken down, ammonia is formed. Since ammonia is extremely toxic to cells, it must be converted into a nitrogen-containing chemical known as urea. When ammonia builds up in excess, it can cause poor coordination, difficulties with balance, tremors, seizures, difficulty breathing, swelling of the brain, and can eventually lead to a coma. A normally functioning liver works to remove excess ammonia by creating urea, which is then filtered into the urine by the kidneys.

Deficiency

Since the body can make its own proline, it is considered non-essential, and deficiency is therefore rare.

Toxicity & Side Effects

Excess proline, like other amino acids, is often broken down and converted into sugars or fats, and used for energy, or stored as fat in the body's fat stores. Excess amino acids can stress the kidneys, stress the bloodstream, and cause dehydration. Furthermore, excess amino acids can cause the kidneys to lose calcium resulting in weakened bones. As with any amino acid, proline in excess in someone with liver disease or with kidney disease may result in accumulation of ammonia or urea in the body, resulting in severe illness (see above).

Interactions with Other Nutrients

Manganese is required for an enzyme that makes proline from other amino acids. Also, vitamin C is required to modify proline that is involved in the formation of collagen. The ultratrace element, silicon, is believed to be required for this vitamin C pathway that modifies proline.

Ideal Dosage

There are no established dosage guidelines or scientifically-based dosage suggestions. In fact, little is known of the bioavailability of proline after ingestion and the body's ability to use proline from the diet. Also, supplementation with proline is not known to increase collagen formation.

Sources (Where to Find It)

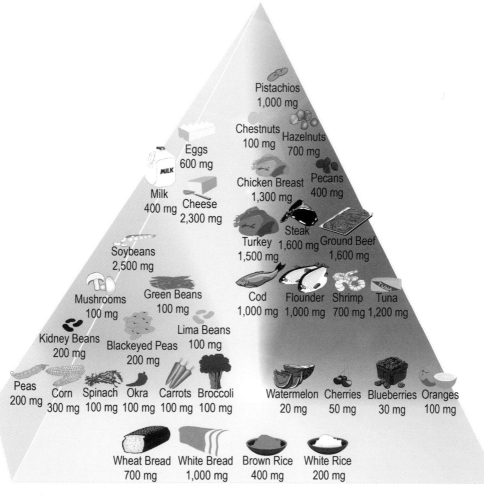

Pistachios
1,000 mg

Chestnuts 100 mg   Hazelnuts 700 mg

Eggs 600 mg

Chicken Breast 1,300 mg   Pecans 400 mg

Milk 400 mg   Cheese 2,300 mg

Steak 1,600 mg   Ground Beef 1,600 mg

Turkey 1,500 mg

Soybeans 2,500 mg

Mushrooms 100 mg   Green Beans 100 mg

Cod 1,000 mg   Flounder 1,000 mg   Shrimp 700 mg   Tuna 1,200 mg

Kidney Beans 200 mg   Blackeyed Peas 200 mg   Lima Beans 100 mg

Peas 200 mg   Corn 300 mg   Spinach 100 mg   Okra 100 mg   Carrots 100 mg   Broccoli 100 mg

Watermelon 20 mg   Cherries 50 mg   Blueberries 30 mg   Oranges 100 mg

Wheat Bread 700 mg   White Bread 1,000 mg   Brown Rice 400 mg   White Rice 200 mg

Pyramid Key:

Fats & Sweets

Dairy   Meats & Nuts

Vegetables   Fruits

Breads & Grains

Top sources of proline are meats, cheeses, and soybeans. Foods that are high in proline, such as chicken skin and cartilage, are not well absorbed, thereby making them poor sources of proline. Grains, wheat, rice, and corn are also relatively high in proline content and perhaps may be absorbed than animal sources of proline.

*See Guides on Pages 467-468.

PYRIDOXAL
(SEE VITAMIN B6)

PYRIDOXAMINE
(SEE VITAMIN B6)

PYRIDOXINE
(SEE VITAMIN B6)

QUERCETIN

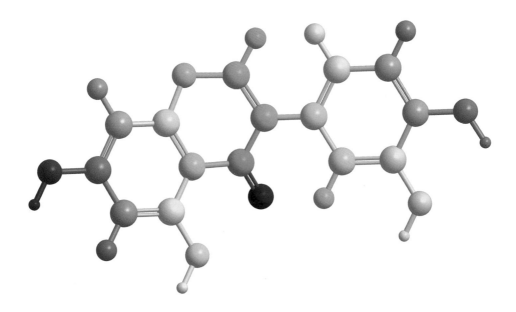

Category

Bioflavonoids are ring-shaped nutrients derived from plant sources (see section on bioflavonoids). There are about 5,000 currently identified bioflavonoids, divided into 6 categories. Quercetin is in the flavonol category. Quercetin is also known as 3,3',4',5,7pentahydroxy-flavone.

Cellular Location

Bioflavonoids are a large group of nutrients, and because they are not required for cellular function, they are concentrated in the bloodstream and delivered to the tissues and organs that need their actions.

Structure

Quercetin is a ring-shaped chemical structure belonging to the group of chemicals, called polyphenols.

Mechanisms of Action

Quercetin is a particularly active bioflavonoid. Quercetin is a powerful antioxidant. It is also believed to inhibit inflammation by blocking inflammatory enzymes.

Biological & Ocular Importance

● Powerful antioxidant

Quercetin is known to be one of the most active bioflavonoids. As the other bioflavonoids, quercetin is highly active as an antioxidant (see section on bioflavonoids).

As an antioxidant, it is believed to be beneficial to retinal diseases, such as macular degeneration and childhood hereditary photoreceptor diseases, in which oxidative damage plays a role in the disease. It may also be beneficial in diseases, such as glaucoma or optic nerve diseases, in which oxidative damage plays a role as well. Furthermore, it may also help prevent cataract formation or corneal disease, again by preventing or decreasing oxidative damage.

● Blocks inflammation as well as allergic pink eye or virus infections in the eye

It is also believed to inhibit inflammation by blocking inflammatory enzymes, such as lipoxygenase and cyclo-oxygenase, popularly known as COX, the target of many new anti-inflammatory COX-inhibitor drugs.

Quercetin also acts as an antihistamine and therefore helps with allergic conjunctivitis (or allergic pink eye). Due to its activity in reducing inflammation, quercetin has been shown to be beneficial in animals with experimental uveitis and retinal inflammation.

In addition, quercetin acts to inhibit herpes virus activities, and, as such, is beneficial during herpes virus infections, such as corneal infections or uveitis, which is inflammation inside the eye.

Quercetin as an antioxidant and anti-inflammatory agent has been recommended for prevention or treatment of a variety of disorders, ranging from heart disease to asthma to arthritis to cancer. In fact, there is good evidence to show its particular benefit in heart disease and blood vessel disease.

● Prevents growth of abnormal blood vessels

There is some thought that quercetin may have some activity in preventing angiogenesis (the growth of abnormal new blood vessels) that can be harmful in the eye. Angiogenesis is particularly harmful in the retina, cornea, and trabecular meshwork (filtration site of the eye) and can cause loss of vision. The problems that result are called choroidal neovascularization (seen in wet macular degeneration), or retinal neovascularization (seen in severe diabetic retinopathy or retinal disease), or corneal neovascularization (seen in corneal injury or disease), or iris neovascularization (seen in angle-closure glaucoma and inflammatory eye disease).

● **Decreases effects of toxic sugar attacks**   There is also some suggestion that quercetin may decrease the damaging effects of high sugars in diabetes. Quercetin may act to block an enzyme that converts blood sugars to sorbitol, thereby preventing the formation of "advanced glycation end products" or AGEs, the toxic products that damage the retina, the lens, and other ocular structures (see introduction).

● **Prevents cataracts, though in extremely high doses, causes cataracts**
Furthermore, quercetin has been shown to reduce enzymes that are associated with cataract formation, particularly in diseases such as diabetes.

Interestingly, in extremely high doses, quercetin has been shown to cause cataracts in mice. Whether this finding represents the toxicity of an additive with the quercetin or represents a toxic effect of the quercetin at high doses, is unknown. Nevertheless, a common theme of ocular nutrition is moderation. Too much of a good thing may be possibly harmful.

Human Studies on Utility

There are no human studies on the use of quercetin in treatment of eye disease reported in the scientifically-reviewed medical literature. Nevertheless, the fact that there are no reported clinical studies does not necessarily imply a benefit or lack of benefit. Looking at the mechanism of action, the use of quercetin in moderation may be possibly of benefit in certain eye diseases.

Body Absorption, Metabolism, & Excretion

Digestion of fruits, vegetables, herbs and other sources of bioflavonoids occurs in the stomach with the assistance of stomach acids that help break down the fruits, vegetables, and herbs to release the bioflavonoids. In the intestines, though, enzymes often further break down the bioflavonoids. Some bioflavonoids, particularly those bound to sugars, are absorbed in the small intestines, while most bioflavonoids pass to the large intestines where they are further broken down.

Overall, a small amount of the bioflavonoids are absorbed in the digestive tract and then into the bloodstream. The majority of bioflavonoids are not absorbed and remain in the digestive tract, where they are either broken down by enzymes or are excreted.

Some reports suggest up to ¼ of ingested quercetin is absorbed into the bloodstream.

Of the bioflavonoids absorbed in the bloodstream, excretion occurs mostly through the kidneys.

Deficiency

There are no known disorders of bioflavonoid deficiency, as bioflavonoids are non-essential nutrients. Instead, any deficiency that ensues is often from a widespread nutritional deficiency.

Toxicity & Side Effects

In general, there are no known toxicities associated with bioflavonoids since the body absorbs relatively little of the bioflavonoids in the digestive tract. Nevertheless, there are some reports of nausea, headaches, and tingling of the hands and feet associated with excess intake of quercetin. There are also suggestions of an increased risk of leukemia in infants born to mothers ingesting high doses of quercetin.

Interactions with Other Nutrients

Bioflavonoids are required to maintain stable vitamin C levels in the blood. A daily dosage of vitamin C should be associated with ingestion of about seven-tenths of that amount of bioflavonoids.

Some nutrients are metal chelators (agents that bind the metals to remove them from action). Such nutrient chelators include bioflavonoids such as quercetin and phytic acid (see section on phytic acid). Chelators can be important in preventing metal toxicity or oxidative damage because they can chelate (bind and remove) metals like iron, copper, lead, mercury, and zinc to prevent them from acting as oxidants or toxins. However, they can also block the absorption of metals needed by the body (some of which are the same metals that cause toxicity in high doses) such as iron or zinc, resulting in iron or zinc deficiency.

Ideal Dosage

There is no established ideal dosage as quercetin is non-essential. A recommend doses is 500 to 1,200 mg per day, divided into multiple smaller dosages each day. It even may be safe in doses up to 4,000 mg per day.

Sources (Where to Find It)

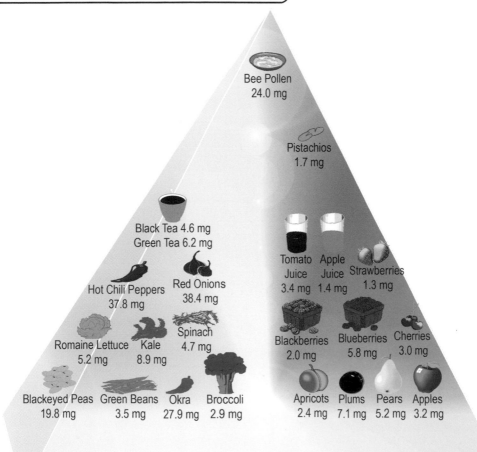

Bee Pollen 24.0 mg

Pistachios 1.7 mg

Black Tea 4.6 mg
Green Tea 6.2 mg

Tomato Juice 3.4 mg   Apple Juice 1.4 mg   Strawberries 1.3 mg

Hot Chili Peppers 37.8 mg   Red Onions 38.4 mg

Spinach 4.7 mg

Blackberries 2.0 mg   Blueberries 5.8 mg   Cherries 3.0 mg

Romaine Lettuce 5.2 mg   Kale 8.9 mg

Blackeyed Peas 19.8 mg   Green Beans 3.5 mg   Okra 27.9 mg   Broccoli 2.9 mg

Apricots 2.4 mg   Plums 7.1 mg   Pears 5.2 mg   Apples 3.2 mg

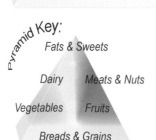

Pyramid Key:

Fats & Sweets

Dairy   Meats & Nuts

Vegetables   Fruits

Breads & Grains

Top sources of quercetin are bee pollen, red onions, hot chili peppers, okra, and blackeyed peas. Of the fruits, the highest sources of quercetin are plums, blueberries, and pears.

*See Guides on Pages 467-468.

RETINOL
(SEE VITAMIN A)

S-ADENOSYL-METHIONINE
(SAMe)

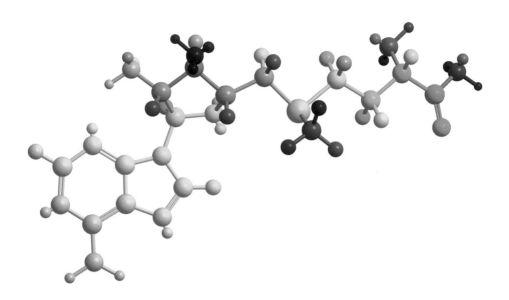

Category

S-adenosyl-methionine is also known as SAMe, a molecule composed through a chemical reaction in which methionine is combined with ATP, the main energy molecule of the cell.

Cellular Location

SAMe is delivered throughout the body for use.

Structure

SAMe is a complex compound that contains three ring structures. The importance of SAMe, however, is in its ability to donate methyl groups, or small groups composed of one carbon and three hydrogen atoms (CH_3).

Mechanisms of Action

SAMe is a chemical donor of methyl groups to many reactions. It participates in the enzymatic activity of hundreds of methyltransferases (enzymes that transfer methyl groups).

Biological & Ocular Importance

● **Donates methyl groups to form antioxidants & energy molecules, to prevent DNA damage, & to regulate light response** SAMe is a potent methylator. Initially discovered to donate methyl groups in order to participate in the formation of creatine, SAMe can also donate sulfur to participate in the formation of the antioxidant lipoic acid (see section on alpha-lipoic acid), or to amino groups in order to participate in the formation of biotin.

Enzymes can be regulated by adding or taking away methyl groups.

Studies have shown that methylation is one step that regulates or controls signaling pathways that are involved in the light response within photoreceptors.

SAMe can also decrease the risk of certain types of cancer by donating methyl groups to DNA to prevent DNA damage. Research suggests that DNA damage is an important precursor to cancer formation. Also, folate is essential in the process of forming SAMe.

● **Blocks inflammation** SAMe may block certain types of inflammation, and therefore has been used to treat arthritis. There is also suggestion that SAMe can help treat inflammation in liver disease.

● **Breaks down neurotransmitter signaling molecules to balance levels** SAMe helps break down brain neurotransmitter signaling molecules. As such, it may be effective as a treatment for depression or mood disorders, as well as for Alzheimer's disease.

SAMe can protect against glutamate toxicity (see section on vitamin B12), which involves the toxic effects of excess glutamate release from the neural cells of the eye. Glutamate is a natural signaling chemical in neural cells that enables signals to transfer from one cell to another. It is the main signal producer in the circuitry of the eye. However, excess glutamate is toxic to surrounding cells. When a cell dies, for example in glaucoma, it can release excess glutamate, resulting in toxic injury and death of surrounding cells.

● **Required to form insulation around nerve fibers**

SAMe is believed to be required for myelin synthesis. Vitamin B12 is required for maintenance of the myelin sheath (the insulation around nerves fibers that enables the signals to be sent efficiently) (see section on vitamin B12). Actually, these myelin sheaths play a critical role in sending information from the eye to the brain through the optic nerve.

Human Studies on Utility

There are no human studies on the use of SAMe in treatment of eye disease reported in the scientifically-reviewed medical literature. Nevertheless, the fact that there are no reported clinical studies does not necessarily imply a benefit or lack of benefit. Looking at the mechanism of action, the use of SAMe in moderation may be possibly of benefit in certain eye diseases.

Body Absorption, Metabolism, & Excretion

Despite the fact that stomach acids and intestinal enzymes break down SAMe, the remaining portion is rapidly absorbed in the intestines and into the bloodstream, through which it is sent to the liver. In the liver, about ½ of SAMe is further broken down.

A large portion of the SAMe that survives the absorption and survives the liver is then distributed throughout the body for use, while the small, remaining portion is filtered out by the kidneys.

The portion of SAMe that is broken down in the liver forms homocysteine, a toxic byproduct (see below).

Deficiency

Since the body can make its own SAMe, deficiency of SAMe is rare. The body makes N-acetyl-cysteine from the amino acid methionine.

Toxicity & Side Effects

Excess SAMe can cause headaches and dry mouth, as well as gastrointestinal side effects, such as upset stomach, nausea, and diarrhea. It can also cause sleeplessness and anxiety. SAMe may also exacerbate manic episodes in people with bipolar disorder. SAMe may also cause manic disorder in people who have had bipolar disorder in the past.

As one can see from the complex circle of interaction of SAMe with other vitamins, SAMe in excess runs the risk of tipping the delicate balance in our cells. When SAMe is in excess, a toxic byproduct called homocysteine is created (see below).

Interactions with Other Nutrients

There are numerous interactions between SAMe and other nutrients. The important concept, however, is that a balance should be achieved between intake of SAMe and other nutrients.

SAMe can provide methyl groups to assist choline in the process of creating cell membrane components, called phospholipids (see section on choline).

SAMe plays a role in providing methyl groups to methionine, which follows a pathway into carnitine (see section on carnitine). Actually, vitamin C plays an important role in two of the steps of formation of carnitine. Vitamins B3 and B6 and iron also play roles in the pathway.

There are several nutrients (SAMe, methionine, vitamin B12, vitamin B6, folate, selenium, and N-acetyl-cysteine) that act in the same complex circular pathway and are all interrelated when it comes to: (1) the toxicity of homocysteine and decreasing its levels, and (2) the activities of SAMe as a donator of methyl groups (see sections on folate, vitamin B12, vitamin B6, selenium, SAMe, and N-acetyl-cysteine). Homocysteine is a toxic chemical that is associated with Alzheimer's disease as well as vascular disease, including blood clots, heart disease, stroke, and vein occlusions in the retina.

Folate plays an important role in the process of converting the toxic chemical homocysteine into methionine. The particular enzyme that converts homocysteine back to methionine is, in fact, one of only two enzymes throughout our body that depend on vitamin B12 for their activity. SAMe participates in this cycle by donating methyl groups (see section on vitamin B12 and SAMe).

Not only do vitamin B12 and folate work together in regulating homocysteine levels, vitamin B6 and zinc regulate homocysteine levels by helping convert homocysteine into glutathione, which ensures lower levels of toxic homocysteine. Selenium is required in this pathway as these glutathione enzymes are selenoproteins, composed of selenium with the protein. N-acetyl-cysteine may lower homocysteine levels as well, by converting homocysteine into the protein building block cysteine, an amino acid.

Choline also interacts in this complex homocysteine pathway. Choline forms a chemical, called betaine, in the body, and betaine works to convert homocysteine to methionine, in order to decrease levels of homocysteine in the body.

SAMe plays a role in providing methyl groups to methionine, which follows a pathway into carnitine.

Ideal Dosage

Dosages of up to 1,600 mg per day have been used in some studies. Some researchers suggest starting out with low doses to avoid the gastrointestinal side effects. A recommended amount may be 200 to 400 mg per day, though others suggest amounts of 600 to 800 mg per day. There is definite concern of increasing quantities of homocysteine by ingesting too much SAMe.

SAMe in its pure form is stable only in sub-zero temperatures (below 0° C). As a salt form, it may be stable at room temperatures.

Sources (Where to Find It)

While SAMe is classified as a dietary supplement, it is not a typical nutrient that is found in food. Because SAMe is unstable at room temperatures, it is available as a nutritional supplement in a synthetic salt form.

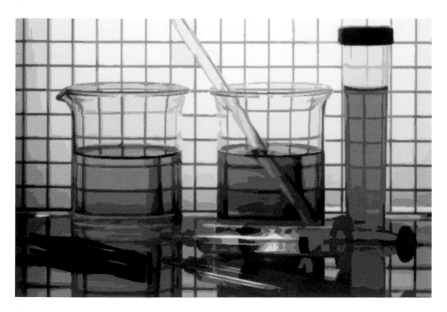

SAINT JOHN'S WORT
(HYPERICIN OR HYPERFORIN)

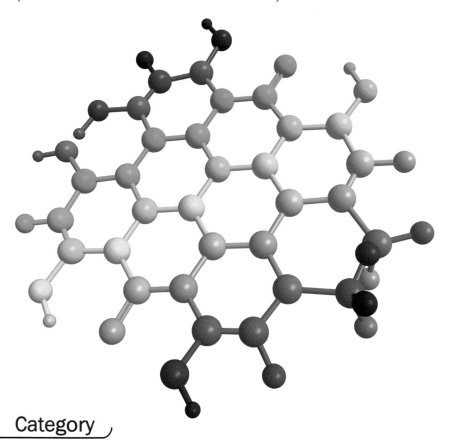

Category

Hypericum perforatum is a flowering herb, known as klamath weed, goat weed, or Saint John's wort. Its name is derived from the fact that it typically blossoms around Saint John's day, the 24th of June, and was used to ward off evil by hanging it over pictures. The active components of Saint John's wort are believed to be hypericin and hyperforin as well as other bioflavonoids, including quercetin (see section on quercetin).

Cellular Location

Saint John's wort is delivered throughout the body for use.

Structure

Hypericin is a quinone with multiple rings that are ringed together themselves.

Mechanisms of Action

Hypericin is a photodynamic or photosensitive agent. In other words, when light strikes the rings of hypericin, it produces an oxidant known as singlet oxygen. It may also produce other reactive oxygen species (toxic chemicals that result in oxidation). In fact, grazing animals that are unfortunate to ingest large quantities of hypericin from plants become ill from the combination of being out in the sunlight with the photodynamic hypericin in their cells.

Biological & Ocular Importance

● **Helps destroy viruses**
Hypericin has been shown to have a strong anti-viral effect. It can inhibit the survival of viruses. In the presence of light, it is particularly effective in staving off and destroying viruses, particularly those viruses with membrane "envelope" walls.

● **Blocks growth of abnormal blood vessels** In animal models, hypericin is believed to block angiogenesis (the formation of abnormal new blood vessels). Angiogenesis is particularly harmful in the retina, cornea, and trabecular meshwork (filtration site of the eye) and can cause loss of vision. The problems that result are called choroidal neovascularization (seen in wet macular degeneration), or retinal neovascularization (seen in severe diabetic retinopathy or retinal disease), or corneal neovascularization (seen in corneal injury or disease), or iris neovascularization (seen in angle-closure glaucoma and inflammatory eye disease). Hypericin may provide this anti-angiogenesis effect by binding to and blocking the effect of inflammatory and cell-signaling enzymes involved in the process of angiogenesis. While some studies have shown that these effects require light to be effective or that light is believed to augment the effects, others have shown that these effects do not require light.

● **Treats wounds & inflammation such as after retinal detachment surgery**
Hypericin has been promoted to

treat wounds and inflammation. Some animal model experiments have shown hypericin's benefits in blocking the inflammation that causes retinal scarring after retinal detachment surgery.

● **Anti-cancer effect** There is growing evidence that hypericin may be useful as a treatment for certain types of cancer cells under certain conditions. Some of this anti-cancer effect may be mediated through the phototoxic effects, the anti-inflammatory effects, and the angiogenesis blocking effects.

● **Balances neurotransmitter signaling molecules** Saint John's wort is believed to work on balancing levels of the neurotransmitter serotonin, thereby acting as an antidepressant. However, there is much conflicting medical literature that casts some doubt on the antidepressant benefits of Saint John's wort, particularly in cases of severe depression. Good evidence shows that it is beneficial in mild to moderate cases of depression. There is evidence that hypericin affects signal transmission at the synapse (the communication junction between neurons). Hypericin also is believed to block uptake of many different types of neurotransmitters (the chemicals that send signals between neurons). It accomplishes this blockade in a very non-specific manner by activating cation channels that interfere with the neurotransmitters. It activates these cation channels by changing the fluidics of the membranes in which these channels sit.

Human Studies on Utility

There are no human studies on the use of hypericin in treatment of eye disease reported in the scientifically-reviewed medical literature. Nevertheless, the fact that there are no reported clinical studies does not necessarily imply a benefit or lack of benefit. Looking at the mechanism of action, the use of hypericin in moderation may be possibly of benefit in certain eye diseases.

Body Absorption, Metabolism, & Excretion

Digestion of fruits, vegetables, herbs and other sources of bioflavonoids occurs in the stomach with the assistance of stomach acids that help break down the fruits, vegetables, and herbs to release the bioflavonoids. In the intestines, though, enzymes often further break down the bioflavonoids. Some bioflavonoids, particularly those bound to sugars, are absorbed in the small intestines, while most bioflavonoids pass to the large intestines where they are further broken down.

Overall, a small amount of the bioflavonoids are absorbed in the digestive tract and then into the bloodstream. The majority of bioflavonoids are not absorbed and remain in the digestive tract, where they are either broken down by enzymes or are excreted.

Some reports suggest up to ¼ of ingested hypericin is absorbed into the bloodstream.

Of the bioflavonoids absorbed in the bloodstream, excretion occurs mostly through the kidneys.

Deficiency

Because Saint John's wort is not an essential nutrient, no deficiency of Saint John's wort is known or believed to occur. However, in people who have used Saint John's wort daily for at least one month, a "withdrawal syndrome" may occur when stopping the Saint John's wort abruptly. Symptoms of the withdrawal syndrome are similar to some of the side effects of Saint John's wort and include dizziness, extreme tiredness, dry mouth, nausea, and chills.

Toxicity & Side Effects

Saint John's wort is known to absorb light and produce toxic oxidants. Therefore, it can increase the risk of sun rashes and sunburns and even skin cancers. Furthermore, it can increase the risk of corneal disease, lens disease, or retinal disease by absorbing light and causing excess oxidative injury.

Human lens surface cells in culture experiments were noted to take up hypericin and degenerate when exposed to ultraviolet light. Similarly, human lens surface cells in culture experiments were noted to take up hypericin and degenerate when exposed to non-ultraviolet visible light, suggesting that even the best UV-protecting sunglasses may not protect against hypericin-induced lens or retinal toxicity. In the lens, the oxidative damage caused by Saint John's wort results in "polymerization" of proteins or clumping of proteins that reduce the clarity of the lens.

Other adverse effects include dizziness, confusion, tiredness as well as restlessness, dry mouth, nausea, constipation, and skin rashes.

There are reports that Saint John's wort also can cause mania.

Interactions with Other Nutrients

Experimental studies have shown that the antioxidant enzyme glutathione-S-transferase can bind to hypericin and block the phototoxic effects of hypericin, as well as blocking the beneficial effects of hypericin (see section on glutathione).

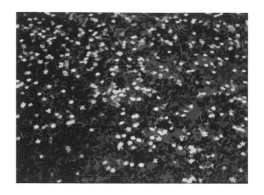

Ideal Dosage

There is a wide-range of dosage guidelines, depending on the concentration of hypericin in the formulation. For formulations that contain about 0.3% hypericin, dosage recommendations range from 300 to 900 mg per day, often in divided doses. A recommended dose may be 300 mg or less per day.

Sources (Where to Find It)

The active components, hypericin and hyperforin, of Saint John's wort are derived from the flowering herb *Hypericum perforatum*.

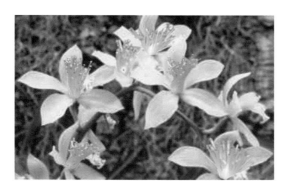

SAMe
(SEE S-ADENOSYL-METHIONINE)

SELENIUM

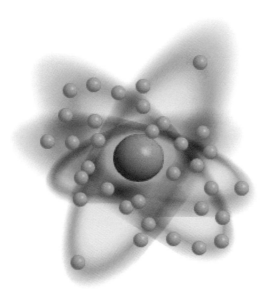

Category

Non-metallic element

Cellular Location

Selenium is distributed throughout the body, though $1/3$ of it becomes incorporated into the bones. Compared to soft tissue and other organs, the kidneys also contain a relatively high concentration of selenium.

Structure

Selenium is found as a non-metallic element. Its symbol on the periodic table of elements is Se, and its atomic number is 34. It is found between arsenic and bromine on the periodic table.

Mechanisms of Action

Selenium is required for the functioning of specific cellular enzymes.

Selenium does not act directly as an antioxidant, but instead provides its functions through enzymes.

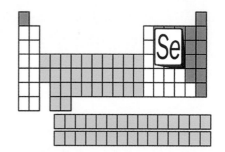

Biological & Ocular Importance

● Acts as a toxic oxidant

Elemental selenium is often found in the oxidized state of selenide or a reduced state of selenite or selenate. A reduced state form of an element often acts as an antioxidant, but in the case of selenium the reduced state is very inert and very resistant to functioning as an antioxidant. In fact, in its reduced state, it can easily react with oxygen to create reactive oxygen species (toxic chemicals that result in oxidation). Oxidation is the process whereby chemical compounds lose electrons resulting in potentially toxic modifications to proteins, lipids, and DNA, that can eventually lead to degeneration and even death of cells (see introduction). Therefore, in high doses, selenium can cause oxidative damage to cells (see below, under toxicity).

● Helps produce antioxidant glutathione
Selenium, along with vitamin B2 and vitamin E, is required for production of glutathione peroxidase, an enzyme involved in the functioning of antioxidant glutathione (see section on glutathione). In fact, glutathione peroxidase is called a selenoprotein as it includes 4 selenium-containing amino acids. Amino acids are the building blocks of proteins.

● Required for antioxidant enzyme thioredoxin reductase
Selenium is also required for the functioning of the enzyme thioredoxin reductase. As with glutathione, the thioredoxin acts as an antioxidant by donating electrons. For example, it "reduces" disulfide bonds of cell proteins that have become oxidized. With the help of the enzyme thioredoxin reductase, it removes free peroxides within the cells, thus preventing lipid peroxidation of, or oxidative damage to, cell membranes. In doing so, it assists vitamin E in its antioxidant activities in saving cell membranes from oxidative damage. Vitamin E performs the first steps of preventing lipid

peroxidation by converting strong and dangerous hydroperoxyl radicals into weaker but still harmful hydroperoxides. Thioredoxin and glutathione perform the second steps, safely removing the hydroperoxides, without which these hydroperoxides would turn back on lipids and cause damage (see sections on glutathione and vitamin E).

Thioredoxin reductase is important for maintaining thioredoxin in its reduced state. Reduced thioredoxin can also prevent or limit the death of cells through its regulation of DNA synthesis and its activity as a transcription factor (a protein that turns specific genes on or off).

● Helps recycle vitamin C
Furthermore, the selenium-containing enzyme thioredoxin reductase is essential for vitamin C recycling. Vitamin C functions as an antioxidant by reducing reactive oxygen species (toxic chemicals that result in oxidation). It donates electrons and in doing so, it oxidizes itself and converts into dehydroascorbic acid or into ascorbyl free radical. These forms cannot act as antioxidants and must be recycled back to vitamin C with the help of the selenium-containing enzyme thioredoxin reductase, glutathione, or the glutathione-dependent enzymes, such as dehydroascorbate reductase (see sections on vitamin C and selenium).

● Required for antioxidant enzymes selenoproteins
Selenium is also required for the enzymes selenoprotein P and W. Selenoprotein W is thought to have a function as an antioxidant in many cell types. Selenoprotein P is believed to function in protecting blood vessel cells from oxidative damage caused by the toxins peroxynitrites. A newly discovered role for selenoprotein P is transportation and storage of selenium in many cell types. Little is known about other selenoproteins, ranging from H to V, which are involved in processes ranging from muscle function to antioxidation.

Selenium also functions in selenophosphate synthetase, an enzyme that is required in order to create selenium-containing proteins and enzymes.

● Protects the retina from oxidation damage
Selenium is 100 times more concentrated in the retinal pigment epithelium. This layer of tissue serves to provide nutrition for the photoreceptors and to remove excess debris and waste from the photoreceptors. This debris and waste includes the discs of the photoreceptors, which are shed each day. In the presence of light and oxygen, excess debris results in the production of reactive oxygen species. Of course light exposure is high in the retina, and the highest amount of oxygen consumption of any tissue in the body occurs in the retina. Therefore, the retina is

particularly susceptible to oxidative damage. The antioxidant glutathione peroxidase is produced by selenium and is essential in protecting the retina from oxidative damage.

Animal studies have shown that selenium can protect the capillaries in the retina from damage during diabetes, such as from oxidation.

● **Prevents cataract formation, though in excess causes cataract formation**
Similarly, light exposure is very high in the lens, and selenium-containing proteins, such as glutathione can protect against cataract formation (see section on glutathione). Levels of glutathione within the lens are the highest of any tissue in the body! With age, though, these levels decrease, and a decrease is associated with increased cataracts.

While selenium can protect against cataract, excess of selenium is associated with cataract formation. However, care must be taken to avoid excess selenium, which can act as a pro-oxidant (see above, under mechanism of action) and cause formation of cataract. In these high doses, selenium may act to oxidize or oxidatively damage calcium channels in the cell membranes in the lens. This damage allows excess calcium to flow into the lens cells causing them to degenerate, resulting in the formation of cataract. Damage to the DNA of lens cells and damage to the clear "crystallin" proteins of the lens may also occur as an additional or concomitant mechanism of cataract formation with excess selenium. In animal models, high doses of selenium are often used to create cataracts to study experimentally.

● **Prevents heart disease as well as blood vessel disease**   There is belief that selenium, by acting as an antioxidant in blood vessels, can protect against atherosclerosis (blood vessel cholesterol clots and plaques that can result in heart disease and stroke, as well as artery or vein clots in the retina or optic nerve strokes).

● **Decreases risk of cancer**
Furthermore, selenium is believed to play a role in preventing or decreasing the risk of numerous types of cancer, ranging from lung cancer to colon cancer. It is also believed to decrease the risk of spread of melanomas. These anti-cancer activities of selenium are believed to be a result of its role as an antioxidant, as a transcription factor (see below), and as an immune system strengthener.

- **Strengthens the immune defense system**   Selenium is thought to strengthen the immune system by its activities as an antioxidant and as a transcription factor, improving the functioning of white blood cells in the body's immune-defense system and improving the ability of immune-defense cells to communicate with each other.

- **Prevents growth of abnormal blood vessels**
There is also evidence that selenium may play a role in preventing angiogenesis (the formation of abnormal new abnormal blood vessels). Angiogenesis is particularly harmful in the retina, cornea, and trabecular meshwork (filtration site of the eye) and can cause loss of vision. The problems that result are called choroidal neovascularization (seen in wet macular degeneration), or retinal neovascularization (seen in severe diabetic retinopathy or retinal disease), or corneal neovascularization (seen in corneal injury or disease), or iris neovascularization (seen in angle-closure glaucoma and inflammatory eye disease). Selenium may help inhibit the expression of enzymes that stimulate new blood vessel growth.

- **Plays a role in thyroid hormones**   Selenium is required for enzymes involved in the activation and inactivation of the thyroid gland hormones. These enzymes are called iodothyronine deiodinases. For example, they can convert inactive thyroxine T_4 into active triiodothyronine T_3.

Human Studies on Utility

Currently, there are only a handful of human studies on selenium use in eye disease reported in the scientifically-reviewed medical literature. These studies involve the following eye diseases: glaucoma, cataract, and macular degeneration. The studies are summarized below. Selenium deficiency, as well as glutathione peroxidase deficiency, has been associated with macular degeneration. Similarly, there are studies that have shown decrease selenium levels in people with cataracts. However, there is actually no clear link between generalized selenium deficiency in the body and macular degeneration or retinitis pigmentosa, nor cataracts because of the ability of the eye to concentrate selenium despite low blood levels of selenium. Nevertheless, looking at the mechanism of action, the use of selenium in moderation may be possibly of benefit in many eye diseases. However, a serious concern is that high dose selenium may increase the risk of glaucoma.

● **Large study found that the use of selenium in moderate-to high-dose increased risk of glaucoma over time**   A study of over 1,300 people who were followed for about 6 years were divided into two groups: one group that took 200 µg of selenium each day and one group that took placebo each day. The group that

Selenium for
Glaucoma
Scale of Benefit

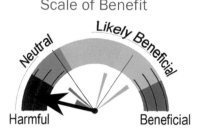

took selenium had lower risks of developing cancer, particularly lung, colorectal, and prostate. However, those that took selenium had a 2-fold increased risk of developing glaucoma over the 6 years, and if they continued to take the selenium after the cancer-investigation portion of the study ended, they had a 10-fold increased risk of developing glaucoma. Women had a higher risk than men to develop the glaucoma when they took 200 µg of selenium each day.[124] Although the mechanism of the selenium-induced glaucoma is unknown, there is thought that selenium affects the trabecular meshwork (the filtration site of the eye). Allowing enough fluid to exit the eye is essential to prevent pressure build-up in the eye, decreasing the risk of glaucoma. Malfunction of

this filtration site is a common mechanism of glaucoma.

Summary of Studies for Macular Degeneration:

Nearly a half-dozen clinical trials have been performed looking at the role of selenium in both preventing and treating macular degeneration. These clinical trials are of various types, some of which are very well-designed and well-performed studies.

As a whole, the clinical studies provide no definitive answer as to whether selenium is beneficial. Some of the studies found no benefit while others found a benefit to selenium for

Selenium for
Macular Degeneration
Scale of Benefit

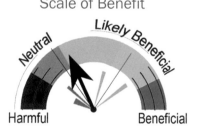

macular degeneration. Looking at the mechanisms of action, there is good reason to use carotenoids in moderation for macular degeneration.

The studies can be summarized as follows: a few studies found no link (neither protective nor harmful) between levels of selenium in the blood and macular degeneration, while one study found that that higher levels of selenium in the blood are associated with a decrease in the risk of macular degeneration.

In following people over time, one small study found that those who took selenium with other antioxidants did not have any benefit in preventing macular degeneration compared to those who did not take selenium with the antioxidants.

● In two studies: no link between blood levels of selenium and macular degeneration

A study of over 100 people, found no difference in the blood levels of selenium, carotenoids, vitamin A, vitamin C, or vitamin E between those with or without macular degeneration. However, the study did find that those who had macular degeneration had lower blood levels of zinc compared to those without macular degeneration.[39]

Another study of nearly 100 people found no difference in the blood levels of selenium, carotenoids, beta-carotene, lutein and zeaxanthin, lycopene, vitamin A, vitamin C, or zinc between those with or without macular degeneration (looking at both early and severe or advanced macular degeneration). However, the study found that those who had severe or advanced macular degeneration had lower blood levels of vitamin E compared to those without macular degeneration. They found no differences in the blood levels of vitamin E between those with or without early macular degeneration.[6]

● In a third study: no link between blood levels of selenium by itself and macular degeneration, but

decreased risk of macular degeneration in those with higher blood levels of a combination of three of four nutrients including selenium

A study of over 1,000 people age 55 to 80 found no link (neither protective nor harmful) between higher blood levels of selenium, vitamin C, or vitamin E by themselves and macular degeneration. [12] However, the study did find that having higher blood levels of carotenoids decreased the risk of having wet macular degeneration by 60% compared to those who had lower blood levels of carotenoids.[11] Looking at specific carotenoids, the study found that having higher blood levels of beta-carotene decreased the risk of having macular degeneration by 70%. Higher blood levels of lutein and zeaxanthin also decreased the risk by 70% and higher blood levels of lycopene decreased the risk by 60%. Also, higher blood levels of a combination of three or more of four nutrients (carotenoids, vitamin C, vitamin E, and selenium) decreased the risk by 70%.[12]

● Though the several studies above found no link, one study found a benefit: decreased risk of macular degeneration in those with higher blood levels of selenium

A study of over 160 people study found that those with macular degeneration had lower blood levels of selenium than those without macular degeneration. However, the study found no differences in the blood levels of vitamin E between those with or without macular degeneration.[122]

● **In one small study: no benefits from the use of selenium with other antioxidants on the future risk of macular degeneration over time**   A small study of 71 people with macular degeneration found no benefit to the macular degeneration or to vision in those who took a daily antioxidant combination, for over 1½ years, that consisted of selenium (50 µg), beta-carotene (20,000 IU), vitamin B2 (25 mg), vitamin C (750 mg), vitamin E (200 IU), chromium (100 µg), zinc (12.5 mg), taurine (100 mg), N-acetyl cysteine (100 mg), glutathione (5 mg), and selected bioflavonoids, compared to placebo.[17] It is impossible, though, to ascertain the individual effect of selenium from this type of study.

 Summary of Studies for Cataract: Three clinical trials have been performed looking at the role of selenium in preventing cataract. As a whole, the clinical studies provide no definitive answer as to whether selenium is beneficial, though all the studies

Carotenoids for Cataract Scale of Benefit

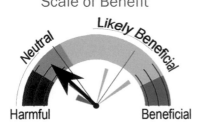

found no benefit to selenium for cataract.

The studies can be summarized as follows: two studies found no link (neither protective nor harmful) between higher levels of selenium in the blood and the risk of cataract. In following people over time, one large study found no link between a diet high in selenium and the risk of developing cataracts.

● **One study found no link between blood levels of selenium and cataract while another study found increased risk of cataract in those with higher blood levels of selenium**   A study of 141 people found no link (neither protective nor harmful) between selenium levels in the blood and cataract. However, the study did find that higher levels of both vitamin A and vitamin E in the blood decreased the risk of developing cataracts a decade or two later.[123]

A study of 165 people found that those who had cataracts had higher levels of selenium in their blood. This study brings to light the double-edged sword of selenium: too little is believed to cause cataract while too much also is believed to cause cataract as well. On the other hand, the study found no link (neither beneficial nor harmful) between cataracts and vitamin A, vitamin E, zinc, copper, and magnesium levels in the blood. However, the study found that those who had cataracts had lower levels of carotenoids and vitamin D in their blood compared to those who did not have cataracts.[41]

● **In one large studies: no benefits from the use of selenium on the future risk of cataract over time** A study of over 2,000 people given a multivitamin or a placebo for 5 years found a 36% decrease in the risk of developing cataracts in those people who were age 65 to 74. Of note, there was no difference in risk in the younger group age 45 to 64. These results exemplify the positive benefit of multivitamins; however, it is difficult to apply these results to a healthy population, as the study was performed on somewhat nutritionally-deprived people in rural China.[33]

The researchers also looked at specific nutrients in a group of over 3,000 people from the same population. They found no link (neither beneficial nor harmful) over the 5-year period between the risk of cataract and those who took selenium with beta-carotene and vitamin E, or those who took vitamin A and zinc, or those who took vitamin C and molybdenum. In contrast, in those who took vitamin B2 (5.2 mg) and vitamin B3 (40 mg) daily for 5 years had a 41% decrease in the risk of developing cataracts, compared to those who took placebo.[33]

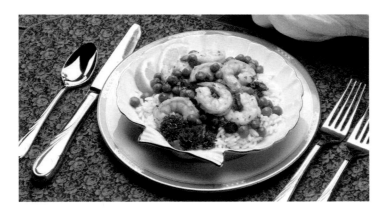

Body Absorption, Metabolism, & Excretion

Selenium is generally well-absorbed, but the absorption depends on the formulation of the selenium. About 90% of selenomethionine, the most common food source of selenium, is absorbed into the bloodstream. Selenate is also well absorbed, and selenite is about 50% absorbed.

In the body, selenium is converted to selenide, which is then converted to seleno-phosphate, which is used to make selenoproteins by turning the amino acids (protein building blocks) such as cysteine into seleno-cysteine.

Excess selenium is filtered out by the kidneys for excretion.

Deficiency

Dietary selenium deficiency is not known to cause cataracts or be associated with cataracts probably because selenium transporters concentrate selenium in the eye and brain. Therefore, even when selenium levels in the body are decreased, the eye and brain receive an appropriate amount of selenium. Only a severe and long-standing selenium deficiency is likely to cause disease in the eye.

Selenium deficiency is rare in the U.S. but can result in muscle weakness, heart disease from inflammation and heart muscle damage, low thyroid levels, and weakened immune protection.

Keshan disease is a degenerative heart disease associated with dietary selenium deficiency that is aggravated by a specific viral infection. Keshan-Beck disease is a presumed fungus-caused disorder in which selenium deficiency results in arthritis of the joints.

Toxicity & Side Effects

Selenium has often been referred to as an environmental pollutant, used in manufacturing of common items, such as electronics, paints, and glass.

Selenium is extremely toxic, though it is necessary for functioning of the body in small doses. Among the first reports of the toxicity of selenium came from the 13th century explorer Marco Polo who noted disease in horses and donkeys, such as shedding of their hair and hooves, in areas of China where the soil is rich in selenium. Recently, there has been controversy as to whether or not these animals were diseased from selenium toxicity or another toxin in the plants they ate.

Excess selenium can cause toxicity to cells resulting in tiredness and irritability, upset stomach and can even result in nerve damage. It often causes hair loss, nail frailty and loss, and garlic breath. Heart attack, kidney failure, and lung failure also can occur. Excess selenium can also cause cataract and glaucoma through oxidative damage.

Interactions with Other Nutrients

There are numerous interactions between selenium and other nutrients. The important concept is that a balance should be achieved between intake of selenium and other nutrients.

Selenium, along with vitamin B2 and vitamin E, is required for production of glutathione peroxidase, an enzyme involved in the functioning of antioxidant glutathione (see section on glutathione). Selenite, selenomethionine, and selenocysteine can be used as dietary supplements in order for cells to produce glutathione peroxidase. Organic selenium and selenomethionine are preferred sources of selenium for raising selenium and glutathione peroxidase levels, unlike the inorganic forms selenate and selenite (see section on glutathione).

There are several nutrients (selenium, vitamin B12, vitamin B6, folate, SAMe, methionine, and N-acetyl-cysteine) that act in the same complex circular pathway and are all interrelated when it comes to: (1) the toxicity of homocysteine and decreasing its levels, and (2) the activities of SAMe as a donator of methyl groups (see sections on vitamin B12, vitamin B6, SAMe, folate, methionine, and N-acetyl-cysteine). Homocysteine is a toxic chemical that is associated with vascular disease including blood clots, heart disease, stroke, and vein occlusions in the retina, as well as Alzheimer's disease.

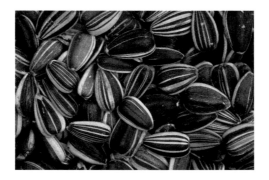

Ideal Dosage

The minimum recommended daily dose is 55 µg per day in children and adults age 14 and older. During pregnancy the minimum recommended dose is increased to 60 micrograms per day, and during lactation the minimum recommended dose is increased to 70 micrograms per day.

Some researchers suggest avoiding doses greater than 55 µg of selenium per day because of the risk of oxidative damage. At 200 µg per day, there may be a risk of developing glaucoma, so a lower dose of 100 µg per day may be more reasonable. Some have recommended doses as high as 400 µg per day, but not higher than 400 µg per day. It is important to note that higher doses should be avoided because of the toxic nature of selenium.

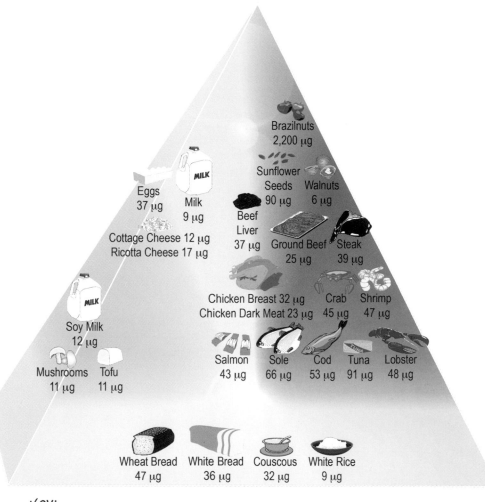

Brazilnuts
2,200 µg

Sunflower
Seeds   Walnuts
90 µg   6 µg

Eggs
37 µg   Milk
9 µg

Beef
Liver
37 µg   Ground Beef   Steak
25 µg   39 µg

Cottage Cheese 12 µg
Ricotta Cheese 17 µg

Chicken Breast 32 µg   Crab   Shrimp
Chicken Dark Meat 23 µg   45 µg   47 µg

Soy Milk
12 µg

Salmon   Sole   Cod   Tuna   Lobster
43 µg   66 µg   53 µg   91 µg   48 µg

Mushrooms   Tofu
11 µg   11 µg

Wheat Bread   White Bread   Couscous   White Rice
47 µg   36 µg   32 µg   9 µg

Pyramid Key:

Fats & Sweets

Dairy   Meats & Nuts

Vegetables   Fruits

Breads & Grains

The top source of selenium is brazilnuts. In fact, a large 4 ounce portion of brazilnuts may contain excess selenium. Other top sources of selenium are meats, grains, and eggs.

ST. JOHN'S WORT
(SEE SAINT JOHN'S WORT)

SULFORAPHANE

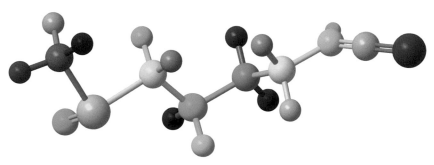

Category

Sulforaphane is a phytochemical, or plant chemical, that is derived from glucosinolates, a group of organic plant compounds that contain glucose-derived sugar that is attached to a nitrogen-and-sulfur-containing chain. Dozens of glucosinolates have been currently identified and dozens or more are likely waiting to be discovered. Glucosinolates play an important protective role in these vegetable plants. The sharp bitter taste of glucosinolates deters animals from eating these vegetables. They can also act as pesticides.

One of the known glucosinolates, known as glucoraphanin, breaks down into sulforaphane, also called 4-methylsulfinylbutyl isothiocyanate (4-MSOB-ITC). Other known important glucosinolates include sinigrin (from broccoli) that breaks down into allyl isothiocyanate (A-ITC), gluconasturtiin (from watercress) that breaks down into phenethyl isothiocyanate (PE-ITC), and glucotropaeolin (also from watercress) that breaks down into benzyl isothiocyanate (B-ITC). These phytochemicals contain a chemical group called isothiocyanate (ITC).

Cellular Location

Because sulforaphane is not required for cellular function, it is concentrated in the bloodstream and delivered to the tissues and organs that need their actions.

Structure

Sulforaphane is a linear shaped chemical structure belonging to the group of chemicals, called isothiocyanates, meaning that it contains a special group of nitrogen, carbon, and sulfur bound together by double bonds.

Mechanisms of Action

Sulforaphane is a particularly bioactive compound, acting to recruit cellular enzymes into action. As such, sulforaphane acts as a powerful antioxidant and powerful cancer-blocking agent.

Biological & Ocular Importance

● **Recruits cell-protecting enzymes into action**

Sulforaphane is a particularly bioactive compound that recruits cellular enzymes into action. These enzymes are called "phase 2" enzymes, and include glutathione S-transferase and quinone reductase. These enzymes act as antioxidants as well as cancer-blocking agents. Sulforaphane may be the most powerful activator of "phase 2" enzymes found in nature.

● **Powerful recruiter of antioxidants** Sulforaphane does not directly act as an antioxidant by donating electrons. In fact, the isothiocyanate group can act in the exact opposite way by attracting electrons. The antioxidant activities of sulforaphane derive from its ability to activate antioxidant enzymes, such as the "phase 2" enzymes.

When sulforaphane enters the bloodstream, it becomes bound to glutathione and is transported into cells in this bound form. This bound form then activates the synthesis of glutathione, glutathione-S-transferase, and glutathione peroxidase. Glutathione is a strong antioxidant, as are the enzymes glutathione-S-transferase and glutathione peroxidase, which act to help glutathione remove free peroxides within cells, thus preventing lipid peroxidation of, or oxidative damage to, cell membranes (see section on glutathione).

However, it is important to note that while sulforaphane increases the production of glutathione and the "phase 2" enzymes, it causes a transient decrease in glutathione levels within cells. Since it binds glutathione, there is a temporary decrease in the free glutathione levels within cells, until more glutathione is produced. This transient decrease does make cells more susceptible to oxidative damage temporarily. However, it is believed that the long-term benefits outweigh the short-term risks.

Sulforaphane also activates the enzyme thioredoxin

reductase. Thioredoxin reductase is important for maintaining thioredoxin in its reduced state. As with glutathione, the thioredoxin acts as an antioxidant by donating electrons. For example, it "reduces" disulfide bonds of cell proteins that have become oxidized. Thioredoxin helps remove free peroxides within the cells (see section on selenium). Reduced thioredoxin can also prevent or limit the death of cells through its regulation of DNA synthesis and its activity as a transcription factor (a protein that turns specific genes on or off).

By helping remove free peroxides, these nutrients and enzymes assists vitamin E in its antioxidant activities in saving cell membranes from oxidative damage. Vitamin E performs the first steps of preventing lipid peroxidation and glutathione and thioredoxin perform the second steps (see section on vitamin E).

Sulforaphane recruits the "phase 2" enzyme quinone reductase. Quinone reductase is an important cellular enzyme that monitors the oxidative balance in the cell and donates electrons to limit oxidative damage from a class of chemicals, called quinones. Furthermore, quinone reductase can recycle coenzyme Q10, a strong antioxidant, back into its active form when its antioxidant ability is used up (see section on coenzyme Q10).

Sulforaphane also activates hemoxygenase-1, an enzyme which increases in stress conditions. Hemoxygenase-1 acts as an antioxidant, and it acts to block inflammation and new blood vessel growth (see below) as well.

As an antioxidant, it is believed to be beneficial to retinal diseases, such as macular degeneration and childhood hereditary photoreceptor diseases, in which oxidative damage plays a role in the disease. It may also be beneficial in diseases, such as glaucoma or optic nerve diseases, in which oxidative damage plays a role as well. Furthermore, it may also help prevent cataract formation or corneal disease, again by preventing or decreasing oxidative damage.

● **Protects retina from oxidative damage**   Several research reports have studied the effects of sulforaphane in animal models of retinal disease. These studies have demonstrated that sulforaphane can protect the retina against oxidative damage. Specifically, the protective effects occur in the photoreceptors and in the retinal pigment epithelium (the layer of cells behind the retina that serve to nourish the retina and remove the excess debris from the retina), suggesting that sulforaphane may be effective in treating or preventing a wide variety of retinal diseases, such as macular degeneration and retinitis pigmentosa.

● Decreases inflammation

Sulforaphane can also act as an anti-inflammatory agent by decreasing a cell's production of enzymes that are involved in sending inflammation signals within cells. One of these inflammation-signaling enzymes is cyclo-oxygenase, popularly known as COX, the target of many new anti-inflammatory COX-inhibitor drugs. Sulforaphane also stimulates the production of hemoxygenase-1, which can also block inflammation (see above). There is belief that inflammatory proteins may play a role in numerous eye diseases, ranging from retinal diseases to glaucoma to cataract.

● Prevents growth of abnormal blood vessels in

the eye   Sulforaphane acts to inhibit the expression of enzymes and cellular growth factors that stimulate angiogenesis (the formation of abnormal new blood vessels) in the eye. Angiogenesis is particularly harmful in the retina, cornea, and trabecular meshwork (filtration site of the eye) and can cause loss of vision. The problems that result are

called choroidal neovascularization (seen in wet macular degeneration), or retinal neovascularization (seen in severe diabetic retinopathy or retinal disease), or corneal neovascularization (seen in corneal injury or disease), or iris neovascularization (seen in angle-closure glaucoma and inflammatory eye disease). Sulforaphane also stimulates the production of hemoxygenase-1, which can block angiogenesis (see above).

● Powerful cancer-blocking

activity   Sulforaphane is known to be a strong cancer-preventing agent. There are several mechanisms of action that are believed to be responsible for its cancer-blocking activity. In addition to its antioxidant activities and its ability to recruit "phase 2" enzymes into action, it also is believed to act by inhibiting damage to DNA. Research suggests that DNA damage is an important precursor to cancer formation.

Furthermore, sulforaphane inhibits "phase 1" enzymes. "Phase 1" enzymes are called cytochrome P450 enzymes that are found inside cells. These "phase 1" enzymes are responsible for converting carcinogens, or cancer-causing toxins, into an active toxic chemical inside cells. By inhibiting "phase 1" enzymes, sulforaphane prevents carcinogens from being converted into the stronger cancer-causing chemicals inside cells.

In addition, sulforaphane can induce cell death in cancer cells and stop cancer cells from dividing by preventing them from entering a cell cycle that results in a cell dividing. This cell death is called apoptosis, and is beneficial in cancer. However, cell death can be harmful in other disorders, such as macular degeneration or retinitis pigmentosa. It is unknown if sulforaphane promotes cell death in those conditions or other eye conditions in which cell death can be harmful. However, while sulforaphane has been shown to promote cell death in certain situations, it has also been shown in a few circumstances to prevent cell death. Although unconfirmed, perhaps it may prevent cell death in non-cancer cells and may cause cell death in cancer cells.

Sulforaphane's anti-cancer activity also derives from its anti-inflammatory and anti-angiogenesis properties (see above).

Human Studies on Utility

There are no human studies on the direct use of sulforaphane in eye disease reported in the scientifically-reviewed medical literature. Nevertheless, the fact that there are no reported clinical studies does not necessarily imply a benefit or lack of benefit. Looking at the mechanism of action, the use of sulforaphane in moderation may be possibly of benefit in certain eye diseases.

Body Absorption, Metabolism, & Excretion

Sulforaphane in dietary sources is often bound to a sugar molecule, in the form: sulforaphane glucosinolate. The vegetables that contain these glucosinolates also contain enzymes that break down these glucosinolates into the active components. Inside the vegetables, the enzymes are located in different compartments from the glucosinolates. Only when the vegetables are thoroughly chewed and digested do the compartments that contain the glucosinolates and the enzymes mix. This mixing allows for the breakdown of the glucosinolates into the active components, releasing the sulforaphane. The normal bacteria that are found in the intestines can also help break down the glucosinolates into the active components.

In the body, sulforaphane becomes bound to glutathione and is transported into cells in this bound form. Excretion of glucosinolates and their breakdown products occurs mostly through the kidneys.

Deficiency

There are no known disorders of sulforaphane deficiency, as sulforaphane is a non-essential nutrient. Instead, any deficiency that ensues is often from a widespread nutritional deficiency.

Toxicity & Side Effects

In general, there are no known toxicities associated with sulforaphane. However, there are reports that extremely high doses (350,000 µg or more per day) of some of the isothiocyanates can actually promote cancer in animals.

Interactions with Other Nutrients

Sulforaphane can help in recycling coenzyme Q10 back into its active form once its antioxidant ability is exhausted (see section on coenzyme Q10).

Ideal Dosage

There is no established ideal dosage as sulforaphane is non-essential. Some sources recommend sulforaphane doses of 200 to 400 µg each day. It is estimated that the typical diet contains about 10,000 to 15,000 µg of total isothiocyanates each day.

Sources (Where to Find It)

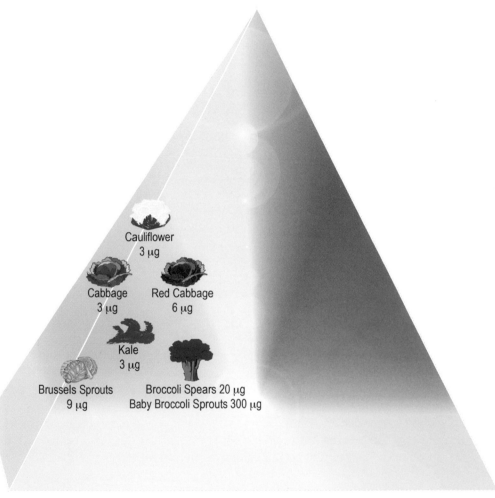

Cauliflower
3 μg

Cabbage
3 μg

Red Cabbage
6 μg

Kale
3 μg

Brussels Sprouts
9 μg

Broccoli Spears 20 μg
Baby Broccoli Sprouts 300 μg

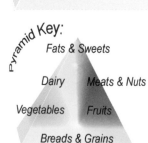

Pyramid Key:

Fats & Sweets

Dairy   Meats & Nuts

Vegetables   Fruits

Breads & Grains

The top source of sulforaphane is baby broccoli sprouts, which are harvested and eaten fresh within a few days of sprouting. Broccoli spears, Brussels sprouts, and red cabbage also contain high amounts of sulforaphane.

*See Guides on Pages 467-468.

TAURINE

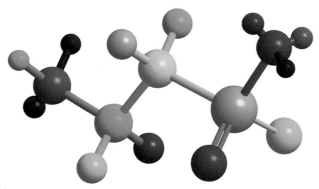

Category

Taurine, also known as 2-amino-ethane-sulfonic acid, is a sulfur amino acid (building block of proteins). However, taurine is not a traditional amino acid, in that it does not participate in the building of proteins.

Taurine was originally discovered in bulls, and is named after Taurus, the Latin word for bull and the constellation that resembles a bull.

Cellular Location

A person of average weight has about 70 grams of taurine throughout the body. In fact, taurine is the second most abundant amino acid in our bodies. Taurine is in particularly high concentration in the brain, retina, heart, skeletal muscle, white blood cells, and platelets. More specifically, high levels of taurine have been shown to be present within the retinal pigment epithelium (the layer of cells behind the retina that serve to nourish the retina and remove the excess debris from the retina) as well as within the photoreceptor cell bodies in the retina. In fact, the amino acid concentration in highest concentration in photoreceptors is taurine.

In pregnancy, taurine is one of the two most abundant amino acids within the placenta. After deliver, taurine is extremely highly concentrated in human breast milk. In fact, in human breast milk, taurine is in 100 to 200 times higher concentration than many other amino acids!

Structure

Taurine is a sulfur-containing amino acid.

Mechanisms of Action

Taurine is a building block of proteins that play many roles in the eye, including regulating fluids, stabilizing cell membranes, helping retinal development, and as a weak antioxidant.

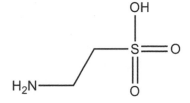

Biological & Ocular Importance

● **Forms gallbladder bile salts**   The first reported role of taurine is in the formation of bile salts in the liver. These bile salts are stored in the gallbladder and secreted into the intestines to assist in the absorption of fats and cholesterols. In doing so, the taurine bile salts help regulate the amount of cholesterol that the body absorbs from our diets. Too little taurine may result in excess cholesterol absorption.

● **Helps in the formation of the retina before birth and rescue of injured retinal cells**
Taurine plays an important role in the generation and development of photoreceptors before birth. One way that taurine may act in this role is by modifying protein phosphorylation (the process of adding a phosphate group to proteins, which activates and de-activates proteins within a cell). Actually, the balance of phosphorylation and de-phosphorylation plays a central role in the development of neural tissues, such as the retina. Phosphorylation modified by taurine helps in the development of photoreceptors before birth; in addition, there is evidence in animal models that phosphorylation modified by taurine helps in portions of the process re-generation of retinal cell components when they are injured in disease. Unfortunately, within the retina, once the neural cells such as the photoreceptors are lost in disease, they cannot be regenerated, but when they are partially injured, they may be rescued.

● **Acts as an antioxidant & helps decrease levels of toxic homocysteine**   Taurine may act as an antioxidant in some conditions, though it is only a weak antioxidant. In actuality, it acts more as an indirect antioxidant by decreasing stress on the protein-building organelles within cells by reducing the toxic activity of homocysteine, an amino acid known to cause atherosclerosis (blood vessel cholesterol clots and plaques that can result in heart disease and stroke, as well as artery or vein clots in the retina or optic nerve strokes). As such, taurine may play a role in mitigating the risks of atherosclerosis as well as vein occlusions and artery occlusions in the eye, particularly the retina. Homocysteine signals stress in the protein-building organelles and causes proteins to be misfolded. Folate, betaine, vitamin B2, and vitamin B12 also help reduce homocysteine levels.

Taurine is also believed to act to stabilize hypochlorous acid by forming taurine-chloramine, which decreases the toxic and scarring effects of hypochlorous acid. Hypochlorous acid also can act as an oxidant, and by binding to hypochlorous acid, taurine in effect acts an antioxidant.

● Stabilizes cell membranes

Taurine stabilizes membranes and assists in maintaining the "integrity" of cell membranes.

● Regulates fluids inside cells

Taurine is one of the most water-soluble amino acid in our bodies. As such, taurine plays an important role in osmoregulation (the maintenance of the fluid concentration of a cell through osmosis, whereby fluids move from areas of low protein and low ionic content to areas of high protein and high ionic content). In addition, in photoreceptor outer segments taurine may play a role in ion transport processes.

● Transporting vitamin A in the retina

Taurine plays a role in assisting in transporting vitamin A into the photoreceptor outer segments. Once vitamin A is used up by the photoreceptors, its metabolites become toxic, and taurine also plays a role in transporting these vitamin A metabolites out of the photoreceptor outer segments and over to the retinal pigment epithelium for recycling. One method by which taurine accomplishes this transport is by binding to vitamin A metabolites and converting these oil-soluble compounds into water-soluble compounds (see section on vitamin A).

● Protects the eye, particularly the retina & lens

These antioxidant, osmo-regulatory, and protective roles of taurine affect not only the primary cells of eye tissues, but also the blood vessel cells that nourish the eye tissues. For example, taurine in these roles helps protect the neural cells in the retina directly, but also indirectly protects the neural cells by protecting the blood vessels that nourish these retinal cells. Other amino acids act in these roles, but because taurine is in particularly high concentration, its role is more prominent (see section on lysine).

Taurine is in particularly high concentration in the retinal pigment epithelium, and may protect photoreceptors from oxidative damage.

Taurine levels are also quite high in the lens, where it serves as an antioxidant and osmoregulator.

● **Protects the eye during diabetes**   As early as the 1930's, taurine was believed to play a role in regulating blood sugars in diabetes. There is some evidence to suggest that taurine has insulin-like actions and acts to stabilize glucose in diabetics. In fact, taurine has been found to be decreased in diabetes through osmolytic effects as well as glucose-mediated downregulation of taurine transport. In laboratory rats with diabetes, dietary taurine supplementation was shown to improve blood flow around nerves and decrease oxidative stress. Therefore, taurine supplementation may decrease the risk of development of retinopathy and cataracts in diabetics. Furthermore, because of its osmoregulator role, taurine may stabilize the intracellular fluid build-up, or swelling of cells, that occurs with elevated blood levels of glucose in diabetes. In addition, taurine may also interact to stabilize carbonyl compounds that are formed as part of excess glucose within cells, preventing the formation of "advanced glycation end products" or AGEs, the toxic

products that damage the retina, the lens, and other ocular structures (see introduction).

● **Decreases inflammation**
Taurine can also decrease expression of genes involved in inflammation. Animal models have demonstrated the role of taurine in both preventing and decreasing inflammation. Recent studies have shown that at sites of inflammation, the toxic chemical hypochlorous acid is produced by active inflammatory cells. Taurine is believed to act to stabilize hypochlorous acid by forming taurine-chloramine, which decreases the toxic and scarring effects of hypochlorous acid. Hypochlorous acid also can act as an oxidant, and by binding to hypochlorous acid, taurine in effect acts an antioxidant. The taurine-chloramine combination also inhibits other mediators of inflammation to decrease the inflammatory side effects.

● **Decreases blood clotting**
Taurine can decrease clumping of platelets involved in blood clotting. Therefore, deficiency of taurine can result in decreased platelet activity and increased platelet clumping. This decrease in the ability of platelets to function properly can lead to vascular disease. In combination with diabetes, which can decrease the taurine levels, the vascular disease and retinopathy can be aggravated. As a result, taurine has been suggested as a treatment to reduce the

complications in diabetes.

● **Balances calcium levels inside cells**   Taurine can maintain appropriate calcium levels inside cells by acting on cell pumps. This characteristic is important because a high level of calcium influxing into cells is associated with injury and degeneration of cells.

● **Regulates cell signaling neurotransmitters**   There is also some evidence to suggest that at high concentrations, taurine acts to stabilize neurotransmission (cell signaling) by inhibiting neurotransmitters.

● **Reduces blood pressure**   Taurine is believed to help reduce hypertension (high blood pressure), which may be a result of its effect on the neural control of blood vessels. Because of this mechanism, taurine may not reduce blood pressure in those without hypertension. It has also been shown to be helpful in people with heart failure.

Human Studies on Utility

Currently, there are only a handful of human studies on taurine use in eye disease reported in the scientifically-reviewed medical literature. These studies involve several eye diseases and are summarized below. Of note, the studies involve only small numbers of people, so the benefits found may be found by chance, and it is difficult to assess the broad applicability of the findings. Nevertheless, looking at the mechanism of action, the use of taurine in moderation may be possibly of benefit in many eye diseases.

● **In one small study: use of taurine decreases visual fatigue**   A study of 25 young healthy adults found that taurine (3,000 mg for 12 days) improved visual system processing during the fatigue of staring at a computer monitor for an extended 2½ hour period of time, as compared to placebo. However, the mechanisms by which this effect occurs were unclear, and the outcome was measured by higher response levels in their brains to visual stimuli. There are questions about whether this study is applicable to real-life situations and whether there is a true physiologic benefit of taurine in visual fatigue. Such a study would have to be reproduced in order to determine applicability of such findings and to assign any value to the results.[125]

● **Some studies find decreased taurine levels in retinitis pigmentosa, while other studies find no differences**   There are a few studies that have shown that taurine levels are decreased in the blood in people with retinitis pigmentosa while other studies have shown no changes. Some researchers believe that it is actually the transport, cellular uptake, and storage of taurine that may be deficient in some forms of retinitis pigmentosa. In fact, there is data to suggest that other amino acids also may be deficient in retinitis pigmentosa; these include aspartate, threonine, and histadine.

● In one small study: use of taurine decreases the future risk of visual field loss over time in retinitis pigmentosa

A study of 62 people with retinitis pigmentosa found that taurine (1,000 mg per day) with vitamin E (800 IU per day) and the calcium-channel blocking anti-hypertension drug diltiazem (30 mg per day) modestly improved peripheral visual fields or slowed the progression of peripheral visual field loss over a period of 3 years.[126]

● In one small study: no benefits from the use of taurine on progression of retinitis pigmentosa over time

An older study of 10 people with retinitis pigmentosa found no link (neither protective nor harmful) between taurine (3,000 mg per day for up to 1 year) and visual acuity, visual field, or retinal function. However, despite the lack of improvement, there was no demonstrable worsening of the visual findings, which often occurs in retinitis pigmentosa. Thus, the study suggests that taurine may be of benefit, though the study did not have a control group to confirm this finding.[127]

● In few studies: no benefits from the use of taurine on diabetes

In animal studies, taurine has been shown to be beneficial in diabetes. However, in the few human studies of taurine in diabetes, generally no beneficial effect has been demonstrated to date, which does not prove necessarily that there is no benefit to taurine. The data simply suggests that there is no conclusive evidence one way or the other. Also, there is evidence from animal tests that taurine taken in infancy and childhood may prevent the onset of diabetes. It is quite an important finding, which remains to be proven.

● In one small study: no benefits from the use of taurine with other antioxidants on the future risk of macular degeneration over time

A small study of 71 people with macular degeneration found no benefit to the macular degeneration or to vision in those who took a daily antioxidant combination, for over 1½ years, that consisted of taurine (100 mg), beta-carotene (20,000 IU), vitamin B2 (25 mg), vitamin C (750 mg), vitamin E (200 IU), chromium (100 μg), selenium (50 μg), zinc (12.5 mg), N-acetyl cysteine (100 mg), glutathione (5 mg), and selected bioflavonoids, compared to placebo.[17] It is impossible, however, to ascertain the individual effect of taurine from this type of study.

Body Absorption, Metabolism, & Excretion

Taurine is digested by the stomach with the help of stomach acids. Digestive enzymes from the pancreas further break down proteins, which are then absorbed into the bloodstream through the intestines.

As proteins are broken down, ammonia is formed. Since ammonia is extremely toxic to cells, it must be converted into a nitrogen-containing chemical known as urea. When ammonia builds up in excess, it can cause poor coordination, difficulties with balance, tremors, seizures, difficulty breathing, swelling of the brain, and can eventually lead to a coma. A normally functioning liver works to remove excess ammonia by creating urea, which is then filtered into the urine by the kidneys.

With taurine, a substantial portion is dumped back into the intestines with bile (a green fluid produced by the liver that is stored in the gallbladder to assist in digestion).

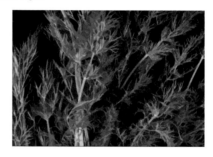

Deficiency

Taurine is considered non-essential since the body can make it by converting other amino acids (methionine and cysteine) into taurine. However, our bodies have only a small amount of the enzyme that can make taurine, and, thus, have only a very limited capacity to convert other amino acids into taurine. Despite these limitations, however, our bodies, in particular our retinas, still require a large amount of taurine.

In healthy individuals, taurine deficiency is uncommon as our diets typically contain sufficient amounts of taurine. However, vegans may not receive enough taurine in their diets because taurine is found almost exclusively from animals, and so they may develop taurine deficiency. Similarly, hospitalized people who are fed long-term parenteral nutrition may develop taurine deficiency. Diabetics with poor kidney function often excrete too much taurine and thus may develop taurine deficiency as well.

Taurine deficiency is also known to occur with the use of chlorpromazine (a tranquilizer) and chloroquine (an anti-malarial drug), both of which have been associated with loss of vision from retinal diseases.

Taurine deficiency has been associated with retinal degeneration. It is also associated with high cholesterol levels (see above).

Toxicity & Side Effects

Excess taurine causes few known side effects. Insomnia, diarrhea, and stomach ulcers have been reported, for example. Eye pain has also been reported as a side effect of high-dose taurine supplementation.

Excess taurine, like other amino acids, is often broken down and converted into sugars or fats, and used for energy, or stored as fat in the body's fat stores. Excess amino acids can stress the kidneys, stress the bloodstream, and cause dehydration. Furthermore, excess amino acids can cause the kidneys to lose calcium resulting in weakened bones. As with any amino acid, taurine in excess in someone with liver disease or with kidney disease may result in build-up of ammonia or urea in the body, resulting in severe illness (see page 308).

In diabetics, excess amino acids can result in an increased sugar load on the body, or increased fat deposits in the body!

Interactions with Other Nutrients

Cysteine and N-acetyl-cysteine are precursors of taurine (see section on N-acetyl-cysteine).

Increased levels of other sulfur-containing nutrients, such as taurine, cysteine, alpha-lipoic acid, and methylsulfonyl-methane, also result in increased levels of glutathione, a sulfur-containing tripeptide.

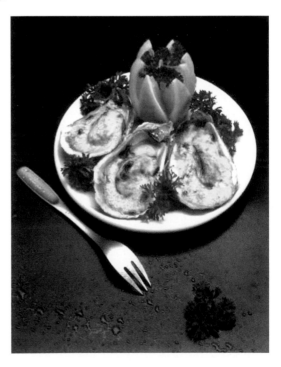

Ideal Dosage

The average dietary intake is around 60 to 200 mg per day, which appears to be a sufficient level of taurine. However, some researchers recommend levels up to 1,000 to 3,000 mg per day. A balanced recommendation may be 1,000 to 1,500 mg per day.

Sources (Where to Find It)

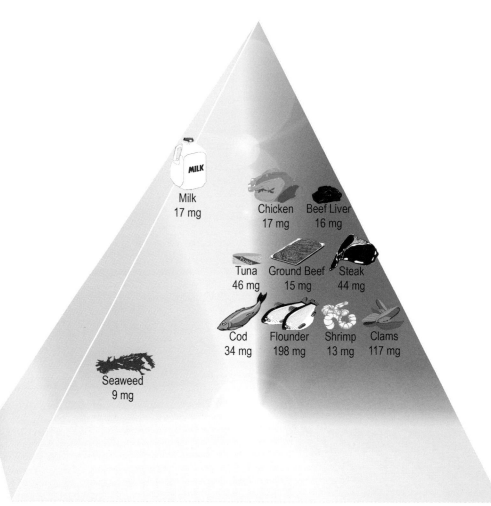

Milk
17 mg

Chicken
17 mg

Beef Liver
16 mg

Tuna
46 mg

Ground Beef
15 mg

Steak
44 mg

Cod
34 mg

Flounder
198 mg

Shrimp
13 mg

Clams
117 mg

Seaweed
9 mg

Pyramid Key:

Fats & Sweets

Dairy   Meats & Nuts

Vegetables   Fruits

Breads & Grains

Taurine is found almost exclusively in animals and animal meats. Plants usually do not contain taurine, though there is taurine in some types of algae. Top sources of taurine are meats, milk, and seaweed.

*See Guides on Pages 467-468.

THIAMIN
(SEE VITAMIN B1)

TOCOPHEROL
(SEE VITAMIN E)

TOCOTRIENOL
(SEE VITAMIN E)

UBIQUINOL
(SEE COENZYME Q10)

UBIQUINONE
(SEE COENZYME Q10)

VANADIUM

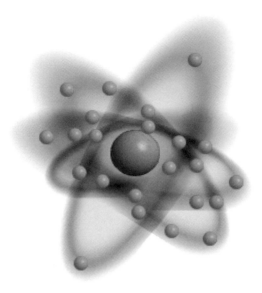

Category

Vanadium is an essential trace metal. Vanadium is also known as its original name, panchromium, as vanadium comes in many different colors. It was originally discovered in 1813 by del Rio, a Spanish mineralogist. Vanadium is quite a hard strong metal and is used to strengthen many metal alloys. It comes in many forms such as vanadyl and vanadate forms.

Cellular Location

Most of the vanadium absorbed is diffusely transported through the body in the bloodstream. A smaller amount of vanadium passes into the brain and the retina as compared to other organs. A higher concentration of vanadium often accumulates in the bones and teeth.

Structure

Vanadium is found as an ionic metal. Its symbol on the periodic table of elements is V, and its atomic number is 23. It is found between titanium and chromium on the periodic table.

Mechanisms of Action

Vanadium acts by blocking the pumping action of a cell-membrane pump, called the sodium-potassium ATPase pump.

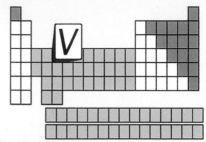

Biological & Ocular Importance

● Causes oxidation

Of concern is the fact that vanadium can actually cause oxidation and oxidative damage, such as causing breaks in DNA. In addition, it interferes with enzymes that are involved in the production of energy by cells.

● Lowers eye pressure to prevent glaucoma

Some of the popularity of vanadium is in lowering the eye pressure, in order to protect against the development of glaucoma or to treat glaucoma. By blocking the sodium-potassium ATPase pump in the fluid-building part of the eye, called the ciliary body, vanadium is believed to decrease the production of fluid inside the eye, which in turn decreases the pressure that the fluid creates in the eye. However, there is concern of the toxicity of vanadium, in its ability to create oxidative damage throughout the eye, and to block energy production in cells throughout the eye.

● Decreases blood sugars in diabetes

Similarly, there has been excitement in the past about vanadium in diabetes. Vanadium is believed to be beneficial in reducing blood sugars in diabetes, perhaps by improving the sensitivity to insulin or by mimicking the actions of insulin.

There is also some suggestion of the beneficial role of vanadium in decreasing cataract formation in diabetics by decreasing glucose levels. Perhaps the same may be said for the role of vanadium in preventing retinal disease in diabetics as well. However, much of the excitement should be tempered by the concerns of the toxicities of vanadium.

● Lowers cholesterol

It has also been shown in one study to lower cholesterol levels in diabetics. In contrast, other studies have suggested that vanadium may actually increase cholesterol levels.

● Lowers blood pressure

There is also some suggestion that it may help lower blood pressure.

● Enhances athletic performance

Vanadium has been used by athletes to enhance performance.

Human Studies on Utility

There are no human studies on the use of vanadium in treatment of eye disease reported in the scientifically-reviewed medical literature. Nevertheless, the fact that there are no reported clinical studies does not necessarily imply a benefit or lack of benefit. Looking at the mechanism of action, the use of vanadium in moderation may be possibly of benefit in certain eye diseases.

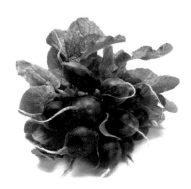

Body Absorption, Metabolism, & Excretion

Only a small portion, often less than 5%, of the ingested vanadium is absorbed by the intestines into the bloodstream. The vanadium that is absorbed is transported in the bloodstream throughout the body.

Of the vanadium that is absorbed and transported into the bloodstream, most of it is filtered out by the kidneys for excretion.

Deficiency

Little is known about vanadium deficiency since most diets include very small amounts of vanadium.

Toxicity & Side Effects

Vanadium may cause fatigue, weakness, upset stomach, nausea, vomiting, diarrhea, and stomach cramps. Other side effects include dry skin, green discoloration of the tongue, and a metallic taste in the mouth.

Anemia (insufficiency of the red blood cells that carry oxygen) has been reported as well as a decrease in the white blood cells of the immune defense system. Some of the symptoms of anemia include fatigue, shortness of breath, increased heart rate, mouth sores or ulcers, tongue soreness, pale skin, and brittle nails.

Kidney and liver failure have been noted to occur in vanadium toxicity as well.

Of concern is the fact that vanadium can actually cause oxidation and oxidative damage, such as causing breaks in DNA. In addition, it interferes with enzymes that are involved in the production of energy by cells.

Interactions with Other Nutrients

There is limited knowledge of the interaction of vanadium with other nutrients.

Ideal Dosage

Athletes have used doses of vanadium as high as 19,000 µg per day from a 60 mg tablet of vanadyl sulfate each day. A study of vanadium use in diabetes used a dose of 31,000 µg per day as a 100 mg tablet of vanadyl sulfate each day. The typical dietary intake of vanadium is 10 to 60 µg per day; though, doses of 50 to 100 µg are sufficient, since the benefits are not well-established while the risks of vanadium are disquieting.

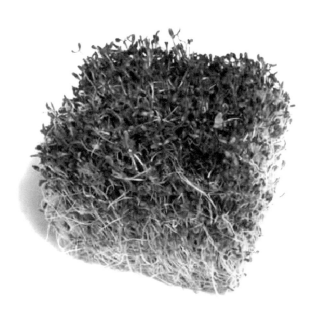

Sources (Where to Find It)

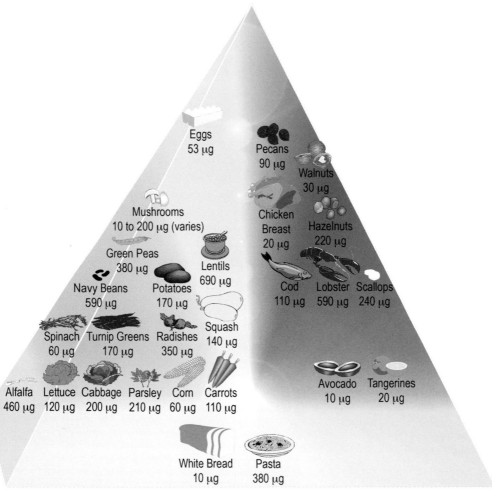

Eggs
53 µg

Pecans
90 µg

Walnuts
30 µg

Mushrooms
10 to 200 µg (varies)

Chicken
Breast
20 µg

Hazelnuts
220 µg

Green Peas
380 µg

Lentils
690 µg

Navy Beans
590 µg

Potatoes
170 µg

Cod
110 µg

Lobster
590 µg

Scallops
240 µg

Spinach
60 µg

Turnip Greens
170 µg

Radishes
350 µg

Squash
140 µg

Alfalfa
460 µg

Lettuce
120 µg

Cabbage
200 µg

Parsley
210 µg

Corn
60 µg

Carrots
110 µg

Avocado
10 µg

Tangerines
20 µg

White Bread
10 µg

Pasta
380 µg

Pyramid Key:

Fats & Sweets

Dairy

Meats & Nuts

Vegetables

Fruits

Breads & Grains

Top sources of vanadium are seafood (particularly lobster), nuts (such as hazelnuts), pasta, and vegetables (peas and beans, radishes, alfalfa, parsley, and cabbage).

*See Guides on Pages 467-468.

VITAMIN A
(RETINOL)

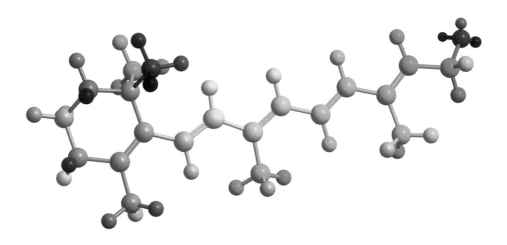

Category

Vitamin A is a fat-soluble vitamin that can also be made by the body from precursors from the carotenoid family of organic pigments that occur naturally in plants (see section on carotenoids). There are many carotenes that can be converted into vitamin A in the liver. These include beta-carotene, alpha-carotene, and beta-cryptoxanthin.

Cellular Location

Vitamin A is often stored in the liver but is also delivered to a variety of organs throughout the body, including bones, body fat, skeletal muscles, lungs, kidneys, and the eye.

Structure

Palmitate and stearate are two forms of vitamin A. There are more than 10,000 retinoids that have been naturally isolated or synthesized in a laboratory. Retinoids are a class of biologically-reactive chemicals made from or related to vitamin A. What makes them a retinoid is the presence of four repeating so-called isoprenoid chemical units.

Mechanisms of Action

Vitamin A is a nutrient that acts by participating in a variety of chemical reactions in our bodies.

Biological & Ocular Importance

● Regulates expression of genes, particularly those involved in cell growth

Vitamin A is a retinol that is converted to retinoic acid and regulates gene expression by activating cell receptors for retinoic acid. These retinoic acid receptors are involving in activating processes that regulate cell growth. In addition, it regulates growth of our bodies as a whole as well.

Vitamin A's regulation of gene expression also enables it to regulate differentiation or maturation of cells. For example, vitamin A can help an immature skin cell to develop, mature, and grow properly. Vitamin A also regulates growth of immune system defense cells as well as bone development.

As such, vitamin A has been recommended for the treatment of acne, psoriasis, skin burns and wounds, and osteoporosis.

● Upregulates cell communication connexin proteins, & prevents cancer

Connexin proteins are important in cell-to-cell communication, and the loss of this communication is thought to play a role in the development of cancer. Vitamin A helps increase expression of the gene to make connexin proteins while also stabilizing connexin proteins as they are being made. Thus, vitamin A has been recommended as a cancer preventing agent.

● Stimulates the immune defense system

Vitamin A is believed to stimulate the immune defense system. Because of its ability to regulate differentiation or maturation of cells, it may also help the cells that line the digestive tract and the airways to mature properly and provide stronger protection against infections.

● Promotes lubrication of the surface of the eye to prevent dry eyes

The surface of the eye is coated by a thin layer of tear, called the tear film, which serves to lubricate and moisturize the eye surface. When this tear film evaporates, the cornea, which is particularly susceptible to dryness, begins to dry and the cells on its surface become damaged.

The tear film is composed of three layers. First, a mucin layer that is closest to the eye allows the tears to adhere more easily to the surface of the eye. This mucin component consists of glycoproteins (proteins conjugated with sugars). Second, an aqueous component consisting of water mixed with electrolytes or salts forms the bulk of the tear film and is the middle layer of the tear film. Third, a lipid component consisting of oils that stabilize the tear layer to prevent its evaporation. This lipid layer is the outermost layer of the tear film.

Vitamin A is required to ensure a proper tear film to lubricate the eye. The tear film is produced from nutrients and other components found in the bloodstream, and vitamin A is required for production of the mucins secreted from the eyelid glands for the natural tear layer. Omega-6 oils are involved in maintaining the lipid component of the tear film. These oils are secreted by oil-secreting glands of the eyelids.

● Forms protective coating on surface of eye to prevent infections
Furthermore, this mucin coating forms a barrier to prevent against infection. Loss of this protective barrier as a result of decreased vitamin A can cause an increased risk of eye infections. For example, vitamin A deficiency has been shown to cause worse corneal infections, such as from bacteria associated with contact lens infections, in animal models. Vitamin A and the carotenoids also play an essential role in immune protection. While vitamin A and the carotenoids assist in maintaining a healthy immune system, there is considerable controversy and unknown mechanism of how they function in this role. A deficiency in carotenoids and vitamin A can impair function of certain types of white blood cells, called neutrophils. The deficiency can also impair the ability of other types of white blood cells, known as macrophages, from ingesting and killing bacteria, while simultaneously causing an increased amount of inflammation (the presence of excess white blood cells). It can also impair the response of other types of white blood cells, called T-cells.

● Promotes proper healing of the surface of the eye
Vitamin A is found in the tears that we secrete to lubricate our eyes. The vitamin A also serves the purpose of maintaining the normal growth of the cells of the surface of the eye and particularly of the surface of the cornea. There is evidence that vitamin A can also stimulate and promote healing of wounds on the surface of the eye, such as those that occur from bacterial or viral infections of the cornea. Vitamin A has been shown to promote regeneration of the surface cells of the cornea as well.

● **Required for production of light sensing pigment in retina**   Vitamin A is required for production of rhodopsin in rod photoreceptors of the retina and for production of iodopsins in the cone photoreceptors of the retina. Vitamin A is a retinol that is converted by the retinal pigment epithelium into retinoic acid or retinal, which is then transported to photoreceptors to be linked to the opsin proteins to form the light sensing pigments of the retina, the rhodopsin and iodopsins. Thus, deficiency of vitamin A is associated with night-blindness and some forms of retinitis pigmentosa.

● **Acts as an antioxidant**
Vitamin A has a long chain of carbons with alternating single and double bonds. In fact, the high number of double bonds is what makes these carotenoids able to function as antioxidants. They are able to donate electrons to free radicals (toxic chemicals that result in oxidation), which prevents the free radicals themselves from accepting electrons and damaging cell components.

As an antioxidant, it is believed to be beneficial to retinal diseases, such as macular degeneration and childhood hereditary photoreceptor diseases, in which oxidative damage plays a role in the disease. It may also be beneficial in diseases, such as glaucoma or optic nerve diseases, in which oxidative damage plays a role as well. Furthermore, it may also help prevent cataract formation or corneal disease, again by preventing or decreasing oxidative damage.

Human Studies on Utility

Currently, there are numerous human studies on vitamin A in eye disease reported in the scientifically-reviewed medical literature. These studies involve several eye diseases, including dry eyes, corneal healing, styes, and retinitis pigmentosa, as well as macular degeneration and cataract. The studies are described below.

Looking at the mechanisms of action, there is good reason to use vitamin A in moderation for dry eyes, macular degeneration, retinitis pigmentosa, and cataract.

● **In a small study: use of multi-vitamin with vitamin A decreases the risk of dry eyes**
A study of 60 healthy young adults found that taking a multivitamin containing vitamins A, C, and E each day improved the stability of

the tear film after just 10 days, compared with those who did not take the multivitamin. The study found that the tears remained stable for an over 40% longer period of time with the multivitamin. The study also found a similar benefit on the stability of the tear film with vitamin C alone.[128 & 147]

● In a small study: use of vitamin A improves healing of the cornea after refractive laser surgery
A study of 40 people found that those people who received vitamin A (25,000 IU) and vitamin E (200 IU in the form of vitamin E nicotinate) each day for one year after refractive laser surgery (the corneal laser treatment designed to do away with the need for eyeglasses) had faster healing of their cornea and decreased haze in their vision compared to those who received placebo.[129]

● In a small study: decreased risk of styes in those with higher blood levels of vitamin A
An older study of 80 people found that higher blood levels of vitamin A decreased the risk of developing styes on the eyelids.[130]

● Used since antiquity to treat night blindness
In a manuscript entitled "The Book of the Eyes" from 3400 years ago, the ancient Egyptians described eating liver to treat night blindness. Hippocrates in the 1st century B.C. used cod liver oil, a natural source of vitamin A, to treat night

blindness. There is a specific genetic defect in about 5% of patients with retinitis pigmentosa, a night-blinding condition, which can be improved with high doses of vitamin A. There is data to show that vitamin A supplementation is beneficial to all forms of retinitis pigmentosa. However, there is toxicity associated with high dose vitamin A (see below).

● In a small study: no benefits from the use of extremely high doses of vitamin A on the future risk of retinitis pigmentosa over time
An older 1968 study of 71 people with retinitis pigmentosa found no link (neither protective nor harmful) between high doses of vitamin A (100,000 IU twice per week) and vision over a period of up to three years.[131] Two concerns with this study are that the high dose of vitamin A is potentially toxic and that the vitamin A was not given daily.

● In a larger study: use of high doses of vitamin A decreases the future risk of retinitis pigmentosa over time
A more recent 1993 study of over 600 people with retinitis pigmentosa found no link (neither protective nor harmful) between vitamin A (15,000 IU per day) and vision or peripheral visual fields over a period of 4 years. However, in those who started the study with less disease, vitamin A decreased the rate of progression of peripheral visual field loss. Also, vitamin A decreased the risk by 32% of having a large decline in

Vitamin A for Retinitis Pigmentosa Scale of Benefit

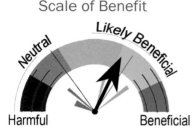

the electrical functioning of photoreceptor cells. However, vitamin E (400 IU per day) increased the risk by 42% of having a large decline in the electrical functioning of photoreceptor cells, suggesting that high doses of vitamin E can be harmful in retinitis pigmentosa. Of note, in this study, the total daily intake of vitamin A was about 18,000 IU per day, with 15,000 IU per day from a pill supplement (in the form of vitamin A palmitate) and 3,000 IU per day from dietary sources; this is how the level of 18,000 IU per day is suggested for people with retinitis pigmentosa.[132]

● **In a small study: use of extremely high doses of vitamin A decreases the future risk of Sorsby's fundus dystrophy over time** High doses of vitamin A also have been shown to be useful in other hereditary retinal diseases that involve night blindness, such as Sorsby's fundus dystrophy. This hereditary retinal disease shares similarities with retinitis pigmentosa, in that people develop night blindness and difficulties with their peripheral vision, and also shares similarities with wet macular degeneration, where

abnormal blood vessels grow in the center of the retina resulting in loss of central vision. One study found that vitamin A (50,000 IU each day) improved the night blindness. However, when the dose was decreased to 5,000 IU each day, the benefit was lost.[133]

Summary of Studies for Macular Degeneration:

Nearly a dozen clinical trials have been performed looking at the role of vitamin A in both preventing and treating macular degeneration. These clinical trials are of many different types, some of which are very well-designed and well-performed studies.

As a whole, the clinical studies provide no definitive answer as to whether vitamin A is beneficial, and, in fact, the majority of studies (11 out of 13) found no benefit to vitamin A for macular degeneration. However,

Vitamin A for Macular Degeneration Scale of Benefit

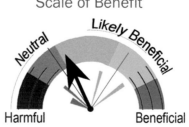

there is some evidence from the studies that it may be beneficial. Looking at the mechanisms of action, there is good reason to use vitamin A in moderation for macular degeneration.

The studies can be summarized as follows: four

large studies found no benefits from the past use of vitamin A on the risk of macular degeneration, while one large study found a benefit in the past use of vitamin A in decreasing the risk of macular degeneration. Several studies have shown no link (neither protective nor harmful) between levels of vitamin A in the blood and macular degeneration.

In following people over time, one large study found that those who took vitamin A did not have any benefit in preventing macular degeneration compared to those who did not take vitamin A, while another large study found that the use of a multi-vitamin with beta-carotene, as a precursor to vitamin A, decreases the future risk of macular degeneration over time.

● **In two large studies: no benefits in past use of vitamin A found on risk of macular degeneration**
Looking forward over time, a study of nearly 3,000 people age 49 and over found no link (neither protective nor harmful) between the risk of having macular degeneration and taking any of the following nutrients (alone or in combination) in the past: vitamin A, vitamin B1, vitamin B2, vitamin B3, vitamin B6, vitamin B12, vitamin C, vitamin E, beta-carotene, folate or zinc.[13]

A study of over 3,500 people age 49 and over found no link (neither protective nor harmful) between the risk of developing macular degeneration over a 5 year period and people who took the following nutrients, alone or in combination, in the past: vitamin A, lycopene, lutein and zeaxanthin, beta-carotene, or zinc. Surprisingly, however, the study found, that those who took vitamin C supplements combined with a diet high in vitamin C had a 2-fold increase in their risk of developing macular degeneration.[2] This finding is quite surprising, as one would expect vitamin C to protect against macular degeneration, as opposed to increasing the risk of macular degeneration. However, the finding highlights the problems associated with these types of studies: namely, that the findings may occur coincidentally and other true findings may be missed. It is sometimes difficult to explain the findings or apply them to real life.

● **In two other large studies: no benefits in past use of *higher amounts* of vitamin A found on risk of macular degeneration**   A study of nearly 3,000 people age 49 and over found no link (neither protective nor harmful) between the risk of having macular degeneration a diet with higher amounts of vitamin A, vitamin C, zinc, or beta-carotene in the past.[4]

A study of nearly 10,000 people found that one daily serving of fruits or vegetables rich in vitamin A decreased the risk of having macular degeneration by 40% compared to less than once per week. However, when the study looked at the actual amount of vitamin A intake from the diet each day, the study found no link (neither protective nor harmful) between higher amounts of dietary vitamin A compared to lower amounts. These findings demonstrate that different results can be obtained from the same group of people depending on how the findings are observed, suggesting that careful interpretation of any result is necessary in order to apply the findings to real life. The study also found no link (neither protective nor harmful) between macular degeneration and more servings of fruits or vegetables rich in vitamin C or higher amounts of dietary vitamin C.[134]

● **Though the four studies above found no link, one large study found a benefit: past use of vitamin A associated with decreased risk of macular degeneration** A study of over 1,000 people age 55 to 80 found that those who consumed a diet high in vitamin A had a greater than 40% decrease in the risk of having wet macular degeneration compared to those who did not consume a diet high in vitamin A. Similarly, dietary beta-carotene decreased the risk by 40% and dietary carotenoids decreased the risk by over 40%, while dietary lutein and zeaxanthin decreased the risk by nearly 60%. The authors found no link (neither protective nor harmful) between macular degeneration and a diet high in vitamin C or E.[5]

● **In several studies: no link between blood levels of vitamin A and macular degeneration** A study in France of over 2,500 people age 60 and over found no link (neither protective nor harmful) between severe or advanced macular degeneration and higher blood levels of vitamin A, vitamin C, or vitamin E. However, the study found that a higher ratio of vitamin E-to-lipid in the blood reduced the risk of severe or advanced macular degeneration by 82% and decreased the risk of early macular degeneration by 18%. It has been suggested that this ratio of vitamin E-to-lipid in the blood is a better measure of how much vitamin E is available in the bloodstream.[135]

A study of over 100 people, found no difference in the blood levels of vitamin A, vitamin C, vitamin E, carotenoids, or selenium between those with or without macular degeneration. However, the study did find that those who had macular degeneration had lower blood levels of zinc compared to those without macular degeneration.[39]

Another study of nearly 100 people found no difference in the blood levels of vitamin A, vitamin C, carotenoids, beta-carotene, lutein and zeaxanthin, lycopene, zinc, or selenium between those with or without macular degeneration (looking at both early and severe or advanced macular degeneration). However, the study found that those who had severe or advanced macular degeneration had lower blood levels of vitamin E compared to those without macular degeneration. They found no differences in the blood levels of vitamin E between those with or without early macular degeneration.[6]

A study of nearly 50 people found no link (neither protective nor harmful) between blood levels of vitamin A, C, or E and wet macular degeneration.[136]

A study of 130 people also found no difference in the blood levels of vitamin A, vitamin E, beta-carotene, lutein, or lycopene between those with or without macular degeneration.[9]

A study of 500 people age 40 and over found no link (neither protective nor harmful) between higher blood levels of vitamin A, vitamin C, or beta-carotene and macular degeneration. However, the study also found that those with higher blood levels of vitamin E had an over 50% decrease in the risk of having macular degeneration when compared to those who had lower blood levels of vitamin E.[10]

● **In one large study: no benefits from the use of vitamin A on the future risk of macular degeneration over time** A study of over 75,000 people (nurses and health professionals) followed over time for up to 18 years found no link (neither protective nor harmful) between the risk of developing macular degeneration (wet or dry) and a diet high in any of the following nutrients: vitamin A, vitamin C, vitamin E, carotenoids, lutein and zeaxanthin, beta-carotene, or lycopene. The study did find that those who consumed more than 3 servings of fruit each day were $1/3$ less likely to develop *wet* macular degeneration over time compared to those who consumed less than 1½ servings of fruit each day. No link (neither protective nor harmful) was found

when looking at increased fruit consumption for dry macular degeneration, nor when looking at increased vegetable consumption for dry or wet macular degeneration.[15]

● **Though the one study above found no link, one large study found a benefit: use of multi-vitamin with beta-carotene as a precursor to vitamin A decreases the future risk of macular degeneration over time** A recent 10-year study of over 3,000 people age 55 and over found that taking a daily antioxidant combination of vitamin C (500 mg), vitamin E (400 IU), and beta-carotene (15 mg), with or without zinc (80 mg) and copper (2 mg) reduced the risk of developing severe or wet macular degeneration, in people with certain features of dry macular degeneration within their retinas. The risk of developing severe or advanced macular degeneration decreased by 34% in people taking the antioxidant combination with zinc and copper, by 24% in people taking the antioxidant combination alone without zinc and copper, and by 30% in people taking the zinc and copper without the antioxidant combination. Looking at vision, the antioxidant combination with zinc and copper decreased the risk of losing vision from macular degeneration by 25% in these people with certain features of dry macular degeneration. There was no benefit to vision for people who took the antioxidant combination alone, without the zinc and copper, or the zinc and copper alone. This study has been used widely to recommend the multivitamin combination for macular degeneration, though the results are only applicable to people with certain features of macular degeneration in their retinas. Moreover, what confounds the interpretation of the data is the use of multivitamins in two-thirds of the people.[19]

Summary of Studies for Cataract:

Over a dozen clinical trials have been performed looking at the role of vitamin A in preventing cataract. These clinical trials are of various types, some of which are very well-designed and well-performed studies.

As a whole, the studies provide no definitive answer that vitamin A is beneficial, though there is suggestion, in 6 out of the 15 studies, that it may be beneficial, particularly in combination with other antioxidant nutrients. Looking at the mechanisms of action, there is reason to use vitamin A in moderation for cataract.

Vitamin A for
Cataract
Scale of Benefit

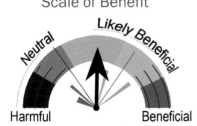

The studies can be summarized as follows: three studies found no benefits from the past use of vitamin A on the risk of cataract, while three larger studies that did find a benefit in the past use of vitamin A in decreasing the risk of cataract. Another large study found mixed results: the past use of vitamin A was associated with decreased risk of certain types of cataract though an increased risk of other types of cataract. However, in this study, one interesting explanation is that there may be an increased lifespan in people on the multivitamins, which may make them more likely to develop cataract as they are living longer. Two studies found no link (neither protective nor harmful) between higher levels of vitamin A in the blood and the risk of cataract, though one study found that higher levels of vitamin A in the blood are associated with a decrease in the risk of cataract.

In following people over time, two large well-performed studies found that those who took vitamin A did not have any benefit in preventing cataract when compared to those who did not take vitamin A. However, one study did show a benefit of the use of vitamin A in decreasing the future risk of cataract over time. Another study found that the use of a multi-vitamin with beta-carotene, as a precursor of vitamin A, decreased the future risk of cataract over time.

● In three studies: no benefits in past use of vitamin A found on risk of cataract   A study of 400 people age 50 to 86 found no link (neither protective nor harmful) between the past use of vitamin A, vitamin E, beta-carotene, lutein, or lycopene and the risk of having cataract.[21]

A study of over 4,000 people found no link (neither protective nor harmful) between the use of vitamin A and the risk of having cataract, as well as no link between the use of vitamin E and the risk of having cataract. The study did find that higher levels of vitamin C in the blood decreased the risk of having cataracts by over 25%.[137]

An Italian study of over 900 people also found no link (neither protective nor harmful) between intake of higher levels of vitamin A, vitamin D, beta-carotene, or methionine and the risk of having cataracts. However, this study found that those who consumed higher dietary levels of folate and vitamin E had a lower risk of developing cataracts that required surgery.[22]

● **Though the studies above found no link, three large study found a benefit: past use of vitamin A associated with decreased risk of**

cataract   A study of nearly 3,000 people found that the past intake of vitamin A, vitamin B1, vitamin B2, vitamin B3, iron, and zinc decreased the risk of having certain types of cataract by 30 to 50%.[62] It is interesting to note that in this study, iron was associated with a decrease in risk of having cataract, and not an increased risk, as some physicians have predicted. Furthermore, it is surprising that no

link (neither protective nor harmful) was found between vitamin C use and cataract, despite other studies showing a benefit.

A large study of nearly 3,000 people age 49 to 97 found that past use of vitamin A in higher doses reduced the risk of having cataracts by 90%. Likewise, the past use of multivitamins was associated with a decreased risk of having cataracts as well. The use of folate reduced the risk of having cataracts by 40 to 60% depending on the type of cataract, the use of vitamin B1 in higher doses reduced the risk of having cataracts by 30 to 40% depending on the type of cataract, the use of vitamin B2 in higher doses reduced the risk of having cataracts by 30%, and the use of vitamin B3 in higher doses reduced the risk of having cataracts by 30%. The study did not find any link (neither protective nor harmful) between the use of vitamin B6 or vitamin B12 and cataract.[51]

A study of nearly 1,800 people found that the past intake of vitamin A, vitamin B1, vitamin B2, vitamin B3, vitamin C, and vitamin E was associated with a decreased risk of having certain types of cataract. This decrease in risk ranged between 40 to 55%. Also, the study found that use of any multivitamin was associated with a 30% decrease in the overall risk of having cataracts. However, the study found no link (neither protective nor harmful) between iron and the risk of having cataract.[61]

● **Another large study found mixed results: past use of**

vitamin A associated with decreased risk of certain types of cataract though an increased risk of other types of cataract A study of over 2,000 people found that the past intake of vitamin A, vitamin B1, vitamin B2, vitamin B3, vitamin B6, vitamin C, vitamin E, and folate were each associated with a decreased risk of having a certain type of cataract (called nuclear sclerosis). However, each of these nutrients was also associated with an increased risk of having another type of cataract (called cortical cataract).[53] The researchers suggest that the finding of increased cortical cataracts reflects the possibility that the presence of nuclear sclerosis cataracts masked the finding of cortical cataracts and skewed the results. This study exemplifies how difficult it is at times to interpret results and make meaningful extrapolations.

● **In two studies: no link between blood levels of vitamin A and cataract**
A study of 165 people found no link (neither beneficial nor harmful) between cataracts and vitamin A, vitamin E, zinc, copper, and magnesium levels in the blood. However, the study found that those who had cataracts had lower levels of carotenoids and vitamin D in their blood compared to those who did not have cataracts. On the other hand, the study found that those who had cataracts had higher levels of selenium in their blood.[41]

A study of over 1,000 people found no link (neither protective nor harmful) between higher levels of vitamin A, beta-carotene, or glutathione in the blood and the risk of having cataracts. However, the study did find that higher levels of vitamin C in the blood decreased the risk of one type of cataract by nearly 50%. Of concern, the study found that higher levels of vitamin E in the blood increased the risk by nearly twice of having cataracts (this finding may be related to increased risks associated with higher doses of vitamin E)![25]

● **Though the two studies above found no link, one study found a benefit: decreased risk of cataract in those with higher blood levels of vitamin A** A study of 141 people found that higher levels of both vitamin A and vitamin E in the blood decreased the risk of developing cataracts a decade or two later. However, the study found no link (neither protective nor harmful) between selenium levels in the blood and cataract.[123]

● **In two large studies: no benefits from the use of vitamin A on the future risk of cataract over time** A recent 10-year study of over 3,000 people found that taking an antioxidant combination of beta-carotene (15 mg), vitamin C (500 mg), and vitamin E (400 IU), with or without zinc and copper each day reduced the risk of macular degeneration over time, but found no link (neither protective nor harmful) to the risk of cataracts over time.[29]

A study of over 2,000 people given a multivitamin or a placebo for 5 years found a 36% decrease in the risk of developing cataracts in those people who were age 65 to 74. Of note, there was no difference in risk in the younger group age 45 to 64. These results exemplify the positive benefit of multivitamins; however, it is difficult to apply these results to a healthy population, as the study was performed on somewhat nutritionally-deprived people in rural China.[33]

The researchers also looked at specific nutrients in a group of over 3,000 people from the same population. They found no link (neither beneficial nor harmful) over the 5-year period between the risk of cataract and those who took vitamin A and zinc, or those who took selenium with beta-carotene and vitamin E, or those who took vitamin C and molybdenum. In contrast, in those who took vitamin B2 (5.2 mg) and vitamin B3 (40 mg) daily for 5 years had a 41% decrease in the risk of developing cataracts, compared to those who took placebo.[33]

● **Though the two studies above found no link, one large study found a benefit: use of vitamin A decreases the future risk of cataract over time** Looking over an 8-year period into the future, a year study of over 50,000 women from a group of over 120,000 participants age 45 to 67 found that a diet with higher amounts of vitamin A decreased the risk by nearly 40%. Similarly, a diet with higher amounts of carotenoids decreased the risk of developing cataracts by over 25%. No such links (neither beneficial nor harmful) were found between diets high in vitamin B2, vitamin C, or vitamin E and cataract. However, the study did find that the duration of vitamin C intake mattered. Those who consumed vitamin C supplements for 10 or more years had a 45% decreased chance of developing cataracts.[42]

However, 7 years later, the same researchers looking forward over time over 12 years at nearly 75,000 women from the previous study found no link (neither protective nor harmful) between vitamin A, C, or E taken for more than 10 years and the risk of cataract.[138]

● **Another large study found a benefit: use of multivitamin with beta-carotene as a precursor to vitamin A decreases the future risk of cataract over time**
A combined British and U.S. study of nearly 300 people found a mild benefit of taking 18 mg beta-carotene, 750 mg vitamin C, and 600 IU of vitamin E each day in reducing the risk of cataract, compared to taking placebo. Interestingly, the results showed that the vitamins were more beneficial to those who lived in the U.S. as compared to those who lived in England, possibly because of genetic, environmental, or dietary differences.[34]

● In one study: increased vitamin A in the lens associated with cataract

Interestingly, vitamin A and vitamin E levels were found to be higher in cataracts than in clear lenses in a study of 27 people and of 22 autopsy cases. These findings are contrary to what one expects, and authors suggest that those who developed cataracts started to supplement their diets with more vitamin A and E compared to those who did not develop cataracts. Alternatively, those who had cataracts were older, and there may be a different mechanism of vitamin utilization or metabolism involved in the lens.[139]

Body Absorption, Metabolism, & Excretion

Vitamin A is easily absorbed orally. It is absorbed from the intestines after it is taken up by fat micelles (spherical soap-bubble-like conglomerates of fat). It is transported to specific tissues with the assistance of fatty-proteins. Carotenoids are also absorbed in this manner. Beta-carotene and other carotenoids such as alpha-carotene and beta-cryptoxanthin are pre-cursors of vitamin A and are converted to vitamin A in the liver (see sections on beta-carotene and carotenoids).

Vitamin A is stored in the liver as an ester. It is often sent from the liver to other parts of the body through the bloodstream on a bloodstream shipping protein, called retinol binding protein, after the ester form of vitamin A is converted to retinol.

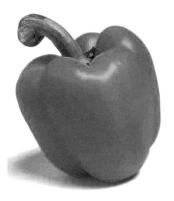

Excretion of vitamin A occurs mostly through the kidneys. Some excretion occurs through the digestive tract and excess carotenoids are often dumped back into the digestive tract through bile (a green fluid produced by the liver that is stored in the gallbladder to assist in digestion).

Deficiency

Vitamin A deficiency is more common in the elderly population, in diabetics, and especially in alcoholics and people with liver disease, as they have a decrease in the ability to convert beta-carotene to vitamin A. In these people, it is recommended that they rely on vitamin A sources more than beta-carotene sources. Vitamin A deficiency can also be caused by decreased absorption from digestive tract diseases, such as Crohn's disease, celiac disease, and pancreatic disease.

Vitamin A deficiency can cause dry skin, skin rash, itching, broken fingernails, and dry hair. Due to vitamin A's involvement in the immune system, vitamin A deficiency is associated with increased susceptibility to infections. Furthermore, severe vitamin A deficiency can cause impaired growth.

Vitamin A deficiency can also cause a range of effects in the eye, grouped under the name xerophthalmia. Xerophthalmia typically and historically refers to a drying out of the surface of the eye, and can range in severity. Mild deficiency results in the formation of foamy spots on the conjunctiva. These foamy spots are called Bitot's spots. Moderate deficiency results in dryness of the surface of the eye from inadequate lubrication. Severe deficiency results in severe dryness of the surface of the eye, including dryness of the cornea that may lead to ulceration. Ulceration is the process in which a break in the surface of the cornea develops, which over time becomes more excavated.

Xerophthalmia also may include night blindness or difficulty adapting to low light conditions. Night blindness from vitamin A deficiency may or may not occur in association with the dryness of xerophthalmia.

Abetalipoproteinemia, or Bazen-Kornzweig disease, is a genetic disorder of poor absorption of fat by the intestines. Certain vitamins, such as vitamins A, D, E, and K are absorbed by intestines by tagging on to the fats. In abetalipoproteinemia, these vitamins are not absorbed properly and the body runs deficient in the vitamins. As a consequence, these people develop degeneration of their retina in a very similar pattern to retinitis pigmentosa, a night-blinding retinal disease. Fortunately though, supplementation with both vitamins A and E has been shown to reverse the process in these people.

Toxicity & Side Effects

Mild vitamin A toxicity can include nausea, vomiting, headaches, and dizziness. Vitamin A in high doses can cause increased pressure in the brain, which can cause headaches, nausea, decreased vision from swelling of the optic nerves, and double vision. Although this association has been known for years and reported by Arctic explorers who consumed excess polar bear liver, which is high in vitamin A, the exact mechanism of vitamin A toxicity is still unknown.

Long-term vitamin A toxicity can include skin problems, including itchy skin or even loss of skin, and also can include hair problems such as hair loss or thickening of the hair. In addition, bone and muscle pains can occur as well as eye pains, fatigue, and anorexia.

There is evidence that high levels of vitamin A may increase the risk of osteoporosis by decreasing bone density. A recent study of over 70,000 women has shown that high doses (greater than 10,000 IU per day) of vitamin A resulted in an increased risk of hip fractures in post-menopausal women.

High doses of vitamin A results in accumulation of debris behind the rod and cone photoreceptors, in a layer of tissue called the retinal pigment epithelium. This layer of tissue serves to provide nutrition for the photoreceptors and to remove excess debris and waste from the photoreceptors. This debris and waste includes the discs of the photoreceptors, which are shed each day. The residue produced is called lipofuscin, which in the presence of light and oxygen, results in the production of reactive oxygen species (toxic chemicals that result in oxidation). Thus, excess lipofuscin can result in oxidative damage to the retina. Of course light exposure is high in the retina, and the highest amount of oxygen consumption of any tissue in the body occurs in the retina. Therefore, the retina is particularly susceptible to oxidative damage. Excess vitamin A may result in excess debris and, thus, toxicity to the retina.

In some people with liver disease, excess vitamin A may be toxic to the liver. The signs and symptoms of this toxicity include brittle nails, dry skin, hair loss, as well as fatigue, irritability, loss of appetite, and nausea. This toxicity occurs at doses of 50,000 IU taken daily over many years, or 100,000 IU taken daily over many months. Even so, the toxicity can be stopped and reversed by stopping the excessive intake of vitamin A. A dose of 15,000 IU daily over as long as 20 years is not known to cause any liver toxicity or to cause skin, hair, or systemic manifestations. However, there are reports that a single ingestion of extremely high doses of vitamin A, such as the high levels found in polar bear liver, can be fatal.

In pregnant people, high doses of vitamin A increase the risk of birth defects and women in the first trimester are at highest risk.

High levels of beta-carotene and/or vitamin A supplementation may be associated with increased risk of lung cancer in both smokers and people with increased exposure to second-hand smoke. The effect is believed to be mediated by the consequences of high levels of vitamin A in the lung. Smoking and second-hand smoke, in the lung, can cause proliferation of cells (an increase in the number of cells) that react to the toxic effects of smoke. Vitamin A can exacerbate this proliferation within the lung, possibly resulting in cancer. A study of over 29,000 smokers, called the

"Alpha Tocopherol (Vitamin E), Beta-carotene Cancer Prevention Study," showed that those smokers who took 20 mg per day beta-carotene supplement were nearly 20% more likely to develop lung cancer, compared to those smokers who did not take the beta-carotene supplement. Another study of over 18,000 smokers, called the "Beta-carotene and Retinol Efficacy Trial," also found that those smokers who took 30 mg per day of beta-carotene and 25,000 IU per day of vitamin A supplementation, were nearly 30% more likely to develop lung cancer, as compared to those who did not take the beta-carotene and vitamin A supplements. These numbers are staggering!

Smoking in itself creates high levels of oxidative stress and injury throughout the body. There is also evidence that vitamin A or beta-carotene supplementation also places smokers, and those who drink alcohol—whether moderately or excessively—at risk for other forms of cancer, such as colon cancer. However, there is conflicting evidence that these nutrients can be beneficial in smokers, especially when obtained from natural sources such as fruits and vegetables. Therefore, for anyone who smokes or is exposed to second hand smoke, it is best avoid high levels of beta-carotene and/or vitamin A supplementation. The best option, of course, is to avoid smoking or second-hand smoke altogether.

There is very controversial evidence on whether or not high doses of vitamin A causes or prevents angiogenesis (the formation of abnormal new blood vessels) because it is debatable whether vitamin A acts to inhibit or to stimulate the expression of the major enzyme that stimulates new blood vessel growth. Angiogenesis is particularly harmful in the retina, cornea, and trabecular meshwork (filtration site of the eye) and can cause loss of vision. The problems that result are called choroidal neovascularization (seen in wet macular degeneration), or retinal neovascularization (seen in severe diabetic retinopathy or retinal disease), or corneal neovascularization (seen in corneal injury or disease), or iris neovascularization (seen in angle-closure glaucoma and inflammatory eye disease).

Vitamin A toxicity is not believed to occur from excessive consumption of beta-carotene. In fact, beta-carotene is metabolized by the liver in a regulated manner such that only the amount of vitamin A needed by the body is produced while excess beta-carotene is stored. The storage of extra beta-carotene occurs in the skin and is commonly known to produce an orange discoloration of the palms and soles. This discoloration is sometimes mistaken for jaundice, though jaundice can be distinguished from beta-carotene storage by the fact that beta-carotene storage does not occur in the whites of the eyes, while jaundice causes discoloration of the whites of the eyes as well.

Much of the toxicity that occurs from excess vitamin A is believed to occur from excess vitamin A being presented to cells in various organs without being carried by the vitamin A carrier protein. In fact, when excess vitamin A is in the bloodstream, it can overwhelm the supply of the vitamin A carrier protein and start being delivered to tissues on other fat-protein carriers, which affects how the cells react to it.

Interactions with Other Nutrients

There are numerous interactions between vitamin A and other nutrients, but the important concept is that a balance should be achieved between intake of vitamin A and the other nutrients.

Excess vitamin E blocks vitamin A conversion in the retina and may cause retinal toxicity. Vitamin E is a non-competitive inhibitor of the enzyme retinyl-esterohydrolase, which is essential in the process of converting vitamin A to retinoic acid or retinal that is then transported to photoreceptors to be linked to the opsin proteins to form the light-sensing pigments of the retina, the rhodopsin and iodopsins. This conversion occurs in the retinal pigment epithelium. Thus, excess vitamin E prevents this conversion of vitamin A to the retinoic acid or retinal and this blockage results in a buildup of vitamin A in the retinal pigment epithelium.

On the other hand, deficiency of vitamin E can also cause photoreceptor damage with vitamin A accumulation in the retinal pigment epithelium. Vitamin E, known to accumulate in high concentrations in the photoreceptors discs, is an antioxidant known to protect photoreceptor disc membranes from oxidative damage. In fact, vitamin E with its antioxidant activities saves any cell membranes from oxidative damage. Vitamin E performs the first steps of preventing oxidative damage to cell membranes, or lipid peroxidation, by converting strong and dangerous hydroperoxyl radicals into weaker, yet still harmful hydroperoxides. Vitamin A as retinoic acid is an essential membrane component of photoreceptors, and oxidative damage to these membranes can result in excess disc debris that must be taken up and ingested by the retinal pigment epithelium.

When zinc levels are extremely low, there is an association with decreased vitamin A metabolism, particularly in photoreceptors. Thus, zinc deficiency has been associated with retinal degeneration, notably night-blindness and retinitis pigmentosa. Zinc is involved in a dehydrogenase enzyme, retinene reductase, which is essential for vitamin A metabolism in photoreceptors (see section on zinc). Zinc also facilitates vitamin A's "mobilization" out of the liver through vitamin A binding proteins. Zinc deficiency has been associated with decreased formation by the liver of these vitamin A binding proteins that carry vitamin A in the bloodstream. Thus, zinc helps maintain appropriate vitamin A levels in the blood. Zinc's role in vitamin A metabolism is not only important for the retina but also for other ocular tissues, such as the surface of the eye, where vitamin A plays an essential role (see above).

Similarly, vitamin A deficiency has been associated with decreases in zinc-binding proteins, which results in decreased zinc absorption and decreased zinc levels in the bloodstream (see section on zinc). A study of over 200 women with night-blindness from vitamin A deficiency who also had zinc deficiency found both vitamin A and zinc were required to treat the night-blindness. Neither vitamin A nor zinc alone could effectively treat the night-blindness.[140]

Taurine plays a role in assisting in transporting vitamin A into the photoreceptor outer segments. Once vitamin A is used up by the photoreceptors, its metabolites become toxic, and taurine also plays a role in transporting these vitamin A metabolites out of the photoreceptor outer segments and over to the retinal pigment epithelium for recycling. One method by which taurine accomplishes this transport is by binding to vitamin A metabolites and converting these oil-soluble compounds into water-soluble compounds (see section on taurine).

Vitamin A deficiency may decrease the amount of iron that can be mobilized out of iron stores in the body, resulting in anemia (insufficiency of the red blood cells that carry oxygen). Some of the symptoms of anemia include fatigue, shortness of breath, increased heart rate, mouth sores or ulcers, tongue soreness, pale skin, and brittle nails.

Ideal Dosage

The minimum recommended daily allowance of vitamin A established by the National Academy of Sciences is 3,333 IU for children and adults. However, many researchers, including the National Cancer Institute recommend a daily dosage of 10,000 IU. Many researchers recommend that 90% of this vitamin A come from beta-carotene, meaning that the dosage should be 1,000 IU per day of vitamin A palmitate or stearate and 5½ to 6 mg per day of beta-carotene.

On the other hand, in Stargardt's disease (a childhood retinal degeneration, see page 13 on hereditary retinal degenerations), there is suggestion that vitamin A should be limited or decreased because the gene defect in Stargardt's results in accumulation of used vitamin A byproducts inside the retina.

Sources (Where to Find It)

Fruits & Vegetables:

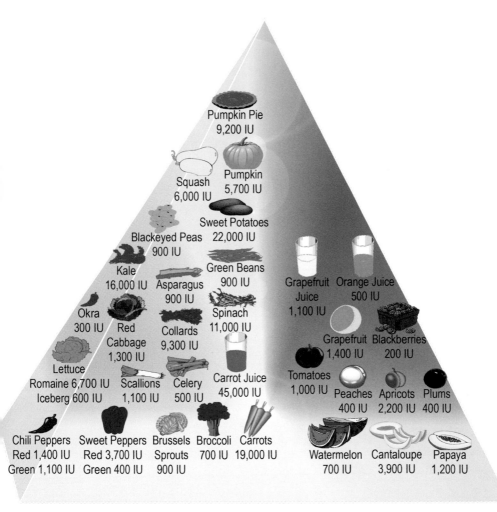

Pumpkin Pie 9,200 IU

Squash 6,000 IU

Pumpkin 5,700 IU

Sweet Potatoes 22,000 IU

Blackeyed Peas 900 IU

Kale 16,000 IU

Asparagus 900 IU

Green Beans 900 IU

Grapefruit Juice 1,100 IU

Orange Juice 500 IU

Okra 300 IU

Red Cabbage 1,300 IU

Collards 9,300 IU

Spinach 11,000 IU

Grapefruit 1,400 IU

Blackberries 200 IU

Lettuce
Romaine 6,700 IU
Iceberg 600 IU

Scallions 1,100 IU

Celery 500 IU

Carrot Juice 45,000 IU

Tomatoes 1,000 IU

Peaches 400 IU

Apricots 2,200 IU

Plums 400 IU

Chili Peppers
Red 1,400 IU
Green 1,100 IU

Sweet Peppers
Red 3,700 IU
Green 400 IU

Brussels Sprouts 900 IU

Broccoli 700 IU

Carrots 19,000 IU

Watermelon 700 IU

Cantaloupe 3,900 IU

Papaya 1,200 IU

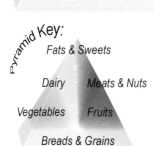

Pyramid Key:

Fats & Sweets

Dairy   Meats & Nuts

Vegetables   Fruits

Breads & Grains

*See Guides on Pages 467-468.

Dairy, Meats, & Grains:

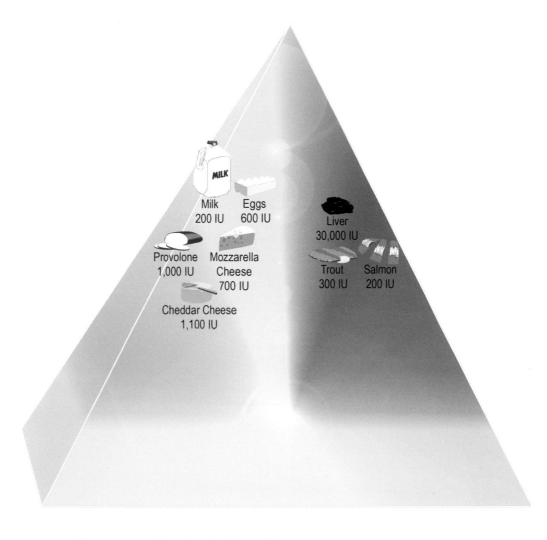

Milk
200 IU

Eggs
600 IU

Liver
30,000 IU

Provolone
1,000 IU

Mozzarella
Cheese
700 IU

Trout
300 IU

Salmon
200 IU

Cheddar Cheese
1,100 IU

Top sources for vitamin A are liver, sweet potatoes, carrots, kale, spinach, and collards. Other sources that are rich in vitamin A include romaine lettuce, squash, pumpkin, red sweet peppers, cantaloupe, and apricots.

VITAMIN B1
(THIAMIN)

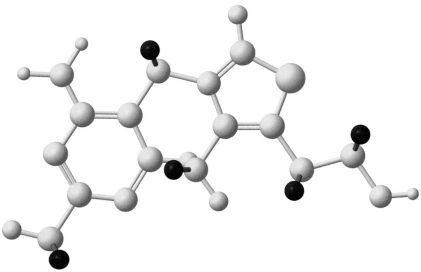

Category

Vitamin B1, also known as thiamin, is a water-soluble vitamin. The Dutch Dr. Christiaan Eijkman, who won the Nobel Prize for discovering vitamins, first described the substance that is now known as vitamin B1. It was found in rice and prevented a disease called beriberi, a form of vitamin B1 deficiency (see below). The Polish Dr. Casimir Funk then characterized this compound as an amine, or a type of nitrogen-containing molecule. Dr. Funk called the substance a "vit-amine," short for vital amine.

Cellular Location

About half of the body's store of vitamin B1 is located in the skeletal muscles and heart. Other storage locations for vitamin B1 include the liver, kidney, and brain. The rest of the vitamin B1 is distributed throughout the body.

Structure

Vitamin B1 is an organic compound known as an amine. It contains two rings: a pyrimidine ring, composed of carbon and nitrogen, and a thiazole ring, composed of sulfur with nitrogen and carbon.

Mechanisms of Action

Vitamin B1 acts to assist enzymes in the formation of energy.

Vitamin B1 also acts in the membranes of nerve fibers to regulate transport of ions, or charged particles.

Biological & Ocular Importance

● **Assists in the formation of energy packets** Vitamin B1 acts to assist enzymes in the formation of energy and is required in certain pathways to make ATP, or energy packets that our cells use. Vitamin B1 is also essential in the creation of nicotinamide adenine dinuclotide phosphate (NADP), another molecule that is required in certain pathways to make ATP.

Vitamin B1 has been suggested to help the heart produce energy during heart disease, such as congestive heart failure. When certain types of medications such as "loop diuretics" are given, they may cause the kidneys to excrete excess vitamin B1, so these people may require higher amounts of vitamin B1.

● **Assists in the formation of energy for the optic nerve** Vitamin B1 plays an important role in maintaining energy for the optic nerve. Of note, because magnesium is essential in maintaining vitamin B1 levels, magnesium plays an important role in the health of the optic nerve.

● **Regulates charged particle transport in nerve fibers** Vitamin B1 also acts in the membranes of nerve fibers to regulate transport of ions, or charged particles, involved in transmitting nerve impulses.

● **Protects neural cells from injury** Vitamin B1 can protect against glutamate toxicity (see under vitamin B12), which involves the toxic effects of excess glutamate release from the neural cells of the eye. Glutamate is a natural signaling chemical in neural cells that enables signals to transfer from one cell to another. It is the main signal producer in the circuitry of the eye. However, excess glutamate is toxic to surrounding cells. When a cell dies, for example in glaucoma, it can release excess glutamate, resulting in toxic injury and death of surrounding cells.

- **Strengthens the immune defense system** Vitamin B1 is believed to strengthen the body's immune defense system.

Human Studies on Utility

Currently, there are only a handful of human studies on vitamin B1 use in eye disease reported in the scientifically-reviewed medical literature. These studies involve the following eye diseases: glaucoma, macular degeneration, and cataract. These studies are summarized below. There are four studies of vitamin B1 in cataract prevention, and suggest a benefit of vitamin B1. Nevertheless, the fact that there are only a few reported clinical studies does not necessarily imply a definite benefit or lack of benefit. Looking at the mechanism of action, the use of vitamin B1 in moderation may be possibly of benefit in many eye diseases.

- **In one small study: no link between blood levels of vitamin B1 and glaucoma**
A study of 50 people found lower blood levels of vitamin B1 decreased the risk of glaucoma. The same study found no link (neither protective nor harmful) between glaucoma and blood levels of vitamin C.[141]

- **In one large study: no benefits in past use of vitamin B1 found on risk of macular degeneration**
Looking forward over time, a study of nearly 3,000 people age 49 and over found no link (neither protective nor harmful) between the risk of having macular degeneration and taking any of the following nutrients (alone or in combination) in the past: vitamin B1, vitamin B2, vitamin B3, vitamin B6, vitamin B12, vitamin A, vitamin C, vitamin E, beta-carotene, folate or zinc.[13]

- **Three large studies found past use of vitamin B1 associated with decreased risk of cataract** A large study of nearly 3,000 people age 49 to 97 found that past use of vitamin B1 in higher doses reduced the risk of having cataracts by 30 to 40% depending on the type of cataract. Likewise, the past use of multivitamins was associated with a decreased risk of having cataracts as well. The use of

Vitamin B1 for
Cataract
Scale of Benefit

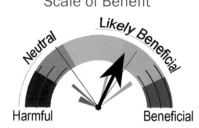

vitamin A in higher doses reduced the risk of having cataracts by 90%, the use of folate reduced the risk of having cataracts by 40 to 60%

depending on the type of cataract, the use of vitamin B2 in higher doses reduced the risk of having cataracts by 30%, and the use of vitamin B3 in higher doses reduced the risk of having cataracts by 30%. The study did not find any link (neither protective nor harmful) between the use of vitamin B6 or vitamin B12 and cataract.[51]

A study of nearly 3,000 people found that the past intake of vitamin B1, vitamin B2, vitamin B3, vitamin A, iron, and zinc decreased the risk of having certain types of cataract by 30 to 50%.[62] It is interesting to note that in this study, iron was associated with a decrease in risk of having cataract, and not an increased risk, as some physicians have predicted. Furthermore, it is surprising that no link (neither protective nor harmful) was found between vitamin C use and cataract, despite other studies showing a benefit.

A study of nearly 1,800 people found that the past intake of vitamin B1, vitamin B2, vitamin B3, vitamin A, vitamin C, and vitamin E was associated with a decreased risk of having certain types of cataract. This decrease in risk ranged between 40 to 55%. Also, the study found that use of any multivitamin was associated with a 30% decrease in the overall risk of having cataracts. However, the study found no link (neither protective nor harmful) between iron and the risk of having cataract.[61]

● **Another large study found mixed results: past use of vitamin B1 associated with decreased risk of certain types of cataract though an increased risk of other types of cataract** A study of over 2,000 people found that the past intake of vitamin B1, vitamin B2, vitamin B3, vitamin B6, vitamin C, vitamin E, vitamin A, and folate were each associated with a decreased risk of having a certain type of cataract (called nuclear sclerosis). However, each of these nutrients was also associated with an increased risk of having another type of cataract (called cortical cataract).[53] The researchers suggest that the finding of increased cortical cataracts reflects the possibility that the presence of nuclear sclerosis cataracts masked the finding of cortical cataracts and skewed the results. This study exemplifies how difficult it is at times to interpret results and make meaningful extrapolations.

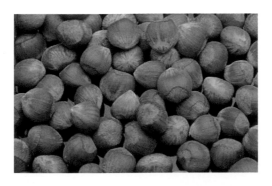

Body Absorption, Metabolism, & Excretion

Vitamin B1 is absorbed by the intestines into the bloodstream, after which it is transported throughout the body.

Excess vitamin B1 is filtered by the kidneys for excretion. And often, excess dietary intake is excreted within 30 minutes, creating very yellow urine.

Deficiency

Specific foods such as blueberries, black currants, Brussels sprouts, and red cabbage contain chemicals called polyhydroxyphenols that can inactivate vitamin B1. However, including vitamin C and citric acid in one's diet can help block the ability of polyhydroxyphenols to inactive vitamin B1.

Raw fish, such as in sushi, has enzymes that can degrade vitamin B1, thus decreasing the amount of thiamine available in a diet. Cooking the fish disables these enzymes.

Vitamin B1 deficiency results in difficulties in a cell's ability to "digest carbohydrates," resulting in build-up of excess pyruvic acid, which is normally used for energy in the body, but in excess, can cause drowsiness, trouble breathing, and heart disease.

Optic nerve disease, manifested as optic atrophy, can occur with vitamin B1 deficiency. Other eye manifestations include disease of the surface of the cornea.

Vitamin B1 causes a disorder called beriberi. The name beriberi comes from the Sri Lankan word that means weakness, or inability to stand up from a sitting position. Literally translated, beriberi means: "I can't, I can't." There are two major types of beriberi: dry and wet.

Dry beriberi often occurs in those with a long-term deficiency of vitamin B1. It is characterized by muscle weakness and wasting, particularly in the legs, resulting in paralysis or inability to walk. Pain, tingling, and burning sensations in the hands and feet have also been described. It is sometimes called "endemic neuritis" because it results from nerve damage caused by long-term deficiency of vitamin B1 and by excess pyruvic acid, which also damages nerves.

Wet beriberi often results in heart failure from improper energy production and excess pyruvic acid. With the heart failure, the heart does not properly pump blood and fluid, so fluid then starts to accumulate in the hands and feet as well as in the lungs, resulting in difficulty breathing. Skin rashes, particularly on the palms of the hands and soles of the feet, have been noted to occur as well, often

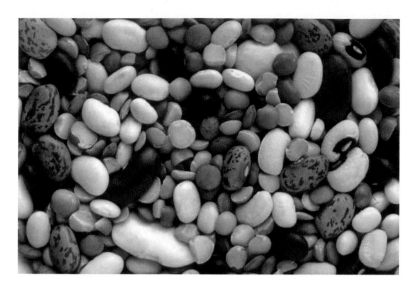

in the early stages of wet beriberi as blood accumulates in the hands and feet.

There is often a lot of overlap between the dry and wet forms, with people having symptoms of both. It is unknown why some people develop more of the dry form and others more of the wet, but it has been suggested that those with the dry form have eaten less carbohydrates and those with the wet form have eaten more carbohydrates.

Beriberi amblyopia refers to decreased visual acuity, blind spots in the center of vision, and decreased peripheral vision that result from degeneration of the neurons of the retina. Beriberi amblyopia occurs with both wet and dry beriberi.

Acute beriberi refers to vitamin B1 deficiency in infants, which is often fatal. It can be caused by lack of vitamin B1 in infant formula or by insufficient vitamin B1 in the breast milk of mothers who are deficient in vitamin B1. They develop signs of both dry and wet beriberi, with muscle wasting and fluid build-up.

Wernicke-Korsakoff syndrome is a vitamin B1 deficiency that is often found in alcoholics with poor nutritional intake. It is characterized by poor coordination, poor balance, confusion, loss of memory, inability to move one's eye from side to side or up and down, and nystagmus or rapid involuntary eye movements that have been described as "jittering" of the eyes.

A rare genetic syndrome known as Rogers' syndrome is caused by defects in vitamin B1 transport into cells. The disease commonly results in anemia (insufficiency of the red blood cells that carry oxygen), deafness caused by ear neural malfunction, and diabetes. Retinal disease characterized by abnormal photoreceptor function has been described in Rogers' syndrome.

Toxicity & Side Effects

Vitamin B1 toxicity is uncommon since most of the excess of vitamin B1 is rapidly excreted in the urine. In extremely high doses, it can cause headaches, seizures, abnormal heart rhythms, and allergic shock.

Interactions with Other Nutrients

When magnesium levels are low, vitamin B1 cannot form thiamine pyrophosphate, an important enzyme involved in metabolism and energy production. An essential function of vitamin B1 is to form the enzyme thiamine pyrophosphate (see section on magnesium). In fact, in states of low magnesium, instead of forming thiamine pyrophosphate, calcium pyrophosphate is formed, which can cause painful crystal formation in the body. In addition to the metabolism and energy problems, low levels of thiamine pyrophosphate are associated with gastrointestinal infections as well as brain disturbances such as hallucinations, confusion, disorientation, and even encephalopathy, a disorder of brain function involving confusion or even coma. Even in the presence of normal vitamin B1 levels in the body, magnesium deficiency can cause low levels of thiamine pyrophosphate, which looks just like vitamin B1 deficiency without an actual deficiency of vitamin B1.

Ideal Dosage

The recommended daily dose ranges from 1.0 to 1.4 mg per day. In boys age 14 to 18, and in men over age 18, the recommended dose is 1.2 mg per day. In girls age 14 to 18, it is 1.0 mg per day, and in women over age 18, it is 1.1 mg per day. During pregnancy and lactation, the recommended dose increases to 1.4 mg per day.

It may be best to obtain a daily dose of 1.5 to 3 mg per day, though some researchers recommend doses up to 10 mg per day.

In cases of vitamin B1 deficiency, doses of up to 200 mg per day are commonly used.

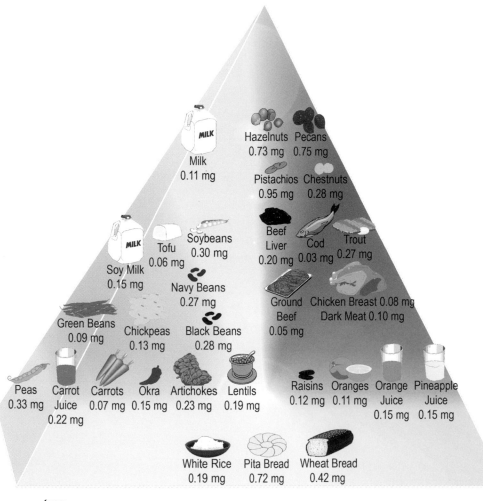

Milk
0.11 mg

Hazelnuts Pecans
0.73 mg 0.75 mg

Pistachios Chestnuts
0.95 mg 0.28 mg

Soy Milk
0.15 mg

Tofu
0.06 mg

Soybeans
0.30 mg

Navy Beans
0.27 mg

Beef Liver
0.20 mg

Cod
0.03 mg

Trout
0.27 mg

Green Beans
0.09 mg

Chickpeas
0.13 mg

Black Beans
0.28 mg

Ground Beef
0.05 mg

Chicken Breast 0.08 mg
Dark Meat 0.10 mg

Peas
0.33 mg

Carrot Juice
0.22 mg

Carrots
0.07 mg

Okra
0.15 mg

Artichokes
0.23 mg

Lentils
0.19 mg

Raisins
0.12 mg

Oranges
0.11 mg

Orange Juice
0.15 mg

Pineapple Juice
0.15 mg

White Rice
0.19 mg

Pita Bread
0.72 mg

Wheat Bread
0.42 mg

Pyramid Key:

Fats & Sweets

Dairy   Meats & Nuts

Vegetables   Fruits

Breads & Grains

Top sources of vitamin B1 are nuts (particularly pistachios, pecans, and hazelnuts), beans (such as soybeans, black beans, and navy beans), artichokes, trout, beef liver, and enriched breads.

*See Guides on Pages 467-468.

VITAMIN B2
(RIBOFLAVIN)

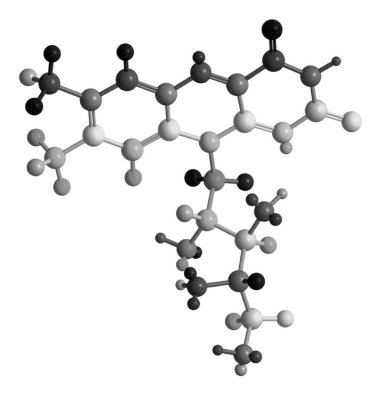

Category

Vitamin B2, also known as riboflavin, is an essential water-soluble vitamin. It was originally called Vitamin G before being reclassified as a B-complex vitamin.

Cellular Location

Vitamin B2 is found throughout the body. However, it is particularly concentrated in the liver, kidneys, and heart. While it is transported as Vitamin B2, inside cells it is present most as its co-enzyme form called flavin mononucleotide (FMN, see below).

Structure

Vitamin B2 is composed of a specialized triple ring called a flavin ring with a sugar alcohol attached to its side.

Mechanisms of Action

Vitamin B2 acts to assist enzymes in the formation of energy, helps in the formation of antioxidant enzymes, and plays a role in some pathways of making amino acids (building block of proteins).

Biological & Ocular Importance

● **Helps in the formation of energy by cells**   Vitamin B2 acts to assist enzymes in the formation of energy and is required in certain pathways to make ATP, or energy packets that our cells use. Vitamin B2 is also essential in the creation of flavin mononucleotide (FMN) and flavin adenine dinucleotide (FAD), molecules that are required in certain pathways to make ATP.

Additionally, vitamin B2 has been suggested as a treatment for migraine headaches because of its role in improving energy production by cells.

● **Helps produce the building blocks of proteins**   Vitamin B2 helps in some pathways of making amino acids (building block of proteins).

● **Helps produce neurotransmitter signaling molecules**   Vitamin B2 is also required in the production of certain neurotransmitters that send communication signals between neurons or brain cells.

● **Supports the formation of antioxidant enzymes**   Vitamin B2 also acts with and / or helps in the formation of antioxidant enzymes. The activation of both folate and vitamin B6 require vitamin B2 in the pathway.

Required for production of glutathione reductase, an antioxidant enzyme, which contains flavin rings (see section on glutathione). Riboflavin is the precursor to flavin adenine dinucleotide, the coenzyme for glutathione reductase.

Vitamin B2 acts with folate as an indirect antioxidant by decreasing stress on protein-building organelles within cells by reducing the activity of homocysteine, an amino acid known to cause atherosclerosis (blood vessel cholesterol clots and plaques that can result in heart disease and stroke, as well as artery or vein clots in the retina or optic nerve strokes). Homocysteine signals stress in the protein-building organelles and causes proteins to be misfolded. High levels of homocysteine have been associated with blood vessel blockages in the retina as well as Alzheimer's disease. Taurine, betaine, and vitamin B12 also help reduce homocysteine levels.

As an antioxidant, it is believed to be beneficial to retinal diseases, such as macular degeneration and childhood hereditary photoreceptor diseases, in which oxidative damage plays a role in the disease. It may also be beneficial in diseases, such as glaucoma or optic nerve diseases, in which oxidative damage plays a role as well. Furthermore, it may also help prevent cataract formation or corneal disease, again by preventing or decreasing oxidative damage.

The role of vitamin B2 in preventing cataracts has been known since at least the 1920's. Its benefits are believed to derive from the actions noted above, particularly its role in the production of glutathione reductase, a major antioxidant in the lens.

Human Studies on Utility

Currently, there are only a handful of human studies on vitamin B2 use in eye disease reported in the scientifically-reviewed medical literature. These studies involve the macular degeneration and cataract, and are summarized below. There are four studies of vitamin B2 in the prevention and treatment of macular degeneration, which do not suggest a benefit of vitamin B2. There are seven studies of vitamin B2 in cataract prevention, and suggest a benefit of vitamin B2. Nevertheless, the fact that there are only a few reported clinical studies does not necessarily imply a definite benefit or lack of benefit. Looking at the mechanism of action, the use of vitamin B2 in moderation may be possibly of benefit in many eye diseases.

● In one large study: no benefits in past use of vitamin B2 found on risk of macular degeneration

Looking forward over time, a study of nearly 3,000 people age 49 and over found no link (neither protective nor harmful) between the risk of having macular degeneration and taking any of the following nutrients (alone or in combination) in the past: vitamin B2, vitamin B3, vitamin B6, vitamin B12, vitamin B1, vitamin A, vitamin C, vitamin E, beta-carotene, folate or zinc.[13]

● In two studies: no benefits from the use of vitamin B2 on the future risk of macular degeneration over time

An older 1964 study of 85 people found no link (neither protective nor harmful) between a multivitamin with vitamins B2, B3, B6, and B12 and progression of macular diseases, such as macular degeneration.[142] Other studies at the time found similar findings.

A small study of 71 people with macular degeneration found no benefit to the macular degeneration or to vision in those who took a daily antioxidant combination, for over 1½ years, that consisted of vitamin B2 (25 mg), beta-carotene (20,000 IU), vitamin C (750 mg), vitamin E (200 IU), chromium (100 µg), selenium (50 µg), zinc (12.5 mg), taurine (100 mg), N-acetyl cysteine (100 mg), glutathione (5 mg), and selected bioflavonoids, when compared to placebo.[17] It is impossible, however, to ascertain the individual effect of vitamin B2 from this type of study.

● **Though the two studies above found no link, one small early study found a benefit: use of vitamin B2 decreases the future risk of macular degeneration over time** A 1974 study of 14 people suggested a benefit of a multivitamin with vitamins B2, B3, B6, and B12, in protecting against progression of macular diseases, such as macular degeneration.[143] However, the study was too small and of too short a duration to provide any conclusive findings.

● **In one study: no benefits in past use of vitamin B2 found on risk of cataract**
A study of 300 women age 56 to

71 from a group of over 120,000 people found no link (neither protective nor harmful) between the use of vitamin B2 or E and cataract. However, the study found that in non-smokers, the past use of beta-carotene in higher doses reduced the risk of having cataracts by over 70%. In fact, carotenoids, as a group, in higher doses reduced the risk of having cataracts by over 80%. The study also found that folate in higher doses reduced the risk of having cataracts by nearly 75%. In addition, past use of higher doses of vitamin C decreased the risk of having cataract by nearly 60% and the use of vitamin C for over 10 years decreased the risk by 60%.[23]

● **Four large studies found a benefit: past use of vitamin B2 associated with decreased risk of cataract**
A study of nearly 3,000 people found that the past intake of vitamin B2, vitamin B1, vitamin B3, vitamin A, iron, and zinc decreased the risk of having certain types of cataract by 30 to 50%.[62] It is interesting to note that in this study, iron was associated with a decrease in risk of having cataract, and not an increased risk, as some physicians have predicted. Furthermore, it is surprising that no link (neither protective nor harmful) was found between vitamin C use and cataract, despite other studies showing a benefit.

A study of nearly 1,800 people found that the past intake of vitamin B2, vitamin B1, vitamin B3, vitamin A, vitamin C, and vitamin E was associated with a decreased risk of having certain types of cataract. This decrease in risk ranged between 40 to 55%. Also, the study found that use of any multivitamin was associated with a 30% decrease in the overall risk of having cataracts. However, the study found no link (neither protective nor harmful) between iron and the risk of having cataract.[61]

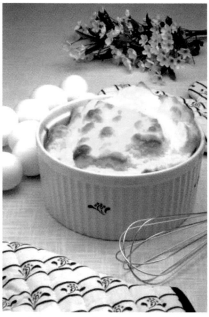

A large study of nearly 3,000 people age 49 to 97 found that past use of vitamin B2 in higher doses reduced the risk of having cataracts by 30%. Likewise, the past use of multivitamins was associated with a decreased risk of having cataracts as well. The use of vitamin A in higher doses reduced the risk of having cataracts by 90%, the use of vitamin B1 in higher doses reduced the risk of having cataracts by 30 to 40% depending on the type of cataract, the use of vitamin B3 in higher doses reduced the risk of having cataracts by 30%, and the use of folate reduced the risk of having cataracts by 40 to 60% depending on the type of cataract. The study did not find any link (neither protective nor harmful) between the use of vitamin B6 or vitamin B12 and cataract.[51]

A study of nearly 500 people age 53 to 73 found that past intake of *higher* amounts of vitamin B2 decreased the risk of having cataracts by over 60%, and past intake of *higher* amounts of folate decreased the risk of having cataracts by about 10%. The study found that the past intake of *higher* amounts of vitamin C decreased the risk of having cataracts by nearly 70%. It also found that long-term intake of vitamin C for over 10 years decreased the risk of having cataracts by nearly 65%. Long-term intake of vitamin E for over 10 years decreased the risk of having cataracts by over 50%, even though the study found no link (neither protective nor harmful) between the past intake of *higher* amounts of vitamin E and the risk of having cataracts. The finding of no beneficial link with higher doses of vitamin E may be related to increased risks associated with the higher doses. Furthermore, the use of a multivitamin for over 10 years reduced the risk of having cataract by over 40%. However, the study found no link (neither protective nor harmful) between the intake of beta-carotene, carotenoids, lutein and zeaxanthin, or lycopene and the risk of having cataracts.[20]

● **Another large study found mixed results: past use of vitamin B2 associated with decreased risk of certain types of cataract though an increased risk of other types of cataract**   A study of over 2,000 people found that the past intake of vitamin B2, vitamin B1, vitamin B3, vitamin B6, vitamin A, vitamin C, vitamin E, and folate were each associated with a decreased risk of having a certain type of cataract (called nuclear sclerosis). However, each of these nutrients was also associated with an increased risk of having another type of cataract (called cortical cataract).[53] The researchers suggest that the finding of increased cortical cataracts reflects the possibility that the presence of nuclear sclerosis cataracts masked the finding of cortical cataracts and skewed the results. This study exemplifies how difficult it is at times to interpret results and make meaningful extrapolations.

● **One large study found a benefit: use of vitamin B2 decreases the future risk of cataract over time**   A study of over 2,000 people given a multivitamin or a placebo for 5 years found a 36% decrease in the risk of developing cataracts in those people who were age 65 to 74. Of note, there was no difference in risk in the younger group age 45 to 64. These results exemplify the positive benefit of multivitamins; however, it is difficult to apply these results to a healthy population, as the study was performed on somewhat nutritionally-deprived people in rural China.[33]

The researchers also looked at specific nutrients in a group of over 3,000 people from the same population. Those who took vitamin B2 (5.2 mg) and vitamin B3 (40 mg) daily for 5 years had a 41% decrease in the risk of developing cataracts, compared to those who took placebo. In contrast, no link was found (neither beneficial nor harmful) over the 5-year period between the risk of cataract and taking selenium with beta-carotene and vitamin E, or taking vitamin A and zinc, or taking vitamin C and molybdenum.[33]

● **One large study found no benefits from the use of vitamin B2 on the future risk of cataract over time**   Looking over an 8-year period into the future, a year study of over 50,000 women from a group of over 120,000 participants age 45 to 67 found no links (neither beneficial nor harmful) between diets high in vitamin B2, vitamin C, or vitamin E and cataract. The study did find that a diet with higher amounts of carotenoids decreased the risk of developing cataracts by over 25%. Similarly, a diet with higher amounts of vitamin A decreased the risk by nearly 40%. In addition, the study did find that the duration of vitamin C intake mattered. Those who consumed vitamin C supplements for 10 or more years had a 45% decreased chance of developing cataracts.[42]

Body Absorption, Metabolism, & Excretion

Dietary vitamin B2 is often bound to protein enzymes and is freed first by the acid in the stomach and then second by secreted enzymes of the pancreas. Animal sources of vitamin B2 are more easily absorbed than plant sources. Once absorbed, vitamin B2 is then transported through the bloodstream throughout the body.

It is excreted through filtration by the kidneys. Like vitamin B1, vitamin B2 is bright yellow in the urine. A small portion of vitamin B2 is excreted by being dumped back into the intestines with bile (a green fluid produced by the liver that is stored in the gallbladder to assist in digestion).

Deficiency

Vitamin B2 deficiency can cause dry scaly skin, cracked lips, mouth irritation, and tongue swelling. Deficiency can also cause malfunction of the nerves of the body, especially those going to the hands and feet. Anemia (insufficiency of the red blood cells that carry oxygen) can also occur, resulting in fatigue, shortness of breath, increased heart rate, mouth sores or ulcers, tongue soreness, pale skin, and brittle nails.

Corneal neovascularization (the abnormal growth of blood vessels across cornea), also has been described in vitamin B2 deficiency, along with dryness or tearing of the eye, burning sensation in the eye, and light sensitivity of the eye.

Long-term vitamin B2 deficiency has been reported to be associated with cancer of the esophagus.

Toxicity & Side Effects

In high levels, vitamin B2 may act as an oxidant, particularly in the presence of light. Vitamin B2 is known as a cellular photosensitizer. In other words, in the presence of light, vitamin B2 can absorb light and become "excited." By becoming energetically excited, it changes its energy conformation such that it pulls in electrons and creates oxidants. As such, excess vitamin B2 can be damaging by increasing oxidative stress on cells. Antioxidants such as vitamin C and alpha-lipoic acid have been shown to be helpful in decreasing the oxidative effects caused by photosensitized vitamin B2.

Excess vitamin B2 may accumulate in the natural lens, and, because sunlight exposure turns it brown, when it is in excess in the natural lens, vitamin B2 can cause the natural lens to turn brown and cataractous.

There is also some evidence that macular degeneration may be exacerbated or even caused by the presence of excess levels of vitamin B2, since its excessive presence in photoreceptors results in oxidation and toxicity when it is exposed to sunlight.

Excess vitamin B2, copper, or iron released into the vitreous may also result in early or accelerated liquefaction of the vitreous gel by increasing hyaluronidase. Hyaluronidase is an enzyme that breaks down hyaluronic acid (the major water-holding matrix compound in the vitreous gel) and increases the liquefaction of the vitreous gel (see section on hyaluronic acid).

Interactions with Other Nutrients

Copper, zinc, iron, and magnesium may inhibit the absorption of vitamin B2.

Additionally, excess boron has been shown to cause excess filtration of vitamin B2 out of the body through the kidneys.

Selenium, along with vitamin B2 and vitamin E, is required for production of glutathione peroxidase, an enzyme involved in the functioning of the antioxidant glutathione. In fact, glutathione peroxidase is called a selenoprotein because it includes 4 selenium-containing amino acids. Selenite, selenomethionine, and selenocysteine can be used as dietary supplements in order for cells to produce glutathione peroxidase. Organic selenium and selenomethionine are preferred sources of selenium for raising selenium and glutathione peroxidase levels, unlike the inorganic forms, selenate and selenite.

Vitamin B2 is also required to make glutathione reductase, which consists of flavin rings.

Ideal Dosage

The recommended daily dose ranges from 1.0 to 1.4 mg per day. In boys age 14 to 18, and in men over age 18, the recommended dose is 1.3 mg per day. In girls age 14 to 18, it is 1.0 mg per day, and in women over age 18, it is 1.1 mg per day. During pregnancy and lactation, the recommended dose increases to 1.4 mg per day.

It may be best to obtain a daily dose of 1.5 to 2.5 mg per day. While some researchers recommend doses up to 10 mg per day, its intake should never surpass 10 mg per day.

For the treatment of migraine headaches, however, some physicians have suggested doses as high as 400 mg per day.

Sources (Where to Find It)

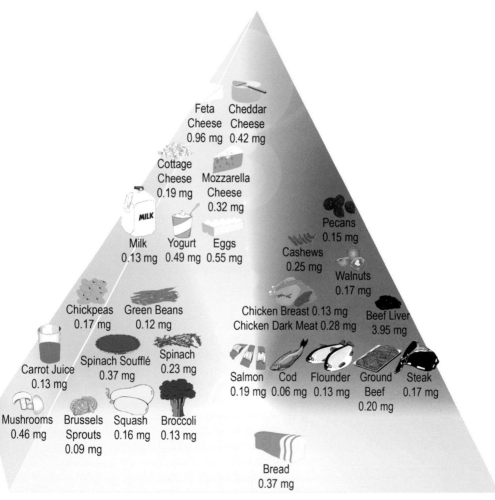

Feta Cheese 0.96 mg
Cheddar Cheese 0.42 mg
Cottage Cheese 0.19 mg
Mozzarella Cheese 0.32 mg
Milk 0.13 mg
Yogurt 0.49 mg
Eggs 0.55 mg
Pecans 0.15 mg
Cashews 0.25 mg
Walnuts 0.17 mg
Chickpeas 0.17 mg
Green Beans 0.12 mg
Chicken Breast 0.13 mg
Chicken Dark Meat 0.28 mg
Beef Liver 3.95 mg
Carrot Juice 0.13 mg
Spinach Soufflé 0.37 mg
Spinach 0.23 mg
Salmon 0.19 mg
Cod 0.06 mg
Flounder 0.13 mg
Ground Beef 0.20 mg
Steak 0.17 mg
Mushrooms 0.46 mg
Brussels Sprouts 0.09 mg
Squash 0.16 mg
Broccoli 0.13 mg
Bread 0.37 mg

Pyramid Key:

Fats & Sweets

Dairy   Meats & Nuts

Vegetables   Fruits

Breads & Grains

The top source of vitamin B2 is beef liver. Other sources rich in vitamin B2 are cheeses (particularly feta cheese), eggs, yogurt, and mushrooms.

*See Guides on Pages 467-468.

VITAMIN B3
(NIACIN)

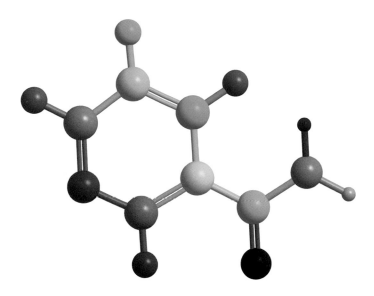

Category

Vitamin B3, also known as niacin, is a water-soluble vitamin. It is sometimes called nicotinic acid, as it was first isolated after chemical modification of the nicotine in tobacco. Although vitamin B4 has some structural similarities to nicotine, it does not act in any way like nicotine and cannot be converted into nicotine in the body in any way. Vitamin B3 was originally known as vitamin PP before it was reclassified as a B-complex vitamin.

Cellular Location

Vitamin B3 is distributed throughout the body via the bloodstream. Inside cells, it is metabolized to energy-forming compounds, called NAD and NADP (see below, in biological & ocular importance). In the liver, small amounts of excess vitamin B3 are also metabolized to NAD and NADP, which can also be stored there.

Structure

Vitamin B3 is a relatively small ring acid. It is a carboxylic acid with a carbon-and-nitrogen ring, called a pyridine ring.

Mechanisms of Action

Vitamin B3 is required for the functioning of several dozen enzymes and is a precursor to molecules involved in energy production.

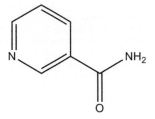

Biological & Ocular Importance

● **Involved in energy production**   Vitamin B3 is a precursor to nicotinamide adenine dinuclotide (NAD) and nicotinamide adenine dinuclotide phosphate (NADP), which are molecules that are involved in certain pathways to make ATP, the energy packets of cells.

In the absence of vitamin B3, NAD and NADP can be made from tryptophan, an amino acid (building block of proteins), with the help of vitamin B2, vitamin B6, and iron.

Because vitamin B3 helps with the utilization and creation of energy resources, it has been suggested to treat fatigue and irritability.

● **Lowers cholesterol**
Vitamin B3 is often used to reduce cholesterol levels in the body. It is believed to act in this role by releasing fatty acids from fat stores, which in turn decreases the demand of the liver to create fatty acids. When the liver does create fatty acids, precursors for LDL cholesterol are formed. There are suggestions that vitamin B3 may also act directly to decrease the liver's

production of cholesterol precursors. As such, it is believed to also prevent atherosclerosis (blood vessel cholesterol clots and plaques that can result in heart disease and stroke, as well as artery or vein clots in the retina or optic nerve strokes). It may also lower blood pressure. Vitamin B3 has been noted to stimulate circulation of blood as well. As such, it has been suggested to treat migraine headaches, leg cramps, and arthritis.

● **Plays a role in diabetes**
There is some inconclusive evidence on whether vitamin B3 functions to decrease blood sugar in diabetes. Some of the suggestions are that it helps decrease the occurrence of insulin-dependent diabetes in children.

● **Protects neural cells from injury**   Vitamin B3 can protect against glutamate toxicity (see section on vitamin B12), or the toxic effects of excess glutamate release from the neural cells of the eye. Glutamate is a natural signaling chemical in neural cells

356

that enables signals to transfer from one cell to another. It is the main signal producer in the circuitry of the eye. However, excess glutamate is toxic to surrounding cells. When a cell dies, for example in glaucoma, it can release excess glutamate, which results in toxic injury and death of surrounding cells.

● **Involved in other functions in the body**   Vitamin B3 plays a role in the creation of red blood cells. It also is involved in the production of steroids and the sex hormones of the body. In addition, it may help with the digestion of food by releasing stomach acids.

Human Studies on Utility

Currently, there are only a handful of human studies on vitamin B3 use in eye disease reported in the scientifically-reviewed medical literature. These studies involve the macular degeneration and cataract, and are summarized below. There are three studies of vitamin B3 in the prevention and treatment of macular degeneration, which do not suggest a benefit of vitamin B3. There are five studies of vitamin B3 in cataract prevention, and suggest a benefit of vitamin B3. Nevertheless, the fact that there are only a few reported clinical studies does not necessarily imply a definite benefit or lack of benefit. Looking at the mechanism of action, the use of vitamin B3 in moderation may be possibly of benefit in many eye diseases.

● **In one large study: no benefits in past use of vitamin B3 found on risk of macular degeneration**
Looking forward over time, a study of nearly 3,000 people age 49 and over found no link (neither protective nor harmful) between the risk of having macular degeneration and taking any of the following nutrients (alone or in combination) in the past: vitamin B3, vitamin B6, vitamin B12, vitamin B1, vitamin B2, vitamin A, vitamin C, vitamin E, beta-carotene, folate or zinc.[13]

● **In one small study: no benefits from the use of vitamin B3 on the future risk of macular degeneration over time**   An older 1964 study of 85 people found no link (neither protective nor harmful) between a multivitamin with vitamins B3, B2, B6, and B12 and progression of macular diseases, such as macular degeneration.[142] Other studies at the time found similar findings.

● **Another small early study found a benefit: use of vitamin B3 decreases the future risk of macular degeneration over time**
A 1974 study of 14 people suggested a benefit of a multivitamin with vitamins B3, B2, B6, and B12, in protecting against

progression of macular diseases, such as macular degeneration.[143] However, the study was too small and of too short a duration to provide any conclusive findings.

● **Three large studies found past use of vitamin B3 associated with decreased risk of cataract**   A large study of nearly 3,000 people age 49 to 97 found that past use of vitamin B3 in higher doses reduced the risk of having cataracts by 30%. Likewise, the past use of multivitamins was associated with a decreased risk of having cataracts as well. The use of vitamin A in higher doses reduced the risk of having cataracts by 90%, the use of vitamin B1 in higher doses reduced the risk of having cataracts by 30 to 40% depending on the type of cataract, the use of vitamin B2 in higher doses reduced the risk of having cataracts by 30%, and the use of folate reduced the risk of having cataracts by 40 to 60% depending on the type of cataract. The study did not find any link (neither protective nor harmful) between the use of vitamin B6 or vitamin B12 and cataract.[51]

A study of nearly 3,000 people found that the past intake of vitamin B3, vitamin B1, vitamin B2, vitamin A, iron, and zinc decreased the risk of having certain types of cataract by 30 to 50%.[62] It is interesting to note that in this study, iron was associated with a decrease in risk of having cataract, and not an increased risk, as some physicians have predicted. Furthermore, it is surprising that no link (neither protective nor harmful) was found between vitamin C use and cataract, despite other studies showing a benefit.

A study of nearly 1,800 people found that the past intake of vitamin B3, vitamin B1, vitamin B2, vitamin A, vitamin C, and vitamin E was associated with a decreased risk of having certain types of cataract. This decrease in risk ranged between 40 to 55%. Also, the study found that use of any multivitamin was associated with a 30% decrease in the overall risk of having cataracts. However, the study found no link (neither protective nor harmful) between iron and the risk of having cataract.[61]

● **Another large study found mixed results: past use of vitamin B3 associated with decreased risk of certain types of cataract though an increased risk of other types of cataract**   A study of over 2,000 people found that the past intake of vitamin A, vitamin B3, vitamin B1, vitamin B2, vitamin B6, vitamin C, vitamin E, and folate were each associated with a decreased risk of having a certain type of cataract (called nuclear sclerosis). However, each of these nutrients was also associated with an increased risk of having another type of cataract (called cortical cataract).[53] The researchers suggest that the finding of increased cortical cataracts reflects the possibility that the presence of nuclear sclerosis cataracts masked the finding of cortical cataracts and skewed the results. This study exemplifies how difficult it is at times to interpret results and make meaningful extrapolations.

● **One large study found a benefit: use of vitamin B3 decreases the future risk of cataract over time** A study of over 2,000 people given a multivitamin or a placebo for 5 years found a 36% decrease in the risk of developing cataracts in those people who were age 65 to 74. Of note, there was no difference in risk in the younger group age 45 to 64. These results exemplify the positive benefit of multivitamins; however, it is difficult to apply these results to a healthy population, as the study was performed on somewhat nutritionally-deprived people in rural China.[33]

The researchers also looked at specific nutrients in a group of over 3,000 people from the same population. Those who took vitamin B3 (40 mg) and vitamin B2 (5.2 mg) daily for 5 years had a 41% decrease in the risk of developing cataracts, compared to those who took placebo. In contrast, no link was found (neither beneficial nor harmful) over the 5-year period between the risk of cataract and taking selenium with beta-carotene and vitamin E, or taking vitamin A and zinc, or taking vitamin C and molybdenum.[33]

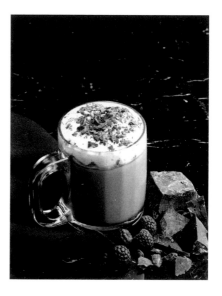

Body Absorption, Metabolism, & Excretion

Nearly the entire amount of vitamin B3 ingested is absorbed easily and rapidly in the stomach and the intestines, after which it is distributed throughout the body via the bloodstream. Inside cells, it is metabolized to NAD and NADP.

In the liver, small amounts of excess vitamin B3 are also metabolized to NAD and NADP, which also can be stored there. Most of the excess vitamin B3, however, is filtered by the kidneys for excretion.

Deficiency

Pure vitamin B3 deficiency is uncommon, because, in the absence of vitamin B3, NAD and NADP can be made from tryptophan, with the help of vitamin B2, vitamin B6, and iron. However, when there is a more generalized nutritional deficiency, vitamin B3 deficiency becomes prominent.

Pellagra is a disorder of vitamin B3 deficiency. Pellagra was first described by Italian Dr. Francesco Frapolli in 1771, who called it "pelle agra" which means rough skin in Italian. Pellagra is characterized by diarrhea, dermatitis, and dementia, and may lead to death. These four characteristics have been termed the "four D's" of pellagra. The dermatitis is a light sensitivity in the skin that results in darkening and increased roughness of the skin in light. This dermatitis is often an early sign of vitamin B3 deficiency. The diarrhea often results from abnormal functioning of the gastrointestinal tract and poor absorption of fat and the fat-soluble vitamins. Lack of adequate stomach acid to properly digest food exacerbates the situation. Other characteristics include dizziness, headaches, and disorientation. People with pellagra are often described as being shiftless, disoriented, lazy, and silly. Loss of appetite, indigestion, and muscle tremors can occur. These features of pellagra can occur in milder forms in people with milder vitamin B3 deficiency.

Toxicity & Side Effects

Most of the toxic effects of vitamin B3 caused by high doses are reversible upon cessation of the high doses of vitamin B3.

There are numerous cases of vitamin B3 toxicity in the eye. Over 70 cases have been reported to the National Registry of Drug-Induced Ocular Side Effects. Most of these cases involve blurred vision and swelling of the retina. Some of the blurred vision is likely caused by swelling of the retina, but other cases of blurred vision may have been caused by other mechanisms. The swelling of the retina, called cystoid macular edema, is fluid build up in the center of the retina, known as the macula, which results in blurred vision. The cause of the swelling is unknown, though it is thought that the swelling results from inflammation from a direct toxic response of the vitamin B3 in the macula.

Other eye side effects that have been reported include dryness of the eyes, swelling of the eyelids, discoloration of the eyelids, bulging out of the eyes, loss of eyelashes, and loss of eyebrows.

Most of the cases of eye toxicity have occurred with doses of 3,000 mg per day, though some have occurred with doses as low as 1,500 mg per day.

In doses of 50 mg or more, vitamin B3 can also cause a red flush through the skin, which is associated with itching and warmth. This flush lasts up to about 15 to 20 minutes and is caused by histamines released by the skin that cause the blood vessels to dilate and initiate the itching.

Vitamin B3 may help the digestion of food by releasing stomach acids. However, in people who are predisposed to stomach ulcers, these stomach acids can cause or exacerbate stomach ulcers. Therefore, vitamin B3 in moderate- to high-doses should be avoided.

Also, there are some reports of liver inflammation from extremely high doses (greater than 500 mg daily) of vitamin B3.

Interactions with Other Nutrients

Vitamin B6 can help form vitamin B3 derivatives, by converting tryptophan into vitamin B3 derivatives. Pure vitamin B3 deficiency is uncommon, because, in the absence of vitamin B3, NAD and NADP can be made from tryptophan, with the help of vitamin B2, vitamin B6, and iron (see page 356).

Vitamin B3, vitamin B6, and iron play roles in the pathway of forming carnitine (see section on carnitine).

Glutathione can be made through a pathway that involves alpha lipoic acid, vitamin B3, and cysteine. The conversion of lipoic acid into dihydrolipoic acid often occurs by one of the co-enzymes (or enzyme helper) NAD or NADP. In this process, the oxidized sulfur amino acid cystine is converted to the biologically-useful sulfur amino acid cysteine. Cysteine can then be recycled into the cell and used to form glutathione (see sections on glutathione and N-acetyl-cysteine).

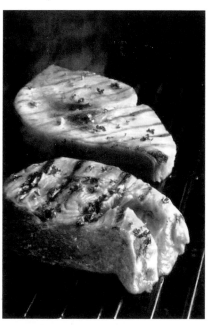

Ideal Dosage

The recommended daily dose ranges from 14 to 18 mg per day. In boys age 14 to 18, and in men over age 18, the recommended dose is 16 mg per day. In girls age 14 to 18, and in women over age 18, it is 14 mg per day. During pregnancy, the recommended dose increases to 18 mg per day, and during lactation, 17 mg per day.

It may be best to obtain a daily dose of about 25 to 50 mg per day in a diet with adequate protein intake. In a low protein diet though, doses of 50 to 100 mg may be more appropriate.

Sources (Where to Find It)

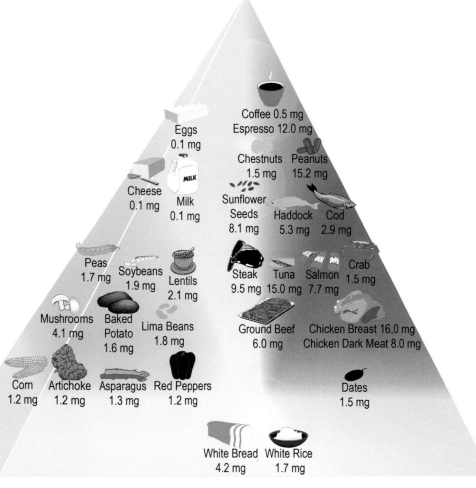

Coffee 0.5 mg
Espresso 12.0 mg

Eggs 0.1 mg

Chestnuts 1.5 mg   Peanuts 15.2 mg

Cheese 0.1 mg   Milk 0.1 mg

Sunflower Seeds 8.1 mg   Haddock 5.3 mg   Cod 2.9 mg

Peas 1.7 mg   Soybeans 1.9 mg   Lentils 2.1 mg

Steak 9.5 mg   Tuna 15.0 mg   Salmon 7.7 mg   Crab 1.5 mg

Mushrooms 4.1 mg   Baked Potato 1.6 mg   Lima Beans 1.8 mg

Ground Beef 6.0 mg   Chicken Breast 16.0 mg   Chicken Dark Meat 8.0 mg

Corn 1.2 mg   Artichoke 1.2 mg   Asparagus 1.3 mg   Red Peppers 1.2 mg

Dates 1.5 mg

White Bread 4.2 mg   White Rice 1.7 mg

Pyramid Key:

Fats & Sweets

Dairy   Meats & Nuts

Vegetables   Fruits

Breads & Grains

The top sources of vitamin B3 are chicken breast, peanuts, and tuna. Other sources rich in vitamin B3 include espresso, steak, sunflower seeds, dark chicken meat, and salmon.

*See Guides on Pages 467-468.

VITAMIN B6
(PYRIDOXINE,
PYRIDOXAL,
PYRIDOXAMINE)

Category

Vitamin B6 is actually a family of similar water-soluble vitamins known as pyridoxine, pyridoxal, and pyridoxamine.

Cellular Location

A large quantity, about ¾, of vitamin B6 is found in muscles as a phosphate derivative of pyridoxal. The liver stores another 10% of vitamin B6, and the remainder is distributed through the body.

Structure

Vitamin B6 is a relatively small-ring alcohol. It is formed by carbon, hydrogen, and oxygen groups attached to a carbon-and-nitrogen ring, called a pyridine ring. It also comes in other forms, such as pyridoxal (the aldehyde form) and pyridoxamine (the amine form).

Mechanisms of Action

The different forms of vitamin B6 act to help enzymes in dozens of essential chemical reactions in the body. Vitamin B6 plays roles in many cellular activities, ranging from energy production to making neurotransmitter signaling molecules.

Biological & Ocular Importance

● **Helps produce energy & protein building blocks**
Vitamin B6 plays a central role in the production of energy from proteins and fat, and also helps in the production of amino acids (building block of proteins).

● **Required for production of neurotransmitter signaling molecules** Vitamin B6 helps in the production of neurotrans-mitters. Many neurotransmitters, compounds that provide signaling between neurons, are made using enzymes that require vitamin B6. These neurotrans-mitters include serotonin, GABA, dopamine, and norepinephrine.

As such, vitamin B6 has been used to treat depression and premenstrual syndrome. It has also been suggested for carpal tunnel syndrome; though the cause of carpal tunnel syndrome is a compression of nerve fibers rather than an imbalance in neurotransmitters.

● **Increases antioxidant glutathione & decreases toxic homocysteine** Vitamin B6 with zinc helps convert the toxic molecule homocysteine into glutathione, and helps ensure lower levels of toxic homocysteine. Elevated levels of homocysteine are associated with Alzheimer's disease as well as vascular disease, including blood clots, heart disease, stroke, and vein occlusions in the retina. This detoxification occurs along with other nutrients (see below under interactions with other nutrients). Because of this role, vitamin B6 has been recommended in the prevention and treatment of the above diseases.

● **Protects neural cells from injury** Vitamin B6 can protect against glutamate toxicity (see section on vitamin B12), which involves the toxic effects of excess glutamate release from the neural cells of the eye. Glutamate is a natural signaling chemical in neural cells that enables signals to transfer from one cell to another. It is the main signal producer in the circuitry of the eye. However, excess glutamate is toxic to surrounding cells. When a cell dies, for example in glaucoma, it can release excess glutamate, resulting in toxic injury and death of surrounding cells.

● **Blocks actions of steroids & hormones** Vitamin B6 can bind to steroid and hormone receptors in the nucleus of cells to prevent the steroid or the hormone from providing its action. Because of its ability to regulate steroids and hormones, it has been used to also treat morning sickness during pregnancy.

● **Helps produce red blood cells** Vitamin B6 helps enzymes in the production of red blood cells that carry oxygen throughout the body.

● **Helps the immune defense system** Vitamin B6 may also help support the immune defense system.

● **Decreases retinal disease in a disorder called gyrate atrophy** The use of vitamin B6 has been reported to be helpful in people with gyrate atrophy.

Gyrate atrophy is a rare inherited disorder of cellular metabolism of ornithine (an amino acid that plays a role in the formation of arginine, another amino acid involved in building proteins). Ornithine also plays a significant role in the removal of excess nitrogen from cells through a process called the urea cycle. Deficiency of the enzyme involved in the cellular metabolism of ornithine results in excess build-up of ornithine and a disease called gyrate atrophy. Gyrate atrophy is a retinal disease resulting in night-blindness and loss of peripheral (or side) vision. One of the enzymes in the metabolism of ornithine works with vitamin B6, a cofactor, or substance that helps in the enzymatic process (see section on vitamin B6). Increasing dietary intake of vitamin B6 results in more metabolism of ornithine and decreased build-up of ornithine in the bloodstream and tissues of concern. Also, these people are asked to decrease their intake of the amino acid arginine, which is a precursor in the ornithine metabolism pathway.

Restriction in arginine along with the use of vitamin B6 has been reported to be helpful in people with gyrate atrophy. (see section on arginine).

Currently, there are only a handful of human studies on vitamin B6 use in eye disease reported in the scientifically-reviewed medical literature. These studies involve the diseases: macular degeneration, diabetic retinopathy, and cataract. These studies are summarized below. Nevertheless, the fact that there are only a few reported clinical studies does not necessarily imply a definite benefit or lack of benefit. Looking at the mechanism of action, the use of vitamin B6 in moderation may be possibly of benefit in many eye diseases.

● One study found a benefit to past use of vitamin B6 on risk of diabetic retinopathy

A 1991 study of 18 diabetic people found that those who took vitamin B6 supplements did not have diabetic retinopathy. However, it is unclear whether they did not have diabetic retinopathy for other reasons, as the study was not controlled (there was no comparison group of diabetics who did not take vitamin B6). Thus, the results are inconclusive.[144]

● One study found no benefit from the use of vitamin B6 for the retinal disease gyrate atrophy

A 1985 study looked at vitamin B6 supplementation for people with gyrate atrophy. Gyrate atrophy is a rare inherited disorder of cellular metabolism of ornithine

(an amino acid that plays a role in the formation of arginine, another amino acid involved in building proteins). Ornithine also plays a significant role in the removal of excess nitrogen from cells through a process called the urea cycle. Deficiency of the enzyme involved in the cellular metabolism of ornithine results in excess build-up of ornithine and a disease called gyrate atrophy. Gyrate atrophy is a retinal disease resulting in night-blindness and loss of peripheral (or side) vision.

The study looked at 2 people with gyrate atrophy who received vitamin B6 supplements, and 4 who received proline supplements. There is no clear evidence of any benefit of vitamin B6 supplementation and in fact the study found no increase in vitamin B6 levels in the bloodstream.[121]

Summary of Studies for Macular Degeneration:

Three clinical trials have been performed looking at the role of vitamin B6 in both preventing and treating macular degeneration.

Vitamin B6 for
Macular Degeneration
Scale of Benefit

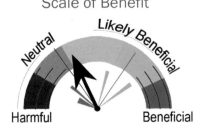

As a whole, the clinical studies provide no definitive answer as to whether vitamin B6 is beneficial. Only one of the three studies found no benefit to vitamin B6 for macular degeneration. Looking at the mechanisms of action, there may be good reason to use vitamin B6 in moderation for macular degeneration.

● In two studies: no benefits in past use of vitamin B6 found on risk of macular degeneration
An older 1964 study of 85 people found no link (neither protective nor harmful) between a multivitamin with vitamins B6, B2, B3, and B12 and progression of macular diseases, such as macular degeneration.[142] Other studies at the time found similar findings.

Looking forward over time, a study of nearly 3,000 people age 49 and over found no link (neither protective nor harmful) between the risk of having macular degeneration and taking any of the following nutrients (alone or in combination) in the past: vitamin B6, vitamin B12, vitamin B1, vitamin B2, vitamin B3, vitamin A, vitamin C, vitamin E, beta-carotene, folate or zinc.[13]

● One study found a benefit to past use of vitamin B6 on risk of macular degeneration
A 1974 study of 14 people suggested a benefit of a multivitamin with vitamins B6, B2, B3, and B12, in protecting against progression of macular diseases, such as macular degeneration.[143] However, the study was too small and of too short a duration to provide any conclusive findings.

Summary of Studies for Cataract: Two clinical trials have been performed looking at the role of vitamin B6 in preventing cataract.

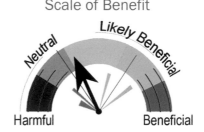

Vitamin B6 for
Cataract
Scale of Benefit

As a whole, the clinical studies provide no definitive answer as to whether vitamin B6 is beneficial. Looking at the mechanisms of action, there may be good reason to use vitamin B6 in moderation for cataract.

● In one study: no benefits in past use of vitamin B6 found on risk of cataract
A large study of nearly 3,000 people age 49 to 97 found no link (neither protective nor harmful) between the use of vitamin B6 or vitamin B12 and cataract. The study did find that past use of folate reduced the risk of having cataracts by 40 to 60% depending on the type of cataract. Likewise, the past use of multivitamins was associated with a decreased risk of having cataracts as well. The use of vitamin A in higher doses reduced the risk of having cataracts by 90%, the use of vitamin B1 in higher doses reduced the risk of having cataracts by 30 to 40% depending on the type of cataract, the use of vitamin B2 in higher doses reduced

the risk of having cataracts by 30%, and the use of vitamin B3 in higher doses reduced the risk of having cataracts by 30%.[51]

● **Another large study found mixed results: past use of vitamin B6 associated with decreased risk of certain types of cataract though an increased risk of other types of cataract** A study of over 2,000 people found that the past intake of vitamin B6, vitamin B1, vitamin B2, vitamin B3, vitamin A, vitamin C, vitamin E, and folate were each associated with a decreased risk of having a certain type of cataract (called nuclear sclerosis). However, each of these nutrients was also associated with an increased risk of having another type of cataract (called cortical cataract).[53] The researchers suggest that the finding of increased cortical cataracts reflects the possibility that the presence of nuclear sclerosis cataracts masked the finding of cortical cataracts and skewed the results. This study exemplifies how difficult it is at times to interpret results and make meaningful extrapolations.

Body Absorption, Metabolism, & Excretion

Vitamin B6 is quickly and easily absorbed in the intestines. About 75% of the vitamin B6 in the diet is absorbed. Since the body is not able to absorb the phosphate derivatives of vitamin B6 in the diet, they must be broken down by the digestive tract to remove the phosphate so that the non-phosphate form then can be absorbed.

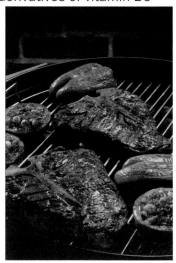

Excess vitamin B6 is excreted through filtration by the kidneys.

Deficiency

Vitamin B6 must be obtained from the diet because the body cannot produce its own supply of it.

Since vitamin B6 assists in forming neurotransmitters, a deficiency of vitamin B6 can be associated with mood disturbances, nervousness, irritability, sleepiness, and depression. Furthermore, disease of the peripheral nerves, such as those to the arms and legs, is often caused by long-term vitamin B6 deficiency.

Mouth sores and tongue swelling have also been reported in vitamin B6 deficiency.

Optic nerve disease has been reported as a rare occurrence in vitamin B6 deficiency.

Toxicity & Side Effects

Side effects of excess vitamin B6 include headaches, and sleepiness. Shooting pains, numbness, difficulties with balance, and other sensory disturbances in the arms and legs can occur from peripheral nerve toxicities from vitamin B6. These nerve toxicities occur at doses of 200 mg or more each day.

Gastrointestinal side effects include upset stomach, nausea, vomiting, and abdominal pains. There is some unconfirmed suggestion that long-term doses of vitamin B6 in amounts of 3½ to 7½ mg each day may increase the chance of developing an inflammatory disease of the gastrointestinal tract, called ulcerative colitis.

Interactions with Other Nutrients

There are numerous interactions between vitamin B6 and other nutrients. The important concept is that a balance should be achieved between intake of vitamin B6 and other nutrients.

Vitamin B6 can help form vitamin B3 derivatives, by converting tryptophan, an amino acid (building block of proteins), into vitamin B3 derivatives: NAD and NADP (see section on vitamin B3).

When the body is producing its own coenzyme Q10, vitamin B6 is required in the first step.

Vitamin B3, vitamin B6, and iron play roles in the pathway of forming carnitine (see section on carnitine). SAMe plays a role in providing methyl groups to methionine, an amino acid, which follows a pathway into carnitine. Vitamin C plays an important role in two of the steps of the formation of carnitine.

The activation of vitamin B6 and folate both require vitamin B2 in the pathway.

There are several nutrients (vitamin B6, vitamin B12, folate, selenium, SAMe, methionine, and N-acetyl-cysteine) that act in the same complex circular pathway and are all interrelated when it comes to: (1) the toxicity of homocysteine and decreasing its levels, and (2) the activities of SAMe as a donator of methyl groups (see sections on folate, vitamin B12, vitamin B6, selenium, SAMe, and N-acetyl-cysteine). Homocysteine is a toxic chemical that is associated with Alzheimer's disease as well as vascular disease, including blood clots, heart disease, stroke, and vein occlusions in the retina.

Folate plays an important role in the process of converting the toxic chemical homocysteine into methionine. The particular enzyme that converts homocysteine back to methionine is, in fact, one of only two enzymes throughout our body that depend on vitamin B12 for their activity. SAMe participates in this cycle by donating methyl groups (see sections on vitamin B12 and SAMe).

Not only do vitamin B12 and folate work together in regulating homocysteine levels, vitamin B6 and zinc regulate homocysteine levels by helping convert homocysteine into glutathione, which ensures lower levels of toxic homocysteine. Selenium is required in this pathway as these glutathione enzymes are selenoproteins, composed of selenium with the protein. N-acetyl-cysteine may lower homocysteine levels as well, by converting homocysteine into the protein building block cysteine, an amino acid.

Choline also interacts in this complex homocysteine pathway. Choline forms a chemical, called betaine, in the body, and betaine works to convert homocysteine to methionine, in order to decrease levels of homocysteine in the body.

SAMe plays a role in providing methyl groups to methionine, which follows a pathway into carnitine.

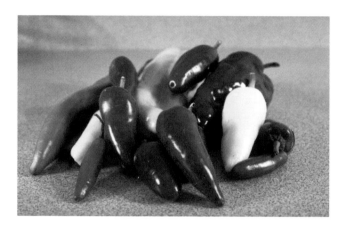

Ideal Dosage

The recommended daily dose ranges from 1.2 to 2.0 mg per day. In boys age 14 to 18, and in men age 19 to 50, the recommended dose is 1.3 mg per day. In men over age 50, the recommended dose is 1.7 mg per day. In girls age 14 to 18, the recommended dose is 1.2 mg per day. In women age 19 to 50, the recommended dose is 1.3 mg per day, and in women over age 50, it is 1.5 mg per day. During pregnancy, the recommended dose increases to 1.9 mg per day, and during lactation, 2.0 mg per day.

It may be best to obtain a daily dose of about 2 to 4 mg per day, with higher doses in those who consume more protein.

The upper limit of what is considered safe for most adults is about 100 mg per day. However, for gyrate atrophy, the recommended dosage of vitamin B6 is 300 to 500 mg per day.

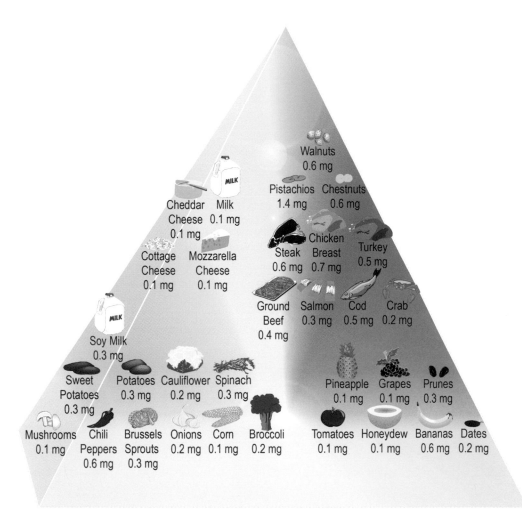

Walnuts
0.6 mg

Pistachios   Chestnuts
1.4 mg   0.6 mg

Cheddar   Milk
Cheese   0.1 mg
0.1 mg

Chicken
Steak   Breast   Turkey
0.6 mg   0.7 mg   0.5 mg

Cottage   Mozzarella
Cheese   Cheese
0.1 mg   0.1 mg

Ground   Salmon   Cod   Crab
Beef   0.3 mg   0.5 mg   0.2 mg
0.4 mg

Soy Milk
0.3 mg

Sweet   Potatoes   Cauliflower   Spinach
Potatoes   0.3 mg   0.2 mg   0.3 mg
0.3 mg

Pineapple   Grapes   Prunes
0.1 mg   0.1 mg   0.3 mg

Mushrooms   Chili   Brussels   Onions   Corn   Broccoli
0.1 mg   Peppers   Sprouts   0.2 mg   0.1 mg   0.2 mg
0.6 mg   0.3 mg

Tomatoes   Honeydew   Bananas   Dates
0.1 mg   0.1 mg   0.6 mg   0.2 mg

Pyramid Key:

Fats & Sweets

Dairy   Meats & Nuts

Vegetables   Fruits

Breads & Grains

Top sources of vitamin B6 are nuts (particularly pistachios), meats (such as chicken breast and steak), bananas, and chili peppers.

*See Guides on Pages 467-468.

VITAMIN B9
(SEE FOLATE)

VITAMIN B12
(COBALAMIN)

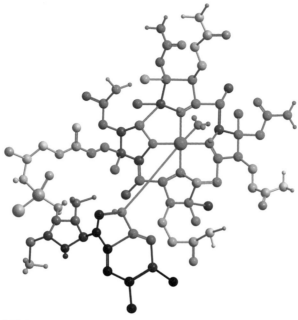

Category

Vitamin B12, also known as cobalamin, is an essential water-soluble vitamin. It is also a cobalt-containing vitamin.

Cellular Location

Extra vitamin B12 is stored primarily in the liver, but it can also be stored in the bones, muscles, heart, kidney, spleen, and brain. The remaining vitamin B12 is delivered via the bloodstream throughout the body.

Structure

Vitamin B12 is a large, complexly-structured vitamin. It contains a cobalt atom in its center surrounded by concentric, smaller rings within a larger ring. Vitamin B12 comes in many similar forms, including hydroxocobalamin, cyanocobalamin, aquacobalamin, nitrocobalamin, methylcobalamin, and 5'-deoxyadenosylcobalamin. The latter two are the active forms in the body. Our cells possess the ability to convert any of the forms into the active forms.

Mechanisms of Action

Vitamin B12 is important for 2 major enzyme reactions. One involves the formation of methionine from a toxin called homocysteine. The other involves the formation of a molecule called succinyl CoA, which is involved in many reactions in the body's cells.

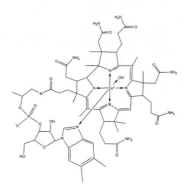

Biological & Ocular Importance

● **Required for making a molecule called succinyl CoA which is essential to many important reactions in the body**   Vitamin B12 is required for the synthesis of the molecule called succinyl CoA, which is involved in the production of amino acids (building block of proteins), membrane phospholipids (unique fatty compounds, see page 228), steroids and hormones, neurotransmitters, large complex cyclic-ring molecules, such as hemoglobin (the molecule in red blood cells that carries oxygen). As such, it plays a major role in the production of red blood cells that carry oxygen. It has also been suggested for other diseases such as Alzheimer's disease and depression, and it is believed to enhance the immune defense system as well.

● **Protects DNA from damage**
Vitamin B12's role in the formation of methionine results in its ability to protect DNA by playing a role in the pathway that eventually provides methyl groups to create DNA. Thus, it is essential in the process of making DNA and also plays a role in repairing damage to DNA. Research suggests that DNA damage is an important precursor to cancer formation. Therefore, vitamin B12 has been suggested to prevent cancer.

● **Required for insulation around nerves including the optic nerve**   SAMe is believed to be required for myelin synthesis. Vitamin B12 is required for maintenance of the myelin sheath (the insulation around nerves fibers that enables the signals to be sent efficiently).

● **Plays a role in production of energy**   Vitamin B12 plays a role in the production of energy during the body's metabolism of protein and fats.

● **Acts indirectly as an antioxidant & decreases toxic**

homocysteine Vitamin B2 acts with folate as an indirect antioxidant by decreasing stress on protein-building organelles within cells by reducing the activity of homocysteine, an amino acid (building block of proteins) known to cause atherosclerosis (blood vessel cholesterol clots and plaques that can result in heart disease and stroke, as well as artery or vein clots in the retina or optic nerve strokes). Homocysteine signals stress in the protein-building organelles and causes proteins to be misfolded. High levels of homocysteine have been associated with blood vessel blockages in the retina as well as Alzheimer's disease. Taurine, betaine, and vitamin B2 also help reduce homocysteine levels.

● **Protects neural cells from injury** Vitamin B12 can protect against the toxic effects of excess glutamate release from the neural cells of the eye. These neural cells include the rod and cone photoreceptors, other retinal circuit neurons, and the retinal ganglion cells that form axons that comprise the optic nerve. Glutamate is a natural signaling chemical in neural cells that enables signals to transfer from one cell to another. It is the main signal producer in the circuitry of the eye. However, excess glutamate is toxic to surrounding cells. When a cell dies, for example in glaucoma, it can release excess glutamate, resulting in toxic injury and death of surrounding cells. Vitamin B12, as well as vitamins B1, B3, B6, and S-adenosyl-methionine (SAMe) may protect against glutamate toxicity.

Human Studies on Utility

Currently, there are only a handful of human studies on vitamin B12 use in eye disease reported in the scientifically-reviewed medical literature. These studies involve glaucoma, macular degeneration, vein occlusions in the retina, and cataract. The studies are summarized below. Nevertheless, the fact that there are only a few reported clinical studies does not necessarily imply a definite benefit or lack of benefit. Looking at the mechanism of action, the use of vitamin B6 in moderation may be possibly of benefit in many eye diseases.

● **In two studies: use of vitamin B12 protects visual fields in glaucoma over time**
A Japanese study in 1982 of over 300 people with glaucoma found that peripheral visual fields improved after supplementation with vitamin B12 (1,500 IU each day for 9 months). While 30% of the glaucoma subjects improved, it remains uncertain whether the improvement represented a natural

fluctuation in the disease process, or true benefit.[145]

Another Japanese study of 64 people with glaucoma found that over a period of 5 years, vitamin B12 (1,500 μg each day) decreased the progression of peripheral visual fields deterioration compared to no vitamin B12 supplementation.[146]

● **In two studies: no benefits in past use of vitamin B12 found on risk of macular degeneration** An older 1964 study of 85 people found no link (neither protective nor harmful) between a multivitamin with vitamins B12, B2, B3, and B6 and progression of macular diseases, such as macular degeneration.[142] Other studies at the time found similar findings.

Looking forward over time, a study of nearly 3,000 people age 49 and over found no link (neither protective nor harmful) between the risk of having macular degeneration and taking any of the following nutrients (alone or in combination) in the past: vitamin B12, vitamin B1, vitamin B2, vitamin B3, vitamin B6, vitamin A, vitamin C, vitamin E, beta-carotene, folate or zinc.[13]

● **One study found a benefit to past use of vitamin B12 on risk of macular degeneration** A 1974 study of 14 people suggested a benefit of a multivitamin with vitamins B12, B2, B3, and B6, in protecting against progression of macular diseases, such as macular degeneration.[143] However, the study was too small

and of too short a duration to provide any conclusive findings.

● **In several studies: no link between blood levels of vitamin B12 and vein occlusions in the retina** An analysis that looked at 4 studies of nearly 300 people with vein occlusions compared to nearly 300 control people found that those who had vein occlusions had lower levels of folate in their blood. The same study did not find any difference in blood levels of vitamin B12 between the two groups.[50]

● **In one small study: no link between blood levels of vitamin B12 and optic nerve disease** A study of 26 people with nutritional amblyopia (a disorder of poor nutrition and optic nerve dysfunction) found that those with nutritional amblyopia had lower levels of folate in their blood than the control groups. Interestingly, vitamin B12 levels were not found to be reduced, even though vitamin B12 is known to be associated with similar optic nerve dysfunction.[52]

● **In one study: no benefits in past use of vitamin B12 found on risk of cataract** A large study of nearly 3,000 people age 49 to 97 found no link (neither protective nor harmful) between the use of vitamin B12 or vitamin B6 and cataract. The study did find that past use of folate reduced the risk of having cataracts by 40 to 60% depending on the type of cataract. Likewise, the past use of multivitamins was associated with a decreased risk of having cataracts as well. The use of vitamin A in higher doses reduced the risk of having cataracts by 90%, the use of vitamin B1 in higher doses reduced the risk of having cataracts by 30 to 40% depending on the type of cataract, the use of vitamin B2 in higher doses reduced the risk of having cataracts by 30%, and the use of vitamin B3 in higher doses reduced the risk of having cataracts by 30%.[51]

Body Absorption, Metabolism, & Excretion

Most of the dietary vitamin B12 is bound to proteins and is digested by stomach acids to remove the proteins. It then becomes bound to a sugar-protein called intrinsic factor, which is required for absorption of vitamin B12. Usually about ¼ to ½ of the vitamin B12 in the diet is absorbed by the intestines into the bloodstream.

Little of the vitamin B12 ingested is excreted; however, the excess that is excreted is dumped back into the gastrointestinal tract with bile (a green fluid produced by the liver that is stored in the gallbladder to assist in digestion).

Deficiency

Because the body stores of vitamin B12 last for years, deficiency is uncommon. However, long-term deficiency can deplete these stores. Vitamin B12 is found in animal products and not in fruits or vegetables. Therefore, vegetarians and those who are malnourished, including alcoholics, are especially prone to vitamin B12 deficiency.

People with a specific disease that causes them not to produce adequate amounts of the sugar-protein intrinsic factor cannot absorb enough vitamin B12 and therefore develop vitamin B12 deficiency.

Vitamin B12 deficiency may be associated with anemia (insufficiency of the red blood cells that carry oxygen), because it plays a role in the production of red blood cells. In people who do not produce the sugar-protein intrinsic factor, the anemia is called pernicious anemia. Some of the symptoms of anemia include fatigue, shortness of breath, increased heart rate, mouth sores or ulcers, tongue soreness, pale skin, and brittle nails.

Neurological changes in vitamin B12 deficiency include numbness or tingling of the hands or feet or difficulties in balance. Other changes include memory loss, disorientation, mood disturbances, and dementia. These changes can often be treated successfully with injections of vitamin B12.

Vitamin B12 deficiency can cause optic neuropathy or decreased vision from optic nerve disease. Visual changes include blind spots and blurred vision. In children, vitamin B12 deficiency may cause amblyopia, (lazy eye).

Gastrointestinal changes that have been reported include loss of appetite, constipation, and a sore tongue.

Folate supplementation can mask the anemia of vitamin B12 deficiency. High-dose folate can correct anemia that is caused by vitamin B12 deficiency, without correcting the neurological disorders caused by vitamin B12 deficiency. Thus, high-dose folate can perpetuate the neurologic disorders that are caused by vitamin B12 deficiency.

Toxicity & Side Effects

Vitamin B12 is generally considered safe with no recommendations for upper limit of dosage. However, it is important to note that vitamin B12 can be detrimental in people with Leber's hereditary optic neuropathy (a genetic form of optic nerve disease characterized by sudden, frequent, and severe decreases in vision). Vitamin B12 has also been reported to worsen acne in those predisposed to acne formation.

Interactions with Other Nutrients

There are numerous interactions between vitamin B12 and other nutrients. The important concept is that a balance should be achieved between intake of vitamin B12 and other nutrients.

There are several nutrients (vitamin B12, vitamin B6, folate, selenium, SAMe, methionine, and N-acetyl-cysteine) that act in the same complex circular pathway and are all interrelated when it comes to: (1) the toxicity of homocysteine and decreasing its levels, and (2) the activities of SAMe as a donator of methyl groups (see sections on vitamin B6, SAMe, selenium, folate, methionine, and N-acetyl-cysteine). Homocysteine is a toxic chemical that is associated with Alzheimer's disease as well as vascular disease, including blood clots, heart disease, stroke, and vein occlusions in the retina.

These nutrients work to convert toxic homocysteine into methionine. However, high levels of methionine can result in increased production of homocysteine (see toxicity & side effects).

Folate plays an important role in the process of converting the toxic chemical homocysteine into methionine. The particular enzyme that converts homocysteine back to methionine is, in fact, one of only two enzymes throughout our body that depend on vitamin B12 for their activity. SAMe participates in this cycle by donating methyl groups (see sections on vitamin B12 and SAMe).

Not only do vitamin B12 and folate work together in regulating homocysteine levels, vitamin B6 and zinc regulate homocysteine levels by helping convert homocysteine into glutathione, which ensures lower levels of toxic homocysteine. Selenium is required in this pathway as these glutathione enzymes are selenoproteins, composed of selenium with the protein. N-acetyl-cysteine may lower homocysteine levels as well, by converting homocysteine into the protein building block cysteine, an amino acid.

Choline also interacts in this complex homocysteine pathway. Choline forms a chemical, called betaine, in the body, and betaine works to convert homocysteine to methionine, in order to decrease levels of homocysteine in the body.

SAMe plays a role in providing methyl groups to methionine, which follows a pathway into carnitine.

In addition to their interactions together in the homocysteine pathway, the activities of vitamin B12 and folate are so intertwined that a deficiency of vitamin B12 can result in a deficiency of folate within cells.

Ideal Dosage

The recommended daily dosage for vitamin B12 in children age 14 to 18 and in adults is 2.4 µg per day. During pregnancy, the recommended dose increases to 2.6 µg per day, and during lactation, 2.8 µg per day.

However, many researchers will recommend doses of 5 to 30 µg per day, while others recommend doses as high as 100 to 400 µg per day. It may be best, however, to obtain a daily dose of around 5 to 20 µg per day.

Cyanocobalamin is the commonly found form of vitamin B12 in dietary supplements. However, methylcobalamin is the more easily absorbable form of vitamin B12. Furthermore, methylcobalamin is an active form of vitamin B12 in our bodies, containing a methyl group attached to the cobalamin. Cyanocobalamin, which contains a cyanide group attached to the cobalamin, must be converted to methylcobalamin in order to be active. Cyanocobalamin is simply a common synthetic form of vitamin B12, a result of the method of making and filtering the vitamin in the laboratory. In addition to being the active form, methylcobalamin is more highly "reduced" than cyanocobalamin, meaning that it is stronger as an antioxidant, and it does not contain the cyanide, which can cause some stress in our cells. Thus, the preferred source of vitamin B12 supplements is the methylcobalamin form.

Sources (Where to Find It)

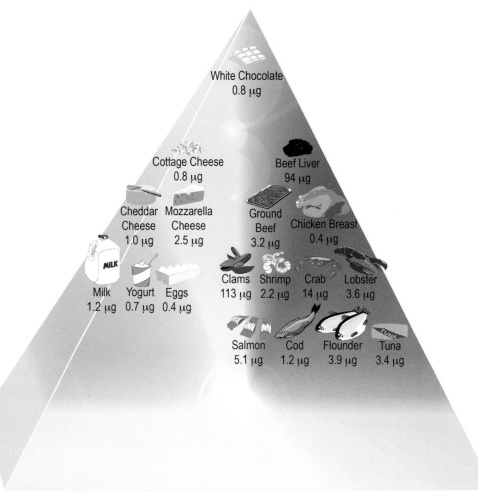

White Chocolate
0.8 µg

Cottage Cheese
0.8 µg

Beef Liver
94 µg

Cheddar   Mozzarella
Cheese   Cheese
1.0 µg   2.5 µg

Ground
Beef
3.2 µg

Chicken Breast
0.4 µg

MILK

Milk   Yogurt   Eggs
1.2 µg   0.7 µg   0.4 µg

Clams   Shrimp   Crab   Lobster
113 µg   2.2 µg   14 µg   3.6 µg

Salmon   Cod   Flounder   Tuna
5.1 µg   1.2 µg   3.9 µg   3.4 µg

Pyramid Key:

Fats & Sweets

Dairy   Meats & Nuts

Vegetables   Fruits

Breads & Grains

The top sources for vitamin B12 are clams, beef liver, and crab. Other sources that are rich in vitamin B12 include fish (particularly salmon and flounder), ground beef, and some cheeses (such as mozzarella cheese).

*See Guides on Pages 467-468.

VITAMIN BT
(SEE CARNITINE)

VITAMIN C
(ASCORBATE OR ASCORBIC ACID)

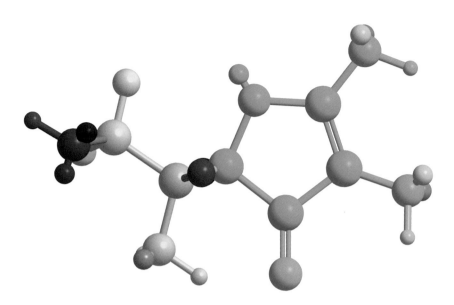

Category

Vitamin C is a hydrophilic or water-soluble vitamin. It is also known as ascorbate or ascorbic acid and was named vitamin C because of the "citrate" form that it is found in citrus fruits.

Cellular Location

Vitamin C is not stored by the body, but it is distributed throughout the body for use.

Vitamin C is found in extremely high concentrations, about 20-times its concentration in the blood levels, in the aqueous fluid behind the cornea that bathes the natural lens. The natural lens has about 10-times the amount of vitamin C levels as that of blood levels. Vitamin C is also in extremely high concentrations in the retina, about 100-fold its concentration found in blood levels!

Structure

Vitamin C is a ring compound with two acidic hydrogen atoms that are available for chemical reactions.

Mechanisms of Action

Vitamin C plays a role in many enzyme processes, including collagen-building. It is a powerful antioxidant as well.

Biological & Ocular Importance

● A very potent antioxidant

As a very potent antioxidant, vitamin C plays an important role in protecting against eye disease. Its chemical structure allows it to function as an antioxidant by donating electrons and reducing reactive oxygen species (toxic chemicals that result in oxidation).

It also acts as antioxidants by binding to metals that cause oxidative damage, such as iron and copper, and stabilizing the number of electrons in these metals. It also binds to heavy metals, such as cadmium, lead, and mercury.

● Protects the eye from oxidative damage

The intake of high doses of vitamin C is believed to decrease the risk of macular degeneration. The cells of the retina are particularly susceptible to oxidative damage. Thus, vitamin C, which is in extremely high concentrations in the retina, is believed to protect the retina from oxidative damage, which thereby decreases the risk of retinal diseases like macular degeneration.

Similarly, vitamin C is believed to play an antioxidant role in protecting the lens from cataract formation. The lens, which has high exposure to light, is at risk for oxidative damage, as light is collected by the lens to be focused on the retina. Vitamin C is found in extremely high concentrations in the aqueous fluid behind the cornea that bathes the natural lens. The intake of high doses of vitamin C over many years may reduce the risk of cataracts.

● As an antioxidant, vitamin C can protect the cells on the surface of the eye

These cells are involved in the process of ensuring that the eye is properly lubricated. The surface of the eye is coated by a thin layer of tear, called the tear film, which serves to lubricate and moisturize the eye surface. When this tear film evaporates, the cornea, which is particularly susceptible to dryness, begins to dry and the cells on its surface become damaged.

The tear film is composed of three layers. First, a mucin layer that is closest to the eye allows the tears to adhere more easily to the surface of the eye. This mucin component consists of glycoproteins (proteins conjugated with sugars). Second, an aqueous component consisting of water mixed with electrolytes or salts forms the bulk of the tear film and is the middle layer of the tear film. Third, a lipid component consisting of oils that stabilize the tear layer to prevent its evaporation. This lipid layer is the outermost layer of the tear film.

Vitamin A and omega oils are also required to ensure a proper tear film to lubricate the eye (see sections on vitamin A and omega-6 oils). The tear film is produced from nutrients and other components found in the bloodstream. Vitamin A is required for production of the mucins secreted from the eyelid glands for the natural tear layer. Omega-6 oils are involved in maintaining the lipid component of the tear film. Vitamin C is required to protect the cells on the surface of the eye that produce components of the tear film. In animal models, vitamin C can also protect corneal cells from oxidative injury.

● **Protects the heart & blood vessels** Vitamin C is believed to play an important role in reducing the risk of coronary heart disease and heart attacks. There is also some suggestion that vitamin C can lower cholesterol levels and decrease hypertension (high blood pressure).

● **Decreases risk of cancer**
Although there is some controversy regarding vitamin C's role in cancer prevention, vitamin C has been found to reduce the risk of development of many types of cancer, including stomach cancer and breast cancer.

● **Important in formation of melanin that protects against light toxicity**   Vitamin C also plays a role in synthesis of carnitine and tyrosine, two amino acids (building blocks of proteins). Tyrosine is important as a precursor to the thyroid hormones as well as to melanin (a pigment, which plays a major role in retinal pigment epithelium by absorbing excess light in order to protect against the light toxicity).

● **Builds collagen**   Vitamin C also works with proline and lysine to build and support collagen. Lysyl oxidase is an important enzyme that helps strengthen collagen, and it requires copper for function (see section on copper).

● **Collagen is essential in many parts of the eye**
Collagen is an important

component of many parts of the eye. It is the major protein of the cornea and its uniformity and pattern of arrangement is essential in maintaining the clarity of the cornea. Along with elastin it forms the layers of Bruch's membrane, a support layer that separates the retinal pigment epithelium from the underlying choroidal blood vessels. In wet macular degeneration as well as in extremely high myopia (near-sightedness), cracks can develop in Bruch's membrane through which new blood vessels grow that can lead to bleeding and scarring as well as detachment and distortion of the retina.

Collagen is essential in maintaining the trabecular meshwork, (the filtration site of the eye) by preventing it from collapsing. Allowing enough fluid to exit the eye is essential to prevent pressure build-up in the eye, decreasing the risk of glaucoma, since malfunction of this filtration site is a common mechanism of glaucoma.

Collagen also forms the lamina cribrosa, a structure that supports individual nerve fibers as they pass from the retina into the optic nerve. One mechanism of glaucoma is damage to these nerve fibers when the lamina cribrosa is unable to support them.

Collagen is also the major structural component of the vitreous. The vitreous gel is water supported by collagen and hyaluronic acid (see section on hyaluronic acid). In fact, the vitreous is 99% water supported in this collagen and hyaluronic acid meshwork. Vitreous floaters, which appear as cobwebs or spiders or spots floating in one's vision, occur when the vitreous begins to shrink. The vitreous shrinks at different ages for different people, often ranging from age 20 to age 70, though more commonly in the elderly. Decrease in collagen is associated with premature shrinking of the vitreous. Vitreous shrinking is associated with tears in the retina as well as detachments of the retina. Excess vitamin B2, excess copper or iron release into the vitreous, along with ultraviolet light, may also result in early or accelerated liquefaction of the vitreous gel.

● Strengthens capillaries

Collagen is also an important protein that forms skin, tendons, ligaments, and blood vessels as well. Vitamin C is also known to strengthen capillaries. Capillaries are where the arteries thin to the point of supplying tissue with nutrients and oxygen from the blood supply, in exchange for waste materials and carbon dioxide that must be transported out in veins. Capillary malfunction can result in tissue swelling, bleeding, and inappropriate control of tissue nutrition and oxygenation.

● Helps with colds?   Despite

common belief, there is little scientific evidence about the role of vitamin C in preventing the common cold! However, as an antioxidant, it can strengthen the body's immune defense system, as there is evidence to suggest its role in activating white blood cells.

● **Plays a role in forming neurotransmitter signaling molecules**   Vitamin C also plays a role in the formation of neurotransmitters, or communication signals that are used to send messages between neurons or brain cells. In fact, neurotransmitters, such as norepinephrine and serotonin, are made through vitamin C pathways.

Human Studies on Utility

Currently, there are numerous human studies on vitamin C in eye disease reported in the scientifically-reviewed medical literature. These studies involve several eye diseases, including dry eyes, glaucoma, macular degeneration, and cataract. The studies are described below.

● **In two studies: use of vitamin C improved stability of tear film to protect against dry eyes**   A study of 60 healthy young adults found that taking a multivitamin containing vitamins A, C, and E each day improved the stability of the tear film after just 10 days, compared with those who did not take the multivitamin. The study found that the tears remained stable for an over 40% longer period of time with the multivitamin. The study also found a similar benefit on the stability of the tear film with vitamin C alone.[128 & 147]

A more recent 2004 study of 60 people who took vitamin C and E found similar improvements in tear stability as well as improvements in the health of the cells on the surface of the eye that maintain adequate lubrication for the surface.[148]

● **Vitamin C associated with decreased pressure in the eye for prevention of glaucoma**   In the 1960's, studies on vitamin C found that its use in extremely high doses of 25,000 to 50,000 mg per day resulted in significant drops in the eye pressure. These doses were then lowered and divided up throughout the day, and similar results were observed. Vitamin C in doses of 500 mg four times a day has been shown in one study to decrease the pressure in the eye by 2 mmHg, probably by acting through collagen formation on

Looking at the mechanisms of action, there is good reason to use vitamin C in moderation for dry eyes, macular degeneration, and cataract.

maintaining the trabecular meshwork.

A study of 50 people found no link (neither protective nor harmful) between glaucoma and blood levels of vitamin C. The same study found lower blood levels of vitamin B1 decreased the risk of glaucoma.[141]

● **Vitamin C and protection of the retina** Studies in animals have also shown that vitamin C can protect photoreceptor cells from degenerating when exposed to high levels of light. There is evidence that lower circulating levels of vitamin C are associated with retinal disease, such as diabetic retinopathy.

A study of nearly 1,000 diabetics found no link (neither protective nor harmful) between vitamin C or vitamin E levels and the amount of retinal disease they had.[149]

Nevertheless, the lack of definitive clinical epidemiological evidence does not necessarily imply the inefficacy of vitamin C, as there is extensive mechanistic and physiologic research on the utility of vitamin C in the health of the eye.

Summary of Studies for Macular Degeneration:
Over a dozen clinical trials have been performed looking at the role of vitamin C in both preventing and treating macular degeneration. These clinical trials are of various types, some of which are very well-designed and well-performed studies.

As a whole, the clinical studies provide no definitive answer as to whether vitamin C is beneficial, and, in fact, the majority of studies found no benefit to vitamin C for macular degeneration. However, there is a little evidence from the studies (4 out of 18) that it may be beneficial, particularly in combination with other antioxidant nutrients. Looking at the mechanisms of action, there is good reason to use vitamin C in moderation for macular degeneration.

The studies can be summarized as follows: several large studies found no benefits or harms to the past use of vitamin C on the risk of macular degeneration, while two studies found a benefit in the past use of vitamin C in decreasing the risk of macular degeneration. However, one study found that the past use of vitamin C can be harmful and associated with an increased risk of macular degeneration. On the other hand, several studies have found no link (neither protective nor harmful) between levels of vitamin C in the blood and macular degeneration. A sixth

Vitamin C for Macular Degeneration Scale of Benefit

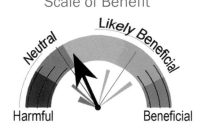

study also found no link between levels of vitamin C in the blood and macular degeneration, though the study did find a decreased risk of macular degeneration in those with higher blood levels of a combination of three of four nutrients including vitamin C.

In following people over time, four studies found that those who took vitamin C did not have any benefit in preventing macular degeneration compared to those who did not take vitamin C. More importantly, another study found that vitamin C by itself did not have any benefit in preventing macular degeneration, but in combination with other nutrients decreased the risk of macular degeneration by one-half! Also, another study found that the use of a multi-vitamin with vitamin C, as a precursor to vitamin C, decreases the future risk of macular degeneration over time.

● In large studies: no benefits in past use of vitamin C found on risk of macular degeneration

Looking forward over time, a study of nearly 3,000 people age 49 and over found no link (neither protective nor harmful) between the risk of having macular degeneration and taking any of the following nutrients (alone or in combination) in the past: vitamin C, vitamin A, vitamin B1, vitamin B2, vitamin B3, vitamin B6, vitamin B12, vitamin E, beta-carotene, folate or zinc.[13]

A study of over 1,000 people age 55 to 80 found no link (neither protective nor harmful) between macular degeneration and a diet high in vitamin C or E. The study did find that those who consumed a diet high in vitamin A had a greater than 40% decrease in the risk of having wet macular degeneration compared to those who did not consume a diet high in vitamin A. Similarly, dietary beta-carotene decreased the risk by 40% and dietary carotenoids decreased the risk by over 40%, while dietary lutein and zeaxanthin decreased the risk by nearly 60%.[5]

Looking at a group of nearly 2,000 people from a study population of nearly 5,000 people, researchers found no link (neither protective nor harmful) between the risk of developing macular degeneration and a diet high in vitamin C, vitamin E, or carotenoids. However, they did find a decreased risk of early-stage macular degeneration for those who consumed diets high in zinc.[3]

● In a large study: no benefits in past use of *higher amounts* of vitamin C found on risk of macular degeneration

A study of nearly 3,000 people age 49 and over found no link (neither protective nor harmful) between the risk of having macular degeneration a diet with higher amounts of vitamin C, vitamin A, zinc, or beta-carotene in the past.[4]

● Though the several studies above found no link, one large study found a harm: past use of vitamin C associated with increased risk of macular degeneration

A study of over 3,500 people age 49 and over, surprisingly found, that those who took vitamin C supplements combined with a diet high in vitamin C had a 2-fold increase in their risk of developing macular degeneration. This finding is quite surprising, as one would expect vitamin C to protect against macular degeneration, as opposed to increasing the risk of macular degeneration. However, the finding highlights the problems associated with these types of studies: namely, that the findings may occur coincidentally and other true findings may be missed. It is sometimes difficult to explain the findings or apply them to real life. The study also found no link (neither protective nor harmful) between the risk of developing macular degeneration over a 5 year period and people who took the following nutrients, alone or in combination, in the past: lycopene, lutein and zeaxanthin, beta-carotene, vitamin A, or zinc.[2]

● **Though the several studies above found no link, two large studies found a benefit: past use of vitamin C associated with decreased risk of macular degeneration**
A study of over 300 people from a group of nearly 5,000 people found that fewer people with macular degeneration use vitamin C than people without macular degeneration. They also found that those who had macular degeneration had lower blood levels of vitamin E compared to those without macular degeneration. However, they found no difference in the blood levels of beta-carotene, lycopene, or lutein and zeaxanthin between those with or without macular degeneration.[7]

A study of nearly 10,000 people found no link (neither protective nor harmful) between macular degeneration and more servings of fruits or vegetables rich in vitamin C or higher amounts of dietary vitamin C. However, the study found that one daily serving of fruits or vegetables rich in vitamin A decreased the risk of having macular degeneration by 40% compared to less than once per week. However, when the study looked at the actual amount of vitamin A intake from the diet each day, the study found no link (neither protective nor harmful) between higher amounts of dietary vitamin A compared to lower amounts. These findings demonstrate that different results can be obtained from the same group of people depending on how the findings are observed, suggesting that careful interpretation of any result is necessary in order to apply the findings to real life.[134]

● **In several studies: no link between blood levels of vitamin C and macular degeneration**   A study of over 100 people, found no difference in the blood levels of vitamin C, vitamin A, vitamin E, carotenoids, or selenium between those with or without macular degeneration. However, the study did find that those who had macular degeneration had lower blood levels of zinc compared to those without macular degeneration.[39]

Another study of nearly 100 people found no difference in the blood levels of vitamin C, vitamin A, carotenoids, beta-carotene, lutein and zeaxanthin, lycopene, zinc, or selenium between those with or without macular degeneration (looking at both early and severe or advanced macular degeneration). However, the study found that those who had severe or advanced macular degeneration had lower blood levels of vitamin E compared to those without macular degeneration. They found no differences in the blood levels of vitamin E between those with or without early macular degeneration.[6]

A study of nearly 50 people found no link (neither protective nor harmful) between blood levels of vitamin C, A, or E and wet macular degeneration.[136]

A study in France of over 2,500 people age 60 and over found no link (neither protective nor harmful) between severe or advanced macular degeneration and higher blood levels of vitamin C, vitamin A, or vitamin E. However, the study found that a higher ratio of vitamin E-to-lipid in the blood reduced the risk of severe or advanced macular degeneration by 82% and decreased the risk of early macular degeneration by 18%. It has been suggested that this ratio of vitamin E-to-lipid in the blood is a better measure of how much vitamin E is available in the bloodstream.[135]

A study of 500 people age 40 and over found no link (neither protective nor harmful) between higher blood levels of vitamin C, vitamin A, or beta-carotene and macular degeneration. However, the study also found that those with higher blood levels of vitamin E had an over 50% decrease in the risk of having macular degeneration when compared to those who had lower blood levels of vitamin E.[10]

● **In a sixth study: no link between blood levels of vitamin C by itself and macular degeneration, but decreased risk of macular degeneration in those with higher blood levels of a combination of three of four nutrients including vitamin C**
A study of over 1,000 people age 55 to 80 found no link (neither protective nor harmful) between higher blood levels of vitamin C, vitamin E, or selenium by themselves and macular degeneration. [12] However, the study did find that having higher blood levels of carotenoids decreased the risk of having wet macular degeneration by 60% compared to those who had lower blood levels of carotenoids.[11] Looking at specific carotenoids, the study found that having higher blood levels of beta-carotene decreased the risk of having macular degeneration by 70%. Higher blood levels of lutein and zeaxanthin also decreased the risk

by 70% and higher blood levels of lycopene decreased the risk by 60%. Also, higher blood levels of a combination of three or more of four nutrients (carotenoids, vitamin C, vitamin E, and selenium) decreased the risk by 70%.[12]

● In several large studies: no benefits from the use of vitamin C on the future risk of macular degeneration over time

Looking over a 5-year period, a study of 2,000 people from a group of nearly 5,000, found no link (neither protective nor harmful) between macular degeneration and a diet high in vitamin C, vitamin E, beta-carotene, carotenoids, lutein and zeaxanthin, or zinc.[14]

A small study of 71 people with macular degeneration found no benefit to the macular degeneration or to vision in those who took a daily antioxidant combination, for over 1½ years, that consisted of vitamin C (750 mg), beta-carotene (20,000 IU), vitamin B2 (25 mg), vitamin E (200 IU), chromium (100 μg), selenium (50 μg), zinc (12.5 mg), taurine (100 mg), N-acetyl cysteine (100 mg), glutathione (5 mg), and selected bioflavonoids, compared to placebo.[17] It is impossible, however, to ascertain the individual effect of vitamin C from this type of study.

A study of over 75,000 people (nurses and health professionals) followed over time for up to 18 years found no link (neither protective nor harmful) between the risk of developing macular degeneration (wet or dry) and a diet high in any of the following

nutrients: vitamin C, vitamin A, vitamin E, carotenoids, lutein and zeaxanthin, beta-carotene, or lycopene. The study did find that those who consumed more than 3 servings of fruit each day were 1/3 less likely to develop *wet* macular degeneration over time compared to those who consumed less than 1½ servings of fruit each day. No link (neither protective nor harmful) was found when looking at increased fruit consumption for dry macular degeneration, nor when looking at increased vegetable consumption for dry or wet macular degeneration.[15]

A similar study of over 20,000 physicians followed for an average of over 12 years found no link (neither protective nor harmful) between the risk of developing macular degeneration (wet or dry) and vitamin C, vitamin E, or a multivitamin.[150]

● In a fifth study: no benefits from the use of vitamin C by itself on the future risk of macular degeneration over time, but use of vitamin C with multiple nutrients decreases future risk of macular degeneration

A study of nearly 4,000 people, looking forward over an average of 8 years, found no link (neither protective nor harmful) between macular degeneration and a diet high in vitamin A, vitamin C, beta-carotene, lutein and zeaxanthin, lycopene, iron, or zinc. However, a diet high in vitamin E decreased the risk of having macular degeneration by 20%. A diet high in multiple nutrients (beta-carotene, vitamin C, vitamin E, and zinc together) decreased the risk of having macular degeneration by about ½![18]

● **Though several studies above found no link, one large study found a benefit: use of vitamin C decreases the future risk of macular degeneration over time**

A recent 10-year study of over 3,000 people age 55 and over found that taking a daily antioxidant combination of vitamin C (500 mg), vitamin E (400 IU), and beta-carotene (15 mg), with or without zinc (80 mg) and copper (2 mg) reduced the risk of developing severe or wet macular degeneration, in people with certain features of dry macular degeneration within their retinas. The risk of developing severe or advanced macular degeneration decreased by 34% in people taking the antioxidant combination with zinc and copper, by 24% in people taking the antioxidant combination alone without zinc and copper, and by 30% in people taking the zinc and copper without the antioxidant combination. Looking at vision, the antioxidant combination with zinc and copper decreased the risk of losing vision from macular degeneration by 25% in these people with certain features of dry macular degeneration. There was no benefit to vision for people who took the antioxidant combination alone, without the zinc and copper, or the zinc and copper alone. This study has been used widely to recommend the multivitamin combination for macular degeneration, though the results are only applicable to people with certain features of macular degeneration in their retinas. Moreover, what confounds the interpretation of the data is the use of multivitamins in two-thirds of the people.[19]

Summary of Studies for Cataract: Over two dozen clinical trials have been performed looking at the role of vitamin C in preventing cataract. These clinical trials are of many different types, some of which are very well-designed and well-performed studies.

As a whole, the studies provide suggestion that vitamin C is beneficial. In 16 out of the 25 studies, vitamin C was found to be of benefit for cataract. Looking at the mechanisms of action, there is reason to use beta-carotene in moderation for cataract. Animal models have confirmed the role of vitamin C in protecting the lens from damage.

The studies can be summarized as follows: while five large, well-performed studies found no benefits from the past use of vitamin C on the risk of cataract, there are 10 studies that did find a benefit in the past use of vitamin C in decreasing the risk of cataract. Two studies found no link (neither protective nor harmful) between levels of vitamin C in the blood and cataract, though three studies found that higher levels of vitamin C in the blood are associated with a decrease in the risk of cataract. Interestingly, one study found the opposite effect: that higher levels of vitamin C in the blood are associated with an increased risk of cataract. This study demonstrates again that results from clinical trials may be difficult to explain and may not be "valid" or applicable to real life. For

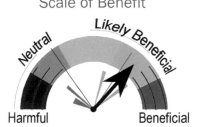

Vitamin C for
Cataract
Scale of Benefit

example, some studies may not have proper adjustments (such as adjusting for differences in the ages of patients), to make them reliable.

In following people over time, three studies found that those who took vitamin C did not have any benefit compared to those who did not take vitamin C. However, three studies did show a benefit of the use of a multi-vitamin in decreasing the future risk of cataract over time.

● **In several studies: no benefits in past use of vitamin C found on risk of cataract** A study of nearly 3,000 people found surprising no link (neither protective nor harmful) between vitamin C use and cataract, despite finding that many other nutrients had a benefit. The study found that past intake of vitamin B1, vitamin B2, vitamin B3, vitamin A, iron, and zinc decreased the risk of having certain types of cataract by 30 to 50%.[62]

A study of over 300 people age

55 or over found no link (neither beneficial nor harmful) between the use of vitamin C and the risk of having cataracts. However, the study found that the past use of higher quantities of tea, which contains high amounts of bioflavonoids, reduced the risk of having cataract by over 60%, and that the past use of vitamin E decreased the risk by nearly 50%.[36]

Another study of over 600 people found no link (neither protective nor harmful) between the past use of vitamin C or vitamin E and the risk of having cataract.[151]

A study of over 1,000 people age 45 to 79 found no link (neither protective nor harmful) between the past use of vitamin C or of vitamin E and the risk of having cataracts.[152]

A study of over 1,300 people age 43 to 84 found no link (neither protective nor harmful) between cataract and the past use of vitamin C or of vitamin E over 10 years. The study did find that higher intake of lutein and zeaxanthin was associated with a decrease in the risk of having cataract by about a ½.[77]

● **Though the several studies above found no link, numerous studies found a benefit: past use of vitamin C associated with decreased risk of cataract** A study of over 2,000 people found that the past intake of vitamin C, vitamin A, vitamin B1, vitamin B2, vitamin B3, vitamin B6, vitamin E, and folate were each associated with a decreased risk of having a certain type of cataract (called nuclear sclerosis). However, each of these nutrients was also associated with an increased risk of having another type of cataract (called cortical cataract).[53] The researchers suggest that the finding of increased cortical cataracts reflects the possibility that the presence of nuclear sclerosis cataracts masked the finding of cortical cataracts and skewed the results. This study exemplifies how difficult it is at times to interpret results and make meaningful extrapolations.

A study of nearly 1,800 people found that the past intake of vitamin C, vitamin A, vitamin B1, vitamin B2, vitamin B3, and vitamin E was associated with a decreased risk of having certain types of cataract. This decrease in risk ranged between 40 to 55%. Also, the study found that use of any multivitamin was associated with a 30% decrease in the overall risk of having cataracts. However, the study found no link (neither protective nor harmful) between iron and the risk of having cataract.[61]

A study of over 100 people age 40 to 70 found that the past use of vitamin C in high amounts decreased the risk of having cataract by 75%. However, the study found no link (neither beneficial nor harmful) between cataract and the past use of carotenoids or vitamin E. This study also found that a diet with at least 3½ servings of fruits and vegetables each day reduced risk of having cataracts by over 80%![40]

Another study of 350 people found that past use of vitamin C supplements decreased the risk of having cataracts by about $2/3$. Also, past use of vitamin E supplements decreased the risk of

having cataracts by over ½.[153]

A study of nearly 500 people age 53 to 73 found that the past intake of higher amounts of vitamin C decreased the risk of having cataracts by nearly 70%. It also found that long-term intake of vitamin C for over 10 years decreased the risk of having cataracts by nearly 65%. The study found that past intake of higher amounts of folate decreased the risk of having cataracts by about 10%, and past intake of higher amounts of vitamin B2 decreased the risk of having cataracts by over 60%. Long-term intake of vitamin E for over 10 years decreased the risk of having cataracts by over 50%, even though the study found no link (neither protective nor harmful) between the past intake of higher amounts of vitamin E and the risk of having cataracts. The finding of no beneficial link with higher doses of vitamin E may be related to increased risks associated with the higher doses. Furthermore, the use of a multivitamin for over 10 years reduced the risk of having cataract by over 40%. However, the study found no link (neither protective nor harmful) between the intake of beta-carotene, carotenoids, lutein and zeaxanthin, or lycopene and the risk of having cataracts.[20]

A study of 165 women found that those who took vitamin C for at least 10 years had a 70 to 80% decrease in their risk of having cataracts.[154]

A study of over 3,000 people found that the use of a multivitamin for more than 10 years decreased the risk of having cataracts by 60%. Similarly, the use of vitamin C or of vitamin E for more than 10 years also decreased the risk of having cataracts by 60%.[155]

A study of 300 women age 56 to 71 from a group of over 120,000 people found that in non-smokers, the past use of higher doses of vitamin C decreased the risk of having cataract by nearly 60% and the use of vitamin C for over 10 years decreased the risk by 60%. In addition, past use of beta-carotene in higher doses reduced the risk of having cataracts by over 70%. In fact, carotenoids, as a group, in higher doses reduced the risk of having cataracts by over 80%. The study also found that folate in higher doses reduced the risk of having cataracts by nearly 75%. However, the study found no link (neither protective nor harmful) between the use of vitamin E or B2 and cataract.[23]

A study of over 1,700 people age 43 to 84 from a population of about 5,000 people found that use of vitamin C in the past for more than 10 years decreased the risk of developing cataracts over the next 5 years by 60%. Similarly, the use of vitamin E in the past for more than 10 years decreased the risk of developing cataracts over the next 5 years by 60%. Also, those who used a multivitamin regularly in the past for more than 10 years decreased the risk of developing cataracts over the next 5 years by 60%.[156]

A study of over 5,000 people found that the past intake of higher amounts of vitamin C reduced the risk of having certain types of cataracts by about 90%, and the use of vitamin C for greater than 5 years decreased the risk by about 85%. Similarly, the past intake of higher amounts of beta-carotene decreased the risk of having cataract by 75 to 90% (depending on the type of cataract). The past intake of higher amounts of vitamin E reduced the risk of having certain types of cataracts by about 80%, and the use of vitamin E for greater than 5 years also reduced the risk by about 80%.[24]

● **In two studies: no link between blood levels of vitamin C and cataract**
A study of nearly 400 people age 66 to 75 found no link (neither protective nor harmful) between higher levels of vitamin C or vitamin E or zeaxanthin and the risk of having any type of cataract. However, the study found that higher levels of beta-carotene and alpha-carotene in the blood decreased the risk of having one type of cataract but not another. Similarly, higher levels of lutein in the blood decreased risk of having one type of cataract, whereas higher levels of lycopene in the blood decreased risk of having another type of cataract.[28]

Another study of over 600 people found no link (neither protective nor harmful) between blood levels of vitamin C and the risk of having cataract, but did find that high blood levels of vitamin E decreased the risk of having certain types of cataract by nearly 50%.[151]

● **Though the two studies above found no link, three studies found a benefit: decreased risk of cataract in those with higher blood levels of vitamin C** A study of over

100 people age 40 to 70 found that higher blood levels of vitamin C decreased risk of having certain types of cataracts. Similarly, higher blood levels of carotenoids decreased risk of having cataracts by over 80%.[40]

A study of over 1,000 people found that higher levels of vitamin C in the blood decreased the risk of one type of cataract by nearly 50%. However, the study found no link (neither protective nor harmful) between higher levels of beta-carotene, vitamin A, or glutathione in the blood and the risk of having cataracts. Of concern, the study found that higher levels of vitamin E in the blood increased the risk by nearly twice of having cataracts (this finding may be related to increased risks associated with higher doses of vitamin E)![25]

A study of over 4,000 people found that higher levels of vitamin C in the blood decreased the risk of having cataracts by over 25%. However, the study found no link (neither protective nor harmful) between the use of vitamin E and the risk of having cataract, as well as no link between the use of vitamin A and the risk of having cataract.[137]

● **Though the several studies above found benefits or no link, one large study found a harm: increased risk of cataract in those with higher blood levels of vitamin C**
A study of over 1,400 people in India found that those who had higher blood levels of vitamin C had an 87% higher risk of having certain types of cataracts. Similarly, the study found that those who had higher blood levels of copper also had a 56% higher risk of having certain types of cataracts. [48]

● **In several large studies: no benefits from the use of vitamin C on the future risk of cataract over time** A study of over 2,000 people given a multivitamin or a placebo for 5 years found a 36% decrease in the risk of developing cataracts in those people who were age 65 to 74. Of note, there was no difference in risk in the younger group age 45 to 64. These results exemplify the positive benefit of multivitamins; however, it is difficult to apply these results to a healthy population, as the study was performed on somewhat nutritionally-deprived people in rural China.[33]

The researchers also looked at specific nutrients in a group of over 3,000 people from the same population. They found no link (neither beneficial nor harmful) over the 5-year period between the risk of cataract and those who took vitamin C and molybdenum, or those who took vitamin A and zinc, or those who took selenium with beta-carotene and vitamin E. In contrast, in those who took vitamin B2 (5.2 mg) and vitamin B3 (40 mg) daily for 5 years had a 41% decrease in the risk of developing cataracts, compared to those who took placebo.[33]

A study of about 20,000 people found that use of a multivitamin decreased the risk of having cataracts by about 25%, but found no link (neither protective nor harmful) between cataract and vitamin C or E.[157]

A recent 10-year study of over

3,000 people found that taking an antioxidant combination of beta-carotene (15 mg), vitamin C (500 mg), and vitamin E (400 IU), with or without zinc and copper each day reduced the risk of macular degeneration over time, but found no link (neither protective nor harmful) to the risk of cataracts over time.[29]

● **Though the several studies above found no link, three studies found a benefit: use of vitamin C decreases the future risk of cataract over time**   Looking over an 8-year period into the future, a year study of over 50,000 women from a group of over 120,000 participants age 45 to 67 found no links (neither beneficial nor harmful) between diets high in vitamin B2, vitamin C, or vitamin E and cataract. In addition, the study found that a diet with higher amounts of carotenoids decreased the risk of developing cataracts by over 25%. Similarly, a diet with higher amounts of vitamin A

decreased the risk by nearly 40%. However, the study did find that the duration of vitamin C intake mattered. Those who consumed vitamin C supplements for 10 or more years had a 45% decreased chance of developing cataracts.[42]

However, 7 years later, the same researchers looking forward over time over 12 years at nearly 75,000 women from the previous study found no link (neither protective nor harmful) between vitamin A, C, or E taken for more than 10 years and the risk of cataract.[138]

A combined British and U.S. study of nearly 300 people found a mild benefit of taking 750 mg vitamin C, 18 mg beta-carotene, and 600 IU of vitamin E each day in reducing the risk of cataract, compared to taking placebo. Interestingly, the results showed that the vitamins were more beneficial to those who lived in the U.S. as compared to those who lived in England, possibly because of genetic, environmental, or dietary differences.[34]

Body Absorption, Metabolism, & Excretion

Vitamin C is easily and rapidly absorbed from the intestines through a sodium-dependent transport system. About 80 to 90% of the vitamin C ingested is absorbed. However, at higher doses, the amount absorbed can decrease to about ¼.

Vitamin C is filtered by the kidneys and recycled back into the bloodstream. However, when vitamin C levels reach a certain threshold in the bloodstream, the kidneys do not recycle the vitamin C back into the bloodstream; instead, they filter it out into the urine.

Therefore, because the intestines limit the amount of vitamin C absorbed and since the kidneys filter out vitamin C when it is in high levels in the bloodstream, it is quite difficult to achieve high levels of vitamin C in the body.

Deficiency

Vitamin C deficiency is also associated with dry hair, splitting of the hair, inflammation of the gums, and bleeding of the gums. Skin problems include dryness, roughness, scaly skin, poor ability to heal wounds, and easy bruising. Nose bleeds and skin bruising are also commonly noted. Vitamin C deficiency is also believed to be associated with increased susceptibility to infections (though there is little evidence that it is associated with increased susceptibility to the common cold).

The overall level of vitamin C needed in the body is 2,000 to 3,000 mg. A minimal dose of 100 mg daily in a healthy individual can maintain an overall level of 2,000 to 3,000 mg in the human body. However, the presence of smoking, excess sunlight exposure, physical disease or stress, or emotional stress, may result in an increased need for vitamin C. A typical diet that does not contain fruits or vegetables may result in daily doses of 60 mg or less. At these daily doses, or at lower daily intakes, the total body level of vitamin C may drop below the 2,000 to 3,000 mg level needed. When the overall body level of vitamin C falls to about 300 mg, a disease called scurvy develops.

Scurvy describes a disease of vitamin C deficiency, which historically was described in malnourished warriors, such as those of the Medieval crusades or of the 16th and 17th century British navy. Symptoms associated with scurvy include skin, hair, and gum disease as noted above, as well as joint pains from swelling of the joints. In addition, bulging or protrusion of the eye has been noted in children with vitamin C deficiency who have been affected with scurvy.

Scurvy is associated with swelling and bleeding in the retina. Bleeding can also occur on the eyelids and conjunctiva (the white of the eye). Bleeding also can occur inside the eye, in the anterior chamber.

It is important to note that when the doctor prescribes steroid eye drops for an eye disease, these drops cause a considerable decrease in vitamin C levels in the anterior chamber (the part of the eye that nourishes the cornea and bathes the lens). In effect, this vitamin C decrease may be one of many factors associated with the common risk of cataract formation in those who take steroid eye drops.

Toxicity & Side Effects

At high doses of vitamin C, some people may complain of abdominal pains, nausea, and diarrhea. Despite these complaints, however, there are only a few isolated reports of toxic effects from high doses of vitamin C. These include vascular disease and kidney stones in adults and birth defects and genetic mutations of the fetus during pregnancy.

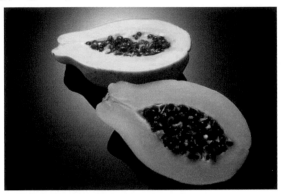

Interactions with Other Nutrients

There are numerous interactions between vitamin C and other nutrients. The important concept is that a balance should be achieved between intake of vitamin C and other nutrients.

Bioflavonoids were initially called vitamin P ("P" for protection) based on a 1936 report of the role in protecting vitamin C. In fact, just as vitamin C can donate electrons to vitamin E to recycle it, bioflavonoids can donate electrons to vitamin C and E when they are used up, so that they can be recycled. In fact, some researchers suggest that a daily dosage of vitamin C should be associated with ingestion of about three-quarters of that amount of bioflavonoids.

Vitamins C and E and glutathione form a highly protective antioxidant team. Vitamin C is able to assist in reforming vitamin E and glutathione when they are used up as antioxidants. When vitamin E or glutathione is used up, it becomes oxidized because it has lost electrons. Vitamin C can donate electrons to vitamin E and to glutathione to regenerate them (see sections on glutathione and vitamin E). In doing so, vitamin C gets used up, since it becomes oxidized and is converted into dehydroascorbic acid or into ascorbyl free radical. These forms cannot act as antioxidants and must be recycled back to vitamin C with the help of the selenium-containing enzyme thioredoxin reductase, glutathione, or the glutathione-dependent enzymes, such as dehydroascorbate reductase (see sections on glutathione and selenium).

Dihydrolipoic acid can also provide electrons to vitamin C to assist in its recycling. The body converts lipoic acid into dihydrolipoic acid, which is a potent antioxidant as well (see section on alpha-lipoic acid).

Vitamin C also plays an important role in two of the steps in the formation of carnitine. Vitamins B3 and B6 and iron also play roles in the pathway.

Moreover, vitamin C is required to modify proline that is incorporated into forming collagen (see section on proline). The ultratrace element silicon is believed to be required for this vitamin C pathway that modifies proline.

Vitamin C is believed to help in the process of chromium absorption (see section on chromium).

Vitamin C in high doses may cause exceedingly high iron levels and low vitamin B12 levels. Thus, people who are on vitamin C should be careful about the amount of iron they ingest.

There is also some controversial evidence that high doses of vitamin C can result in copper deficiency. While this finding has been observed in animals, it has not been demonstrated in humans. Nevertheless, balancing vitamin C intake with appropriate mineral intake is necessary.

Specific foods such as blueberries, black currants, Brussels sprouts, and red cabbage contain chemicals, called polyhydroxyphenols, which can inactivate vitamin B1. Vitamin C and citric acid in the diet, however, can help block the ability of polyhydroxyphenols to inactive vitamin B1.

Ideal Dosage

The recommended daily dosage for vitamin C ranges from 65 to 120 mg per day. In boys age 14 to 18, the recommended daily dose is 75 mg per day, and in men over age 18, the recommended daily dose is 90 mg per day. In girls age 14 to 18, the recommended daily dose is 65 mg per day, and in women over age 18, the recommended daily dose is 75 mg per day. During pregnancy, the recommended dose increases to 85 mg per day, and during lactation, 120 mg per day is suggested.

Many researchers, however, will recommend minimum daily doses of 300 mg per day. It may be best to obtain a daily dose of around 500 to 800 mg per day, which should be divided into several smaller doses throughout the day for maximized efficacy.

Some researchers recommend doses of 2,000 mg per day, since that is the level human bodies used to receive thousands of years ago, when the human body used to produce its own vitamin C before a gene mutation occurred that made us unable to produce our own vitamin C. Humans depend on vitamin C intake from dietary sources. Most animals, incidentally, can produce their own vitamin C and do not rely on fruits and vegetables for vitamin C. It is important to note, however, that there is concern that levels of over 2,000 mg per day may be associated with toxicity.

Vegetables, Nuts, & Seafood:

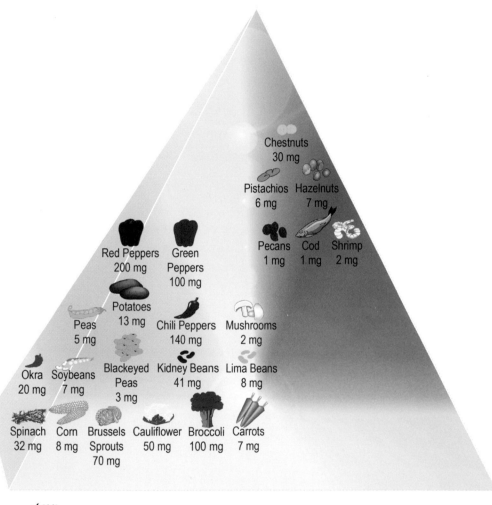

Chestnuts
30 mg

Pistachios   Hazelnuts
6 mg   7 mg

Pecans   Cod   Shrimp
1 mg   1 mg   2 mg

Red Peppers   Green
200 mg   Peppers
              100 mg

Potatoes
Peas   13 mg   Chili Peppers   Mushrooms
5 mg   140 mg   2 mg

Okra   Soybeans   Blackeyed   Kidney Beans   Lima Beans
20 mg 7 mg   Peas   41 mg   8 mg
                  3 mg

Spinach   Corn   Brussels   Cauliflower   Broccoli   Carrots
32 mg   8 mg   Sprouts   50 mg   100 mg   7 mg
                 70 mg

Pyramid Key:

Fats & Sweets

Dairy   Meats & Nuts

Vegetables   Fruits

Breads & Grains

*See Guides on Pages 467-468.

Fruits:

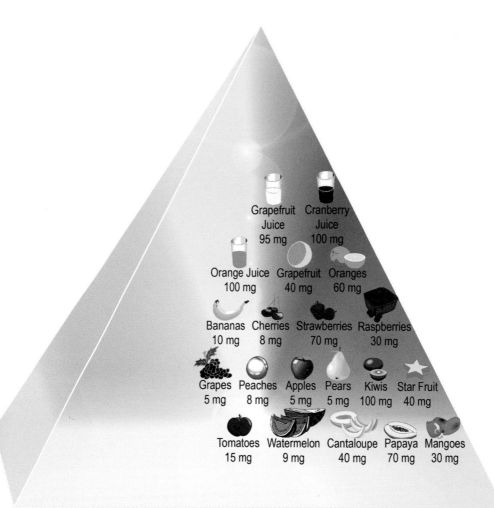

Top sources of vitamin C are peppers (red peppers, green peppers, and chili peppers), broccoli, and kiwis. Other vegetables that are rich in vitamin C are Brussels sprouts, cauliflower, kidney beans, and spinach. Other fruits that are rich in vitamin C are papaya, strawberries, oranges, grapefruit, star fruit, cantaloupe, raspberries, and mangoes.

VITAMIN D
(CALCIFEROL, CALCITRIOL)

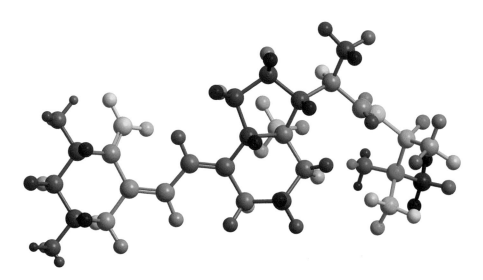

Category

Vitamin D is not a true vitamin, but rather a steroid hormone, known as calciferol. Activated vitamin D is called calcitriol. It is often referred to as a fat-soluble vitamin. Also, it is non-essential, as the body can produce its own vitamin D with sunlight exposure, specifically ultraviolet UV exposure.

Cellular Location

Most of the vitamin D is found in the bloodstream, circulating to various tissues throughout the body where it performs its actions. Some vitamin D is stored in the liver, skin, and bones.

Structure

Two forms of vitamin D are vitamin D2, known as ergocalciferol, which is the most common type found in dietary supplements, and vitamin D3, known as cholecalciferol, which is the type made by the body. Since it is a steroid hormone, it shares a common ring structure with other steroids.

Mechanisms of Action

Vitamin D itself actually does not and cannot perform any actions. It is converted through a series of reactions into a molecule called 1,25(OH)2D. This molecule goes into the nucleus of cells and turns on the expression of certain genes. In fact, there about 50 genes in the body that are turned on by the vitamin D metabolite 1,25(OH)2D.

Biological & Ocular Importance

● **Development & strengthening of bones**
Vitamin D maintains the calcium levels in the body and promotes the development and strengthening of bones. Vitamin D is essential for the normal growth of bones and for prevention of osteoporosis.

● **Promotes proper growth of cells**   By acting on genes in the nucleus of cells, vitamin D promotes the proper growth and development of cells and prevents proliferation (an increase in the number of cells). In this role, vitamin D is thought to help prevent the development of cancer, which is characterized by uncontrolled growth or proliferation of cells.

● **Regulates calcium in neurons to improve their ability to send signals**
Vitamin D-dependent calcium-binding proteins are found throughout the neurons of the brain and the retina and are involved in regulating calcium levels within these cells. The regulation of calcium in these cells plays a role in their functions, including their ability to send signals and communicate neuronal messages.

● **Enhances the immune defense system**   By acting on genes in the nucleus of cells, vitamin D enhances the immune defense system. There is also suggestion that vitamin D may help prevent the immune defense system from attacking cells that belong to the person's body. This type of attack is called an autoimmune attack, and occurs in many diseases, such as lupus or certain types of arthritis or even certain types of diabetes. There is also some suggestion that vitamin D can decrease the risk of multiple sclerosis.

- **Decreases high blood pressure**   Vitamin D may also play a role in decreasing hypertension (high blood pressure) by decreasing expression of a kidney gene. This gene results in the kidney retaining fluid, which leads to high blood pressure. By decreasing expression of this gene, vitamin D has been called a natural ACE-inhibitor, referring to a type of medication that acts to reduce high blood pressure. Thus, vitamin D has been recommended to treat hypertension.

- **Decreases the winter season "blues"**   Because of the decreased sunlight exposure in the wintertime, it has been suggested that the winter-season "blues" that develop are perhaps partly related to vitamin D deficiency and it is therefore recommended that dietary vitamin D be increased in the winter season.

Human Studies on Utility

Currently, there are only two human studies on vitamin D use in eye disease reported in the scientifically-reviewed medical literature. Nevertheless, the fact that there are only two reported clinical studies does not necessarily imply a benefit or lackof benefit. Looking at the mechanism of action, the use of vitamin D in moderation may be possibly of benefit in many eye diseases.

- **In one study: no benefits in past use of vitamin D found on risk of cataract**   An Italian study of over 900 people also found no link (neither protective nor harmful) between intake of higher levels of vitamin D, vitamin A, beta-carotene, or methionine and the risk of having cataracts. However, this study found that those who consumed higher dietary levels of folate and vitamin E had a lower risk of developing cataracts that required surgery.[22]

- **One small study found decreased risk of cataract in those with higher blood levels of vitamin D**   A study of 165 people found that those who had cataracts had lower levels of vitamin D and carotenoids in their blood compared to those who did not have cataracts. However, the study found no link (neither beneficial nor harmful) between cataracts and vitamin A, vitamin E, zinc, copper, and magnesium levels in the blood. On the other hand, the study found that those who had cataracts had higher levels of selenium in their blood.[41]

It is difficult to draw conclusions from such types of

clinical trials, because those who had already developed cataracts may have started certain supplements in their diets compared to those who did not develop cataracts. It is not known how vitamin D can decrease the risk of cataract, so the authors of this study provide the following explanation: those with cataracts may be at risk for vitamin D deficiency because of lifestyle issues that may be related to having cataracts. In other words, having a cataract led to more glare and other cataract-related sensitivity to the sunlight. These people may then have spent less time in the sun, putting them at risk for vitamin D deficiency, since the body's production of vitamin D is dependent on sunlight.

Body Absorption, Metabolism, & Excretion

Vitamin D is absorbed from the intestines after it is taken up by fat micelles (spherical soap-bubble-like conglomerates of fat). About ½ of the dietary vitamin D is absorbed into the bloodstream and taken to the liver, which is where the first step in its activation occurs. Then, the kidneys perform the second step in the activation of vitamin D, which converts it to calcitriol.

Excess vitamin D is dumped back into the digestive tract for excretion with bile (a green fluid produced by the liver that is stored in the gallbladder to assist in digestion).

Deficiency

Vitamin D deficiency can cause muscle pains and weakness.

Rickets is a disorder characterized by decreased bone formation in children and is caused by vitamin D deficiency. A common manifestation of rickets is bowed legs. Osteomalacia, also known as adult rickets, is a similar condition in which bones soften and become painful.

Toxicity & Side Effects

Excess vitamin D ingestion is associated with excess calcium in the bloodstream. This excess level of calcium can cause kidney stones and calcium build-up in organs, such as in the heart and kidneys. Interestingly, it also can cause bone loss! Of importance, excess vitamin D can cause a build-up of calcium on the surface of the cornea. While this excess calcium on the cornea, often seen in a pattern called band keratopathy, is often reversible, it can cause symptoms such as decrease in vision and irritation of the eye.

Interactions with Other Nutrients

Vitamin D assists in the conversion of phytic acid (or inositol hexaphosphate) into inositol triphosphate (see section on phytic acid). Inositol triphosphate functions as a cell-signal compound that signals the retinal pigment epithelium to increase its clean up of debris from photoreceptors. The retinal pigment epithelium serves to provide nutrition for the photoreceptors and to remove excess debris and waste from the photoreceptors. This debris and waste includes the discs of the photoreceptors, which are shed each day. Photoreceptors contain up to 1,000 discs arranged in layers to detect photons, or light particles. Each retinal pigment epithelial cell cleans up by packaging and ingesting 2,000 to 4,000 discs each day from an average of 30 to 40 adjacent photoreceptor cells. On a cellular level, this task is mammoth and complex, though it can be easily overwhelmed by debris. In the presence of light and oxygen, excess debris results in the production of reactive oxygen species (toxic chemicals that result in oxidation). Oxidation is the process whereby chemical compounds lose electrons, which results in potentially toxic modifications to proteins, lipids, and DNA that can eventually lead to degeneration and even death of cells. Thus, excess debris can result in oxidative damage to the retina. Of course light exposure is high in the retina, and the highest amount of oxygen consumption of any tissue in the body occurs in the retina. Therefore, the retina is particularly susceptible to oxidative damage, and vitamin D assists in promoting the clean up of the debris that leads to oxidative damage.

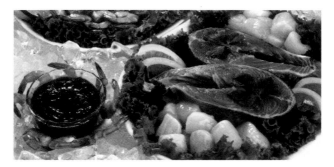

Ideal Dosage

The recommended dose of vitamin D is about 200 IU to 600 IU, depending on age. In children and adults up to the age of 50, the recommended dose is 200 IU per day. In those between the ages of 50 to 70, 400 IU is the recommended dose, while in those over the age of 70, 600 IU is the recommended dose.

Doses above 2,000 IU per day are not recommended, however.

Sources (Where to Find It)

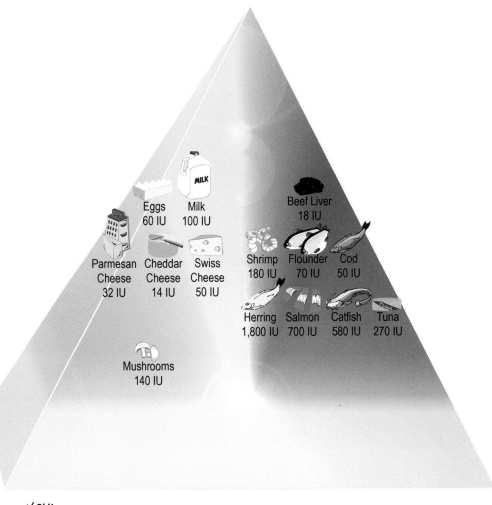

Eggs
60 IU

Milk
100 IU

Beef Liver
18 IU

Parmesan
Cheese
32 IU

Cheddar
Cheese
14 IU

Swiss
Cheese
50 IU

Shrimp
180 IU

Flounder
70 IU

Cod
50 IU

Herring
1,800 IU

Salmon
700 IU

Catfish
580 IU

Tuna
270 IU

Mushrooms
140 IU

Pyramid Key:

Fats & Sweets

Dairy   Meats & Nuts

Vegetables   Fruits

Breads & Grains

The top sources of vitamin D are seafood, particularly herring, salmon, and catfish. Other top sources of vitamin B are mushrooms, milk, and eggs.

*See Guides on Pages 467-468.

VITAMIN E
(ALPHA-TOCOPHEROL)

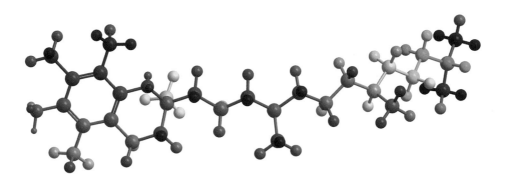

Category

Vitamin E is a family of fat-soluble vitamins.

Cellular Location

Vitamin E is distributed in the bloodstream throughout the body. Vitamin E is found in high concentrations in the aqueous fluid behind the cornea that bathes the natural lens, and also within the natural lens. It is also in high concentrations in the retina, particularly within photoreceptor cells and retinal pigment epithelial cells.

Structure

There are several forms of vitamin E: alpha-, beta-, delta-, and gamma-tocopherol and tocotrienols. Alpha-tocopherol is the form of vitamin E found in the highest concentration in the human body. It is a ring compound with a long chain and contains a hydroxyl group that is available for chemical reactions.

Mechanisms of Action

Vitamin E acts as a strong antioxidant, particularly in cell membranes.

Biological & Ocular Importance

● Powerful antioxidant

Vitamin E is a powerful antioxidant, and plays an essential role in protecting lipids, the major component of cell membranes, from oxidation. Vitamin E's chemical structure allows it to function as an antioxidant by reducing reactive oxygen species (toxic chemicals that result in oxidation). In fact, because of its hydroxyl group on its ring, it reduces reactive oxygen species more quickly than they can attack lipids. Therefore, it is extremely potent in protecting against oxidation of lipids, which are the predominant component of cell membranes.

● Protects the retina & photoreceptors from oxidative injury
Photoreceptor discs have a very high lipid content and are very susceptible to oxidative damage. Photoreceptors contain up to 1,000 discs arranged in layers to detect photons, or light particles. Within these discs are the light-sensing compounds, the chromophores, of the retina that are necessary for visual transduction (the process whereby a light signal is converted into a chemical signal that is sent through the retina and eventually to the brain). These photoreceptor discs contain exceedingly low levels of cholesterol and high levels of unsaturated fatty acids, particularly the omega-3s. In fact, anywhere from 50 to 90% of the lipid content of the disc membranes is composed of unsaturated fatty acids. This membrane composition is essential in providing the right microenvironment for visual transduction to occur, allowing for proper membrane component interactions and proper membrane fluidics (the movement of compounds within the membranes).

What makes these fatty acids unsaturated is the presence of an increased proportion of double bonds. However, it is the high number of double bonds that makes these fatty acids prone to oxidation and oxidative damage. The presence of light and oxygen results in the production of reactive oxygen species. Of course light exposure is high in the retina, and the highest amount of oxygen consumption of any tissue in the body occurs in the retina. Therefore, the photoreceptor discs are particularly susceptible to oxidative damage.

Vitamin E, known to accumulate in high concentrations in the photoreceptors discs, is an antioxidant known to protect photoreceptor disc membranes from oxidative damage. In fact, vitamin E with its antioxidant activities saves any cell membranes from oxidative damage. Vitamin E performs the first steps of preventing oxidative damage to cell membranes, or lipid peroxidation, by converting strong and dangerous hydroperoxyl radicals into weaker, though still harmful hydroperoxides. Thioredoxin and glutathione perform the second steps, safely removing the hydroperoxides, without which these hydroperoxides would turn back on lipids and cause damage (see sections on selenium and glutathione).

● **Produces the antioxidant enzyme glutathione peroxidase** Furthermore, vitamin E, with the help of selenium and vitamin B2, produce a naturally occurring antioxidant enzyme called glutathione peroxidase, which functions with glutathione to protect cell structures, especially lipids, from oxidation (see sections on selenium and glutathione).

● **Protects the lens from cataract formation** Similarly, vitamin E is believed to play an antioxidant role in protecting the lens from cataract formation. The lens, which has high exposure to light, is at risk for oxidative damage, as light is collected by the lens to be focused on the retina. Vitamin E is found in high concentrations in the aqueous fluid behind the cornea that bathes the natural lens.

● **Protects the cornea from oxidative injury** In animal models, vitamin E can also protect corneal cells from oxidative injury.

● **Protects the eye from oxidative injury causing glaucoma** As an antioxidant, vitamin E is thought to protect the trabecular meshwork (the filtration site of the eye). Allowing enough fluid to exit the eye is essential to prevent pressure build-up in the eye, decreasing the risk of glaucoma, since malfunction of this filtration site is a common mechanism of glaucoma.

● **Blocks pathways of harmful inflammation** In addition to its functions as an antioxidant, vitamin E functions to block the activity of the cell-signaling molecule protein kinase C. It also has an affect on white blood cells involved in inflammation and allergy, and is believed to enhance the body's immune response. This pathway is also believed to play a role in the disease process in diabetic retinopathy.

These anti-inflammatory properties of vitamin E suggest

that it may play a useful role in both inflammations of the eye and following the inflammation that develops after eye surgery. Animal models of glaucoma surgery have found a potential role for vitamin E in certain types of glaucoma surgery. Similar animal models have demonstrated its role in protecting against the damage during inflammatory disorders of the retina. Similarly, animal models have shown that vitamin E can slow down scar tissue formation after vitreous and retinal surgery.

It also is believed to enhance the function of the immune defense system and has been suggested for diseases such as asthma.

● Improves blood flow

In addition, animal studies have shown that vitamin E can block the enzymes that play a role in some of the abnormal blood flow that occurs in diabetic retinopathy. In fact, in other studies of diabetic animals, giving vitamin E has been shown to improve blood flow in the retina compared to not giving the vitamin E. Similarly, in animal models of stroke in the eye, vitamin E given prior to the stroke demonstrated a protective effect on the retinas.

● Blocks blood vessel disease
In addition to encouraging the dilation of blood vessels, vitamin E has an effect on blood clotting by blocking the clumping or aggregation of platelets. It has been recommended for preventing or decreasing atherosclerosis (blood vessel cholesterol clots and plaques that can result in heart disease and stroke, as well as artery or vein clots in the retina or optic nerve strokes).

Additionally, vitamin E is believed to play an important role in reducing the risk of coronary heart disease and heart attacks, though there is some conflicting data. Similarly, vitamin E has been believed to reduce the risk of development of many types of cancer, but there has not been much that has demonstrated this beneficial aspect of vitamin E. Its role in preventing cancer is believed to be derived from its antioxidant effects.

● Prevents or slows down neurologic diseases
It has also been suggested to prevent or slow down neurologic diseases such as Alzheimer's disease. It has been suggested for many other diseases as well, ranging from Parkinson's disease to Lou Gehrig's disease to seizures.

Human Studies on Utility

Currently, there are numerous human studies on vitamin E in eye disease reported in the scientifically-reviewed medical literature. These studies involve several eye diseases, including glaucoma, dry eyes, corneal healing, diabetic retinopathy, retinopathy of prematurity, retinal swelling, retinitis pigmentosa, macular degeneration, and cataract. The studies are described below.

> Looking at the mechanisms of action, there is good reason to use vitamin E in moderation for dry eyes, macular degeneration, and cataract.

● **In a small study: use of vitamin E improves healing of the cornea after refractive laser surgery** A study of 40 people found that those people who received vitamin A (25,000 IU) and vitamin E (200 IU in the form of vitamin E nicotinate) each day for one year after refractive laser surgery (the corneal laser treatment designed to do away with the need for eyeglasses) had faster healing of their cornea and decreased haze in their vision compared to those who received placebo.[129]

● **In two studies: use of vitamin E improved stability of tear film to protect against dry eyes** A study of 60 healthy young adults found that taking a multivitamin containing vitamins E, A, and C each day improved the stability of the tear film after just 10 days, compared with those who did not take the multivitamin. The study found that the tears remained stable for an over 40% longer period of time with the multivitamin. The study also found a similar benefit on the stability of the tear film with vitamin C alone.[128 & 147]

A more recent 2004 study of 60 people who took vitamin C and E found similar improvements in tear stability as well as improvements in the health of the cells on the surface of the eye that maintain adequate lubrication for the surface.[148]

● **In a small study: use of vitamin E decreases oxidative damage and improves visual fields in glaucoma** A Russian study of 122 people with glaucoma found that vitamin E (100 IU each day for 2 weeks followed by 30 IU each day for 1 week) decreased the amount of oxidative damage in the bloodstream. It remains unknown, however, whether or not this decrease in oxidative damage in the bloodstream is beneficial to the person's glaucoma. Interestingly, the 17 of the 122 people who were treated with vitamin E had an improvement in their visual fields.[158] However, this improvement is likely a chance occurrence, since fluctuations in the visual field can occur naturally.

● Several studies found a benefit of vitamin E in retinopathy of prematurity, while others found no benefit

A 1949 report suggested that a possible benefit of vitamin E in retinopathy of prematurity (a blinding retinal disease in new born infants who are born premature and exposed to oxygen in their incubator).

A report in 1982 of 12 years of experience with retinopathy of prematurity suggested that vitamin E prevented serious complications of retinopathy of prematurity and decreasing the severity of the disease.[159] Since then, some studies have found no benefit of vitamin E in preventing retinopathy of prematurity,[160] while others have found strong benefit.[161, 162, & 163]

Another study of 200 infants found no benefits from vitamin E, but did find a higher incidence of retinal bleeding in those infants given vitamin E![164]

In a series of 6 studies on over 500 preterm infants with retinopathy of prematurity, the use of vitamin E at birth decreased the progression to severe blinding forms of retinopathy of prematurity by 50%. This action is believed to result from vitamin E's ability to inhibit precursors of the blood vessel capillaries in the retina.

● In one study: vitamin E improved blood flow in the retina in diabetes, though another study found that vitamin E did not reduce

retinal disease in diabetes

In a study of 45 diabetics with mild or no retinal disease, high doses of vitamin E (1,800 IU per day) over 4 months restored back to normal the abnormal blood flow in the retina that occurs in diabetes, compared to placebo.[165] The benefits found by this study are believed to be derived from the antioxidant and anti-inflammatory mechanisms of vitamin E as well as the cellular messaging pathway activated by vitamin E that help improve blood flow through vessels. Inositol triphosphate is involved in this pathway (see section on phytic acid). This mechanism is particularly important in maintaining appropriate blood flow in the eye, especially in the retina in disorders such as diabetes or hypertension (high blood pressure).

A study of nearly 1,000 diabetics found no link (neither protective nor harmful) between vitamin C or vitamin E levels and the amount of retinal disease they had.[149]

● In one study: no benefits from the use of vitamin E on decreasing swelling of the retina

A study of 17 people with fluid swelling in their retinas from inflammation found no link (neither protective nor harmful) between high doses of vitamin E (1,600 IU per day over 4 months) and vision or swelling in the retina compared to placebo.[166]

● One study found harm in use of vitamin E in future risk of retinitis pigmentosa over

time, while another study found benefit in use of vitamin E with other nutrients over time A 1993 study of over 600 people with retinitis pigmentosa found that vitamin E (400 IU per day) increased the risk by 42% of having a large decline in the electrical functioning of photoreceptor cells, suggesting that high doses of vitamin E can be harmful in retinitis pigmentosa.

Vitamin E for
Retinitis Pigmentosa
Scale of Benefit

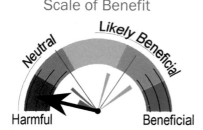

However, vitamin A decreased the risk by 32% of having a large decline in the electrical functioning of photoreceptor cells. The study found no link (neither protective nor harmful) between vitamin A (15,000 IU per day) and vision or peripheral visual fields over a period of 4 years. However, in those who started the study with less disease, vitamin A decreased the rate of progression of peripheral visual field loss. Of note, in this study, the total daily intake of vitamin A was about 18,000 IU per day, with 15,000 IU per day from a pill supplement (in the form of vitamin A palmitate) and 3,000 IU per day from dietary sources; this is how the level of 18,000 IU per day is suggested for people with retinitis pigmentosa.[132]

A more recent study of 62 people with retinitis pigmentosa found that taurine (1,000 mg per day) with vitamin E (800 IU per day) and the calcium-channel blocking anti-hypertension drug diltiazem (30 mg per day) modestly improved peripheral visual fields or slowed the progression of peripheral visual field loss over a period of 3 years.[126]

While these two studies provide conflicting results, the more recent study did not look at visual acuity or the electrical functioning of photoreceptor cells, like the older study did. Also, in the recent study, all people who took vitamin E also took taurine as well; it is possible that the benefits of taurine may counteract any harms of vitamin E. Until proven otherwise, there is reason to be concerned with high dose vitamin E in retinitis pigmentosa.

Summary of Studies for Macular Degeneration: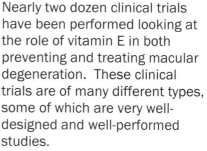

Nearly two dozen clinical trials have been performed looking at the role of vitamin E in both preventing and treating macular degeneration. These clinical trials are of many different types, some of which are very well-designed and well-performed studies.

As a whole, the clinical studies provide no definitive answer as to whether vitamin E is beneficial, and, in fact, the majority of studies found no benefit to vitamin E for macular degeneration. However, there is some evidence from 8 of the 23 studies that it may be beneficial, particularly in combination with other antioxidant nutrients.

Looking at the mechanisms of action, there may be good reason to use vitamin E in moderation for macular degeneration.

Vitamin E for Macular Degeneration Scale of Benefit

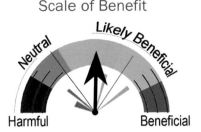

The studies can be summarized as follows: three large studies found no benefits from the past use of vitamin E on the risk of macular degeneration. Also, several studies have shown no link (neither protective nor harmful) between levels of vitamin E in the blood and macular degeneration. Another study also found no link between levels of vitamin E in the blood and macular degeneration, though it did find a decreased risk of macular degeneration in those with higher blood levels of a combination of three of four nutrients including vitamin E. Several studies have shown a decreased risk of macular degeneration in those with higher blood levels of vitamin E.

In following people over time, several studies found that those who took vitamin E did not have any benefit in preventing macular degeneration compared to those who did not take vitamin E. Two studies found that the use of vitamin E decreases the future risk of macular degeneration over time.

• In large studies: no benefits in past use of vitamin E found on risk of macular degeneration

Looking forward over time, a study of nearly 3,000 people age 49 and over found no link (neither protective nor harmful) between the risk of having macular degeneration and taking any of the following nutrients (alone or in combination) in the past: vitamin E, vitamin A, vitamin B1, vitamin B2, vitamin B3, vitamin B6, vitamin B12, vitamin C, beta-carotene, folate or zinc.[13]

Similarly, a study of over 1,000 people age 55 to 80 found no link (neither protective nor harmful) between macular degeneration and a diet high in vitamin C or E. The study did find that those who consumed a diet high in vitamin A had a greater than 40% decrease in the risk of having wet macular degeneration compared to those who did not consume a diet high in vitamin A. Similarly, dietary beta-carotene decreased the risk by 40% and dietary carotenoids decreased the risk by over 40%, while dietary lutein and zeaxanthin decreased the risk by nearly 60%.[5]

Looking at a group of nearly 2,000 people from a study population of nearly 5,000 people, researchers found no link (neither protective nor harmful) between the risk of developing macular degeneration and a diet high in vitamin E, vitamin C, or carotenoids. However, they did find a decreased risk of early-stage macular degeneration for those who consumed diets high in zinc.[3]

● **In several studies: no link between blood levels of vitamin E and macular degeneration**   A study of over 100 people, found no difference in the blood levels of vitamin E, vitamin A, vitamin C, carotenoids, or selenium between those with or without macular degeneration. However, the study did find that those who had macular degeneration had lower blood levels of zinc compared to those without macular degeneration.[39]

A study of 300 people from a group of nearly 4,000 people found no link (neither protective nor harmful) between the risk of having macular degeneration and higher blood levels of vitamin E or of beta-carotene.[8]

A study of 130 people also found no difference in the blood levels of vitamin E, vitamin A, beta-carotene, lutein, or lycopene between those with or without macular degeneration.[9]

And yet another study of over 160 people found no differences in the blood levels of vitamin E comparing those with or without macular degeneration. However, the study found that those with macular degeneration had lower blood levels of selenium, compared with those without macular degeneration.[122]

A study of nearly 50 people found no link (neither protective nor harmful) between blood levels of vitamin E, A, or C and wet macular degeneration.[136]

A study in France of over 2,500 people age 60 and over found no link (neither protective nor harmful) between severe or advanced macular degeneration and higher blood levels of vitamin E, vitamin A, or vitamin C. However, the study found that a higher ratio of vitamin E-to-lipid in the blood reduced the risk of severe or advanced macular degeneration by 82% and decreased the risk of early macular degeneration by 18%. It has been suggested that this ratio of vitamin E-to-lipid in the blood is a better measure of how much vitamin E is available in the bloodstream.[135]

● **In another study: no link between blood levels of vitamin E by itself and macular degeneration, but decreased risk of macular degeneration in those with higher blood levels of a combination of three of four nutrients including vitamin E**
A study of over 1,000 people age 55 to 80 found no link (neither protective nor harmful) between higher blood levels of vitamin E, vitamin C, or selenium by themselves and macular degeneration. [12] However, the study did find that having higher blood levels of carotenoids decreased the risk of having wet macular degeneration by 60% compared to those who had lower blood levels of carotenoids.[11] Looking at specific carotenoids, the study found that having higher blood levels of beta-carotene decreased the risk of having macular degeneration by 70%. Higher blood levels of lutein and zeaxanthin also decreased the risk by 70% and higher blood levels of

lycopene decreased the risk by 60%. Also, higher blood levels of a combination of three or more of four nutrients (carotenoids, vitamin C, vitamin E, and selenium) decreased the risk by 70%.[12]

● **Though the several studies above found no link, several studies found a benefit: decreased risk of macular degeneration in those with higher blood levels of vitamin E** Another study of nearly 100 people found that those who had severe or advanced macular degeneration had lower blood levels of vitamin E compared to those without macular degeneration. They found no differences in the blood levels of vitamin E between those with or without early macular degeneration. Also, the study no difference in the blood levels of carotenoids, beta-carotene, lutein and zeaxanthin, lycopene, vitamin A, vitamin C, zinc, or selenium between those with or without macular degeneration (looking at both early and severe or advanced macular degeneration).[6]

Another study of 40 people found that those who had macular degeneration had lower blood levels of vitamin E and lower levels of zinc compared to those without macular degeneration.[167]

There are also studies that have shown that higher circulating blood levels of vitamin E are associated with a lower risk of macular degeneration. One such study was a large clinical trial of nearly 1,000 people.[168]

A study of 500 people age 40 and over found that those with higher blood levels of vitamin E had an over 50% decrease in the risk of having macular degeneration when compared to those who had lower blood levels of vitamin E. However, the study also found no link (neither protective nor harmful) between higher blood levels of vitamin A, vitamin C, or beta-carotene and macular degeneration.[10]

A study of over 300 people from a group of nearly 5,000 people found that those who had macular degeneration had lower blood levels of vitamin E compared to those without macular degeneration. However, they found no difference in the blood levels of beta-carotene, lycopene, or lutein and zeaxanthin between those with or without macular degeneration. Interestingly, they did find that fewer people with macular degeneration use vitamin C than people without macular degeneration.[7]

● **In several large studies: no benefits from the use of vitamin E on the future risk of macular degeneration over time** A study of over 75,000 people (nurses and health professionals) followed over time for up to 18 years found no link (neither protective nor harmful) between the risk of developing macular degeneration (wet or dry) and a diet high in any of the following nutrients: vitamin E, vitamin A, vitamin C, carotenoids, lutein and zeaxanthin, beta-carotene, or lycopene. The study did find that those who consumed more than 3 servings of fruit each day were $1/3$ less likely to develop *wet* macular degeneration over time compared to those who consumed less than 1½ servings of fruit each day. No link (neither protective nor harmful) was found when looking at increased fruit consumption for dry macular degeneration, nor when looking at increased vegetable consumption for dry or wet macular degeneration.[15]

A similar study of over 20,000 physicians followed for an average of over 12 years found no link (neither protective nor harmful) between the risk of developing macular degeneration (wet or dry) and vitamin E, vitamin C, or a multivitamin.[150]

Looking over a 5-year period, a study of 2,000 people from a group of nearly 5,000, found no link (neither protective nor harmful) between macular degeneration and a diet high in vitamin E, vitamin C, beta-carotene, carotenoids, lutein and zeaxanthin, or zinc.[14]

A small study of 71 people with macular degeneration found no benefit to the macular degeneration or to vision in those who took a daily antioxidant combination, for over 1½ years, that consisted of vitamin E (200 IU), beta-carotene (20,000 IU), vitamin B2 (25 mg), vitamin C (750 mg), chromium (100 µg), selenium (50 µg), zinc (12.5 mg), taurine (100 mg), N-acetyl cysteine (100 mg), glutathione (5 mg), and selected bioflavonoids, compared to placebo.[17] It is impossible, however, to ascertain the individual effect of vitamin E from this type of study.

One study of over 29,000 smokers looked at whether or not supplements of vitamin E (70 IU) and/or beta-carotene (20 mg) taken daily for 6 years could prevent cancer. The study also looked at macular degeneration and found no link (neither protective nor harmful) between taking vitamin E, beta-carotene, or the two together and the risk of developing macular degeneration. Because the study looked only at smokers, its applicability to the general population is limited. Such limitations are always concerns of clinical trials.[16]

Another study of nearly 1,200 healthy people age 55 to 80 found no link (neither protective nor harmful) between vitamin E (500 IU each day over 4 years) and preventing the onset of macular degeneration.[169]

● **Though the several studies above found no link, two studies found a benefit: use of vitamin E decreases the future risk of macular degeneration over time** A study of nearly 4,000 people, looking forward over an average of 8 years, found that a diet high in vitamin E decreased the risk of having macular degeneration by 20%. However, the study found no link (neither protective nor harmful) between macular degeneration and a diet high in vitamin C, vitamin A, beta-carotene, lutein and zeaxanthin, lycopene, iron, or zinc. A diet high in multiple nutrients (beta-carotene, vitamin C, vitamin E, and zinc together) decreased the risk of having macular degeneration by about ½![18]

A recent 10-year study of over 3,000 people age 55 and over found that taking a daily antioxidant combination of vitamin C (500 mg), vitamin E (400 IU), and beta-carotene (15 mg), with or without zinc (80 mg) and copper (2 mg) reduced the risk of developing severe or wet macular degeneration, in people with certain features of dry macular degeneration within their retinas. The risk of developing severe or advanced macular degeneration decreased by 34% in people taking the antioxidant combination with zinc and copper, by 24% in people taking the antioxidant combination alone without zinc and copper, and by 30% in people taking the zinc and copper without the antioxidant combination. Looking at vision, the antioxidant combination with zinc and copper decreased the risk of losing vision from macular degeneration by 25% in these people with certain features of dry macular degeneration. There was no benefit to vision for people who took the antioxidant combination alone, without the zinc and copper, or the zinc and copper alone. This study has been used widely to recommend the multivitamin combination for macular degeneration, though the results are only applicable to people with certain features of macular degeneration in their retinas. Moreover, what confounds the interpretation of the data is the use of multivitamins in two-thirds of the people.[19]

● One small study found no benefit in adding vitamin E during laser treatment for macular degeneration

A small study of 35 people with advanced wet macular degeneration found no benefit in adding vitamin E and omega oils to a treatment of photodynamic therapy (a laser-based treatment for wet macular degeneration). People were divided into two groups: both received the photodynamic therapy, but only one also received vitamin E and omega oils for 3 months after the photodynamic therapy.[98]

Summary of Studies for Cataract: 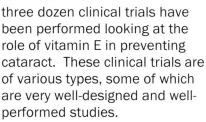 Over three dozen clinical trials have been performed looking at the role of vitamin E in preventing cataract. These clinical trials are of various types, some of which are very well-designed and well-performed studies.

As a whole, the clinical studies provide no definitive

Vitamin E for
Cataract
Scale of Benefit

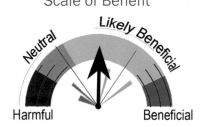

answer as to whether vitamin E is beneficial, and, in fact, half of the studies found no benefit to vitamin E for cataract, while the other half found benefit. Looking at the mechanisms of action, there may be good reason to use vitamin E in moderation for cataract.

The studies can be summarized as follows: several studies found no benefits from the past use of vitamin E on the risk of cataract, while are even more studies found a benefit in the past use of vitamin E in decreasing the risk of cataract. Two studies have found no link (neither protective nor harmful) between levels of vitamin E in the blood and cataract, though several studies found that higher levels of vitamin E in the blood are associated with a decrease in the risk of cataract. Interestingly, one study found the opposite effect: that higher levels of vitamin E in the blood are associated with an increased risk of cataract. This study demonstrates again that results from clinical trials may be difficult to explain, and sometimes they may not be "valid" or applicable to real life.

In following people over time, several studies found that those who took vitamin E did not have any benefit compared to those who did not take vitamin E. However, two large studies did show a benefit of the use of a vitamin E in decreasing the future risk of cataract over time.

● **In several studies: no benefits in past use of vitamin E found on risk of cataract** Another study of over 600 people found no link (neither protective nor harmful) between the past use of vitamin E or vitamin C and the risk of having cataract.[151]

A study of over 100 people age 40 to 70 found no link (neither beneficial nor harmful) between cataract and the past use of vitamin E or carotenoids. However, the past use of vitamin C in high amounts decreased the risk of having cataract by 75%. This study also found that a diet with at least 3½ servings of fruits and vegetables each day reduced risk of having cataracts by over 80%![40]

A study of over 1,000 people age 45 to 79 found no link (neither protective nor harmful) between the past use of vitamin E or of vitamin C and the risk of having cataracts.[152]

A study of over 4,000 people found no link (neither protective nor harmful) between the use of vitamin E and the risk of having cataract, as well as no link between the use of vitamin A and the risk of having cataract. The study did find that higher levels of vitamin C in the blood decreased the risk of having cataracts by over 25%.[137]

A study of 300 women age 56 to 71 from a group of over 120,000 people found no link (neither protective nor harmful) between the use of vitamin E or B2 and cataract. However, the study found that in non-smokers, the past use of beta-carotene in higher doses reduced the risk of having cataracts by over 70%. In fact, carotenoids, as a group, in higher doses reduced the risk of having cataracts by over 80%. The study also found that folate in higher doses reduced the risk of having cataracts by nearly 75%. In addition, past use of higher doses of vitamin C decreased the risk of having cataract by nearly 60% and the use of vitamin C for over 10 years decreased the risk by 60%.[23]

A study of 400 people age 50 to 86 found no link (neither protective nor harmful) between the past use of vitamin E, vitamin A, beta-carotene, lutein, or lycopene and the risk of having cataract.[21]

A study of over 1,300 people age 43 to 84 found no link (neither protective nor harmful) between cataract and the past use of vitamin E or of vitamin C over 10 years. The study did find that higher intake of lutein and zeaxanthin was associated with a decrease in the risk of having cataract by about a ½.[77]

● **Though the several studies above found no link, numerous studies found a benefit: past use of vitamin E associated with decreased risk of cataract**   A study of over 2,000 people found that the past intake of vitamin E, vitamin A, vitamin B1, vitamin B2, vitamin B3, vitamin B6, vitamin C, and folate were each associated with a decreased risk of having a certain type of cataract (called nuclear sclerosis). However, each of these nutrients was also associated with an increased risk of having another type of cataract (called cortical cataract).[53] The researchers suggest that the finding of increased cortical cataracts reflects the possibility that the presence of nuclear sclerosis cataracts masked the finding of cortical cataracts and skewed the results. This study exemplifies how difficult it is at times to interpret results and make meaningful extrapolations.

A study of over 300 people age 55 or over found that the past use of vitamin E decreased the risk of having cataract by nearly 50%, and that the past use of higher quantities of tea, which contains high amounts of bioflavonoids reduced the by over 60%. However, there was no link (neither beneficial nor harmful) between the use of vitamin C and the risk of having cataracts.[36]

Another study of 350 people found that past use of vitamin C supplements decreased the risk of having cataracts by over ½. Also, past use of vitamin E supplements decreased the risk of having cataracts by about $2/3$.[153]

A study of nearly 1,800 people found that the past intake of vitamin E, vitamin A, vitamin B1, vitamin B2, vitamin B3, and vitamin C was associated with a decreased risk of having certain types of cataract. This decrease in risk ranged between 40 to 55%. Also, the study found that use of any multivitamin was associated with a 30% decrease in the overall risk of having cataracts. However, the study found no link (neither protective nor harmful) between iron and the risk of having cataract.[61]

A study of over 5,000 people found that the past intake of higher amounts of vitamin E reduced the risk of having certain types of cataracts by about 80%, and the use of vitamin E for greater than 5 years also reduced the risk by about 80%. Similarly, the past intake of higher amounts of vitamin C decreased the risk of having certain types of cataracts by about 90%, and the use of vitamin C for greater than 5 years decreased the risk by about 85%. The past intake of higher amounts of beta-carotene reduced the risk of having cataract by 75 to 90% (depending on the type of cataract).[24]

A study of nearly 500 people age 53 to 73 found that long-term intake of vitamin E for over 10 years decreased the risk of having cataracts by over 50%, even though the study found no link (neither protective nor harmful) between the past intake of *higher* amounts of vitamin E and the risk of having cataracts. The finding of no beneficial link with higher doses of vitamin E may be related to increased risks associated with the higher doses. The study also found that past intake of *higher* amounts of folate decreased the risk of having cataracts by about 10%, and past intake of *higher* amounts of vitamin B2 decreased the risk of having cataracts by over 60%. The study found that the past intake of *higher* amounts of vitamin C decreased the risk of having cataracts by nearly 70%. It also found that long-term intake of vitamin C for over 10 years decreased the risk of having cataracts by nearly 65%. Furthermore, the use of a multivitamin for over 10 years reduced the risk of having cataract by over 40%. However, the study found no link (neither protective nor harmful) between the intake of beta-carotene, carotenoids, lutein and zeaxanthin, or lycopene and the risk of having cataracts.[20]

A study of over 3,000 people found that the use of a multivitamin for more than 10 years decreased the risk of having cataracts by 60%. Similarly, the use of vitamin E or of vitamin C for more than 10 years also decreased the risk of having cataracts by 60%.[155]

Another study of over 750 people found that vitamin E in the past decreased the risk of having cataracts by over 50%, and multivitamin supplements in the past decreased the risk of having cataracts by over 30%.[170]

Another study of over 1,100 people age 55 and over found that vitamin E with or without a multivitamin decreased the risk of having certain types of cataracts compared by nearly 50%. This study is difficult to interpret, sort out, and determine if the benefit was due to multivitamin use or to vitamin E by itself.[171]

An Italian study of over 900 people found that those who consumed higher dietary levels of vitamin E and folate had a lower risk of developing cataracts that required surgery. However, no link (neither protective nor harmful) was found between intake of higher levels of beta-carotene, methionine, vitamin A, or vitamin D and the risk of having cataracts.[22]

● In two studies: no link between blood levels of vitamin E and cataract

A study of 165 people found no link (neither beneficial nor harmful) between cataracts and vitamin E, vitamin A, zinc, copper, and magnesium levels in the blood. However, the study found that those who had cataracts had lower levels of carotenoids and vitamin D in their blood compared to those who did not have cataracts. On the other hand, the study found that those who had cataracts had higher levels of selenium in their blood.[41]

A study of nearly 400 people age 66 to 75 found no link (neither protective nor harmful) between higher levels of vitamin E or vitamin C or zeaxanthin and the risk of having any type of cataract. However, the study found that higher levels of beta-carotene and alpha-carotene in the blood decreased the risk of having one type of cataract but not another. Similarly, higher levels of lutein in the blood decreased risk of having one type of cataract, whereas higher levels of lycopene in the blood decreased risk of having another type of cataract.[28]

● **Though the two studies above found no link, several studies found a benefit: decreased risk of cataract in those with higher blood levels of vitamin E**   A study of nearly 1,800 people found that increased blood levels of either iron or vitamin E were associated with an over 50% decrease in the risk of having certain types of cataracts.[63]

A study of 141 people found that higher levels of both vitamin E and vitamin A in the blood decreased the risk of developing cataracts a decade or two later. However, the study found no link (neither protective nor harmful) between selenium levels in the blood and cataract.[123]

Another study of over 600 people found that high blood levels of vitamin E decreased the risk of having certain types of cataract by nearly 50%, but found no link (neither protective nor harmful) between blood levels of vitamin C and the risk of having cataract.[151]

Looking forward over time, a study of over 400 people found that higher blood levels of vitamin E decreased the risk of developing cataract over time by over 70%.[172]

A study of over 750 people found that higher blood levels of vitamin E decreased the risk of having cataracts by over 40%.[170]

Looking at blood levels in 400 people, from a population of about 5,000 people age 43 to 84, found that those with higher blood levels of vitamin E had a 60% decrease in the risk of having cataracts, but they found no link (neither protective nor harmful) between blood levels of beta-carotene, lutein, or lycopene and the risk of having cataracts.[26]

● **Though the several studies above found benefits or no link, one large study found a harm: increased risk of cataract in those with higher blood levels of vitamin E**
A study of over 1,000 people found that higher levels of vitamin E in the blood increased the risk by nearly twice of having cataracts (this finding may be related to increased risks associated with higher doses of vitamin E)! The study found no link (neither protective nor harmful) between higher levels of beta-carotene, vitamin A, or glutathione in the blood and the risk of having

cataracts. However, the study did find that higher levels of vitamin C in the blood decreased the risk of one type of cataract by nearly 50%.[25]

● **In several large studies: no benefits from the use of vitamin E on the future risk of cataract over time**   A recent 10-year study of over 3,000 people found that taking an antioxidant combination of beta-carotene (15 mg), vitamin C (500 mg), and vitamin E (400 IU), with or without zinc and copper each day reduced the risk of macular degeneration over time, but found no link (neither protective nor harmful) to the risk of cataracts over time.[29]

An Australian study of nearly 1,200 people found no link (neither protective nor harmful) between vitamin E (500 IU per day over 4 years) and reducing the risk of developing cataract or progression of cataract, compared to placebo.[173]

Another study of nearly 2,000 people randomly sampled from a study of over 20,000 people found no link (neither protective nor harmful) between taking 20 mg of vitamin E each day for 5 to 8 years and the risk of cataracts over time. Also, there was no link between taking 20 mg of beta-carotene with vitamin E, or taking beta-carotene alone, each day for 5 to 8 years and the risk of cataracts over time.[30]

A study of about 20,000 people found that use of a multivitamin decreased the risk of having cataracts by about 25%, but found no link (neither protective nor harmful) between cataract and vitamin E or C.[157]

A study of over 2,000 people given a multivitamin or a placebo for 5 years found a 36% decrease in the risk of developing cataracts in those people who were age 65 to 74. Of note, there was no difference in risk in the younger group age 45 to 64. These results exemplify the positive benefit of multivitamins; however, it is difficult to apply these results to a healthy population, as the study was performed on somewhat nutritionally-deprived people in rural China.[33]

The researchers also looked at specific nutrients in a group of over 3,000 people from the same population. They found no link (neither beneficial nor harmful) over the 5-year period between the risk of cataract and those who took selenium with beta-carotene and vitamin E, or those who took vitamin A and zinc, or those who took vitamin C and molybdenum. In contrast, in those who took vitamin B2 (5.2 mg) and vitamin B3 (40 mg) daily for 5 years had a 41% decrease in the risk of developing cataracts, compared to those who took placebo.[33]

Looking over an 8-year period into the future, a year study of over 50,000 women from a group of over 120,000 participants age 45 to 67 found no links (neither beneficial nor harmful) between diets high in vitamin E, vitamin B2, or vitamin C and cataract. The study did find that a diet with higher amounts of carotenoids decreased the risk of developing cataracts by over 25%. Similarly, a diet with higher amounts of vitamin A decreased the risk by nearly 40%.

In addition, the study did find that the duration of vitamin C intake mattered. Those who consumed vitamin C supplements for 10 or more years had a 45% decreased chance of developing cataracts.[42]

However, 7 years later, the same researchers looking forward over time over 12 years at nearly 75,000 women from the previous study found no link (neither protective nor harmful) between vitamin A, C, or E taken for more than 10 years and the risk of cataract.[138]

An interesting, but small, study of 15 people with cataracts found that those who took about 14 IU of vitamin E each day did not do any better or worse than those who took placebo. Of note, the study also found that vision actually modestly improved in the group that took about 7 mg of lutein each day over a period of 2 years, compared to placebo.[78] This study is remarkable in that it shows an improvement in vision in those people on lutein. However, the study was problematic because of its small size (only 15 people enrolled) and the fact that the some people dropped out to have cataract surgery. Furthermore, it is inconclusive in the study whether the improvement in visual acuity was related to the cataracts or the retina.

● **Though the several studies above found no link, two large studies found a benefit: use of vitamin E decreases the future risk of cataract over time** A combined British and U.S. study of nearly 300 people found a mild benefit of taking 600 IU of vitamin E, 18 mg beta-carotene, and 750 mg vitamin C each day in reducing the risk of cataract, compared to taking placebo. Interestingly, the results showed that the vitamins were more beneficial to those who lived in the U.S. as compared to those who lived in England, possibly because of genetic, environmental, or dietary differences.[34]

A study of over 1,700 people age 43 to 84 from a population of about 5,000 people found that use of vitamin E in the past for more than 10 years decreased the risk of developing cataracts over the next 5 years by 60%. Similarly, the use of vitamin C in the past for more than 10 years decreased the risk of developing cataracts over the next 5 years by 60%. Also, those who used a multivitamin regularly in the past for more than 10 years decreased the risk of developing cataracts over the next 5 years by 60%.[156]

● **In one study: increased vitamin E in the lens associated with cataract**
Interestingly, vitamin A and vitamin E levels were found to be higher in cataracts than in clear lenses in a study of 27 people and of 22 autopsy cases. These findings are contrary to what one expects, and authors suggest that those who developed cataracts started to supplement their diets with more vitamin A and E compared to those who did not develop cataracts. Alternatively, those who had cataracts were older, and there may be a different mechanism of vitamin utilization or metabolism involved in the lens.[139]

Body Absorption, Metabolism, & Excretion

Vitamin E is absorbed from the intestines after it is taken up by fat micelles (spherical soap-bubble-like conglomerates of fat). The amount absorbed varies from ¼ to ¾. It is transported to specific tissues with the assistance of fatty-proteins.

Most of the excess or used vitamin E is dumped back into the gastrointestinal tract to be excreted with bile (a green fluid produced by the liver that is stored in the gallbladder to assist in digestion).

Deficiency

Vitamin E deficiency can result in neurological problems, such as difficulty with balance and decreased sensitivity of peripheral nerves. It can also cause muscle weakness. In the retina, chronic vitamin E deficiency can cause a retinal disease with pigment deposits or debris deposits that appear similar to other retinal diseases such as macular degeneration or retinitis pigmentosa.

Abetalipoproteinemia, or Bazen-Kornzweig disease, is a genetic disorder of poor absorption of fat by the intestines. Certain vitamins, such as vitamins A, D, E, and K are absorbed by intestines by tagging on to the fats. In abetalipoproteinemia, these vitamins are not absorbed properly, so the body runs deficient in the vitamins. As a consequence, these people develop degeneration of their retina in a very similar pattern to retinitis pigmentosa (a night-blinding retinal disease). Supplementation with both vitamins A and E has been shown to reverse the process in these people.

Toxicity & Side Effects

High doses of vitamin E may cause nausea, diarrhea, bloating, fatigue, and muscle weakness. Importantly, vitamin E in high doses is associated with an increased risk of bleeding because it blocks the clumping or aggregation of platelets and inhibits vitamin K clotting activities. The risk of bleeding complications in those taking moderate or high doses of vitamin E may be exacerbated if combined with ginkgo or high dose omega-3 oils. Vitamin K, however, may mediate some of the bleeding complications. Some of the serious consequences of bleeding have included stroke.

Because of the risk of bleeding, some eye surgeons suggest that high doses of vitamin E should be stopped at least one month prior to eye surgery.

At high doses, vitamin E may be an oxidant and it may block the action of antioxidant systems. It may also block the actions of other vitamins, such as vitamin A. Furthermore, it may prevent the absorption of other fat-soluble vitamins (vitamin A, D, and K) in the intestines.

In 2004, a review of over 135,000 people enrolled in 19 different clinical trials showed that vitamin E in doses over 400 IU per day is associated with a moderate increase in the risk of early death. These studies demonstrate that some of the mortality from high doses of vitamin E may be due to increases in the risk of heart failure or cancer.

A recurring theme in ocular nutrition is moderation. Too much of a good nutrient may end up being detrimental.

Interactions with Other Nutrients

There are numerous interactions between vitamin E and other nutrients. The important concept is that a balance should be achieved between intake of vitamin E and other nutrients.

Excess vitamin E blocks vitamin A conversion in the retina and may cause retinal toxicity. Vitamin E is a non-competitive inhibitor of the enzyme retinyl-esterohydrolase, which is essential in this process of converting vitamin A into retinoic acid or retinal, which is then transported to photoreceptors to be linked to the opsin proteins to form the light-sensing pigments of the retina, the rhodopsin and iodopsins. This conversion occurs in the retinal pigment epithelium. Excess vitamin E, however, prevents this conversion of vitamin A into the retinoic acid or retinal and causes a blockage that results in a buildup of vitamin A in the retinal pigment epithelium.

Deficiency of vitamin E can also cause photoreceptor damage because of vitamin A accumulation in the retinal pigment epithelium. Vitamin E performs the first steps of preventing lipid peroxidation (oxidative damage to cell membranes), by converting strong and dangerous hydroperoxyl radicals into weaker, yet still harmful hydroperoxides. Vitamin A as retinoic acid is an essential membrane component of photoreceptors, and oxidative damage to these membranes can result in excess disc debris that must be taken up and ingested by the retinal pigment epithelium.

Bioflavonoids in combination with vitamin E are more effective as antioxidants than each one is on its own. Bioflavonoids were initially called vitamin P based on a 1936 report of their vitamin C protective role. In fact, just as vitamin C can donate electrons to vitamin E to recycle it, bioflavonoids can donate electrons to vitamin E and C when they are used up and recycle them (see sections on vitamin C and bioflavonoids).

Vitamins C and E and glutathione form a highly protective antioxidant team. Vitamin C is able to assist in recycling or reforming vitamin E when it is used up as an antioxidant. When vitamin E used up, it becomes oxidized because it has lost electrons. Vitamin C can donate electrons to vitamin E to regenerate it. In doing so, vitamin C gets used up, since it becomes oxidized, and is converted into dehydroascorbic acid or into ascorbyl free radical. Vitamin C must then be recycled itself (see section on vitamin C).

Coenzyme Q10 is also able to assist in reforming vitamin E when it is used up as an antioxidant (see section on coenzyme Q10). Coenzyme Q10 often plays such an antioxidant role in cell membranes, where vitamin E is also present.

Selenium, along with vitamin B2 and vitamin E, is required for production of glutathione peroxidase, an enzyme involved in the functioning of antioxidant glutathione. In fact, glutathione peroxidase is called a selenoprotein since it includes 4 selenium-containing amino acids (building blocks of proteins). Selenite, selenomethionine, and selenocysteine can be used as dietary supplements in order for cells to produce glutathione peroxidase. Organic selenium and selenomethionine are preferred sources of selenium to be used in raising selenium and glutathione peroxidase levels, unlike the inorganic forms, selenate and selenite.

Ideal Dosage

An average American diet contains about 10 to 15 IU of vitamin E. The recommended dose of vitamin E for children age 14 to 18 and adults is 22 IU per day. Some studies have shown that the ideal dosage may be around 500 IU per day.

It may be best to obtain a dose of around 150 to 200 IU per day. There is concern that levels over 1,500 IU per day in adults may cause toxicity, including bleeding complications.

Most food sources are labeled in mg. About 1 IU of natural dietary vitamin E is about $2/3$ mg. Alternatively, about 1 mg of natural dietary vitamin E is about 1½ IU.

Alpha-tocopherol is the form of vitamin E found in the highest concentration in the human body, and the most potent form. Synthetic forms of vitamin E often contain all 8 forms of vitamin E (see page 409), whereas the natural sources of vitamin E are often more concentrated in the alpha-tocopherol form. Therefore, our bodies may benefit more from the natural sources of vitamin E than from the synthetics forms.

Sources (Where to Find It)

Fruits & Vegetables:

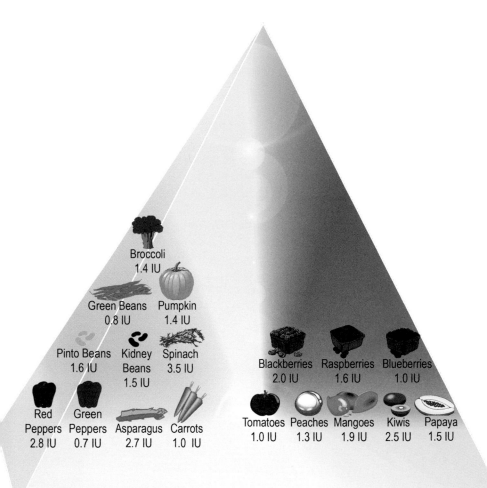

Broccoli
1.4 IU

Green Beans
0.8 IU

Pumpkin
1.4 IU

Pinto Beans
1.6 IU

Kidney Beans
1.5 IU

Spinach
3.5 IU

Red Peppers
2.8 IU

Green Peppers
0.7 IU

Asparagus
2.7 IU

Carrots
1.0 IU

Blackberries
2.0 IU

Raspberries
1.6 IU

Blueberries
1.0 IU

Tomatoes
1.0 IU

Peaches
1.3 IU

Mangoes
1.9 IU

Kiwis
2.5 IU

Papaya
1.5 IU

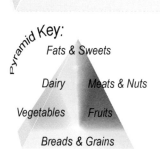

Pyramid Key:

Fats & Sweets

Dairy   Meats & Nuts

Vegetables   Fruits

Breads & Grains

*See Guides on Pages 467-468.

Dairy, Meats & Nuts:

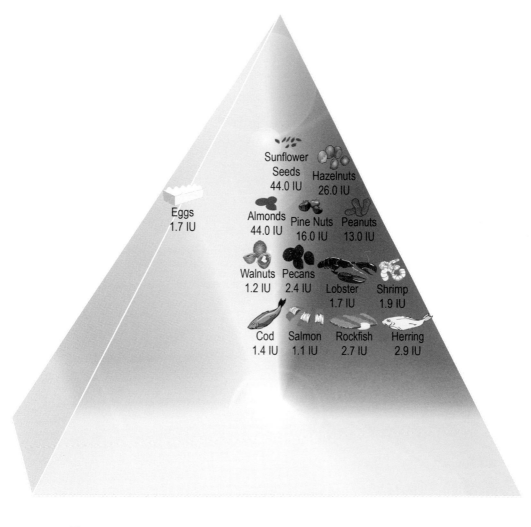

The top source of vitamin E is nuts, particularly almonds, sunflower seeds, and hazelnuts. Other sources high in vitamin E include seafood (such as herring and rockfish), spinach, red peppers, asparagus, kiwis, and blueberries.

VITAMIN G
(SEE VITAMIN B2)

VITAMIN K
(PHYLLOQUINONE, MENAQUINONE, MENADIONE)

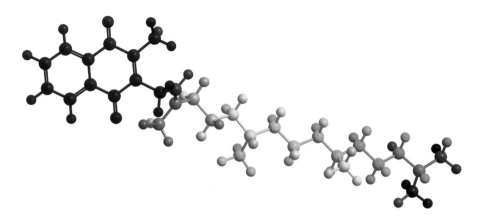

Category

Vitamin K is a fat-soluble vitamin. Its name comes from the German word for coagulation, "koagulation," which means blood clotting. There are three forms of vitamin K. Plants make a form known as vitamin K1, or phylloquinone. Bacteria make a group of forms known as vitamin K2, or menaquinones. Menadione is a synthetic form of vitamin K, and is sometimes called vitamin K3.

Cellular Location

Vitamin K is found in its highest concentrations in the liver. It is distributed in the bloodstream.

Structure

Vitamin K is composed of a double-ring, called a naphthoquinone ring with a long side chain that is composed of units called isoprenoid.

Mechanisms of Action

Vitamin K is required for an enzyme that converts glutamic acid, an amino acid (building blocks of proteins), into gamma-carboxyglutamic acid, which in turns forms very specific proteins that play roles in blood clotting and bone maintenance.

Biological & Ocular Importance

● **Assists in normal blood clotting** The gamma-carboxyglutamic acid formed by vitamin K forms very specific proteins that play roles in blood clotting. Thus, vitamin K has been used to treat bleeding complications. Vitamin K has also been suggested as being beneficial in preventing atherosclerosis (blood vessel cholesterol clots and plaques that can result in heart disease and stroke, as well as artery or vein clots in the retina or optic nerve strokes).

● **Plays a role in the risk of bleeding in wet macular degeneration** There is some evidence that vitamin K may reduce the incidence of bleeding in people with wet macular degeneration, which is the form of macular degeneration in which new blood vessels that are prone to bleeding start to grow beneath the retina.

● **Important for bone maintenance** The specific proteins formed by vitamin K also play roles in bone maintenance and cell growth. As such, vitamin K has been recommended to prevent osteoporosis as well.

Human Studies on Utility

There are no human studies on the use of vitamin K in treatment of eye disease reported in the scientifically-reviewed medical literature. Nevertheless, the fact that there are no reported clinical studies does not necessarily imply a benefit or lack of benefit. Looking at the mechanism of action, the use of vitamin K in moderation may be possibly of benefit in certain eye diseases.

Body Absorption, Metabolism, & Excretion

Vitamin K is absorbed from the intestines after it is taken up by fat micelles (spherical soap-bubble-like conglomerates of fat). Then, it is transported to specific tissues with the assistance of fatty-proteins.

The excess or used vitamin K is filtered by the kidneys for excretion and is also dumped back into the gastrointestinal tract to be excreted with bile (a green fluid produced by the liver that is stored in the gallbladder to assist in digestion).

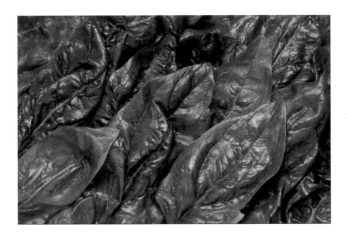

Deficiency

Vitamin K deficiency is characterized by excess bleeding, such as nosebleeds, gum bleeding, skin bruising. Bruising and bleeding can occur in or around the eye. Additionally, intestinal bleeding and bloody stools can occur as well as kidney bleeding and bloody urine. In addition, menstruation in women can be particularly heavy during vitamin K deficiency.

Toxicity & Side Effects

There are no known toxicities or side effects of naturally occurring forms of vitamin K. However, the synthetic form of vitamin K, menadione, may interfere with the functioning of glutathione, an important antioxidant in the body. Furthermore, the synthetic form of vitamin K can build-up in high concentrations in the bloodstream, whereas the natural forms are easily stored or excreted.

Interactions with Other Nutrients

Vitamins A and E may interfere with the absorption of vitamin K.

The synthetic form of vitamin K, called menadione, may interfere with the functioning of glutathione. Thus, it may be better to avoid this synthetic form of vitamin K.

The risk of bleeding complications is higher in those taking ginkgo, high doses of vitamin E, high dose omega-3 oils, or a combination of these nutrients together. Thus, vitamin K may decrease some of the risk of bleeding complications.

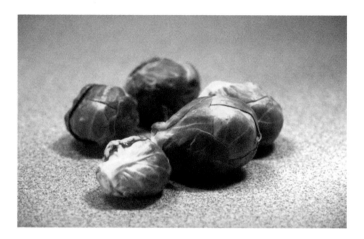

Ideal Dosage

The recommended dose is 45 to 80 µg per day. In children age 11 to 14, the recommended dose is 45 µg per day. In children age 15 to 18, the recommended dose is 55 µg per day in girls and 65 µg per day in boys. The recommended dose for adults age 19 to 24 is 60 µg per day in women and 70 µg per day in men. For adults age 25 and over, the recommended dose is 65 µg per day in women and 80 µg per day in men.

It may be best, however, to obtain a dose of around 90 to 120 µg per day; although, a dose of 300 µg per day from natural sources may be recommended in those taking ginkgo, high doses of vitamin E, high doses of omega-3 oils, or a combination of these nutrients together.

Also, natural sources of vitamin K are superior to synthetic sources because of the interference with glutathione (see above).

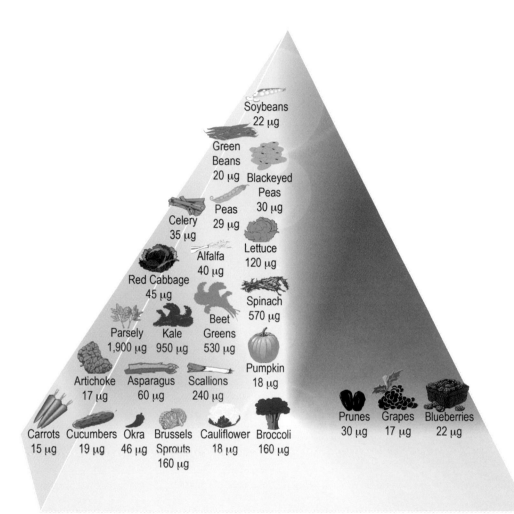

Soybeans 22 μg
Green Beans 20 μg
Blackeyed Peas 30 μg
Peas 29 μg
Celery 35 μg
Lettuce 120 μg
Alfalfa 40 μg
Red Cabbage 45 μg
Spinach 570 μg
Parsely 1,900 μg
Kale 950 μg
Beet Greens 530 μg
Pumpkin 18 μg
Artichoke 17 μg
Asparagus 60 μg
Scallions 240 μg
Prunes 30 μg
Grapes 17 μg
Blueberries 22 μg
Carrots 15 μg
Cucumbers 19 μg
Okra 46 μg
Brussels Sprouts 160 μg
Cauliflower 18 μg
Broccoli 160 μg

Pyramid Key:

Fats & Sweets

Dairy   Meats & Nuts

Vegetables   Fruits

Breads & Grains

Top sources of vitamin K are greens, particularly parsley, kale, spinach, and beet greens. Other sources rich in vitamin K include scallions, Brussels sprouts, broccoli, and lettuce.

VITAMIN M
(SEE FOLATE)

VITAMIN P
(SEE BIOFLAVONOIDS)

VITAMIN PP
(SEE VITAMIN B3)

VITAMIN Q
(SEE COENZYME Q10)

ZEAXANTHIN

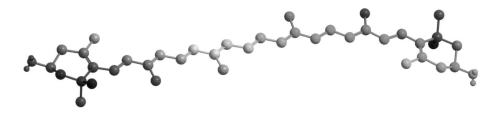

Category

Carotenoids are organic pigments that occur naturally in plants, but that cannot be made by animals (see section on carotenoids).

The yellow carotenoids are zeaxanthin and lutein, both also known as xanthophylls. They are structurally nearly identical, differing only in the position of a double bond in one of their hydroxyl groups.

Cellular Location

The highest concentration of the xanthophylls, lutein and zeaxanthin, are found within the retina, predominantly in the macula (the central portion of the retina), where their concentration is 100 times that of the peripheral retina. Lutein is found throughout all areas of the retina from the peripheral retina to the central retina, while zeaxanthin is concentrated within the macula, and predominantly within the fovea (the center of the macula where images are focused).

The xanthophylls, lutein and zeaxanthin, are also concentrated in the nerve fiber layer that serves as the connection between the photoreceptors and the processing neurons of the retina, and within the outer segments of photoreceptor cells, where the photoreceptor discs are located. There are numerous reports that increased dietary consumption of lutein and zeaxanthin increase blood levels of lutein and zeaxanthin, and that increased blood levels of lutein and zeaxanthin are associated with increased levels of lutein and zeaxanthin in the macula. As a matter of fact, researchers as early as 1941 have shown that the amount of lutein and zeaxanthin in the macula is related to the amount in the diet.

Interestingly, lutein and zeaxanthin are also found to become concentrated in the lens, following a diet with higher levels of the nutrients. This finding suggests a protective role for lutein and zeaxanthin in the lens, likely as antioxidants. In past studies, other carotenoids have not been observed in the lens.

Structure

The xanthophylls lutein and zeaxanthin are polar because they have hydroxyl groups on both ends, unlike other carotenoids. This structure makes them particularly effective as retinal pigments since this polarity can enable them to lay in the photoreceptor discs with their ends sticking out, which enables them to function more effectively in their antioxidant role.

The long chain contains many double bonds that give zeaxanthin its characteristic yellow color. Additionally, its structure causes it to be insoluble in water, so it prefers to be in the presence of oils and fats.

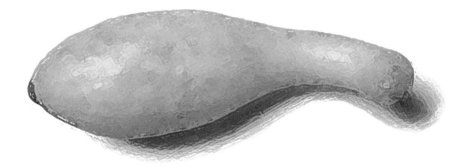

Mechanisms of Action

The carotenoids can function as antioxidants as well as light filters.

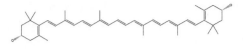

Biological & Ocular Importance

● **Acts as a powerful antioxidant**   The carotenoids have a long chain of carbons with alternating single and double bonds. In fact, the high number of double bonds is what makes these carotenoids able to function as antioxidants. They are able to donate electrons to free radicals (toxic chemicals that result in oxidation), which prevents the free radicals themselves from accepting electrons and damaging cell components. Lycopene is known as the most potent antioxidant of the carotenoids.

Light exposure is high in the retina, and the highest amount of oxygen consumption of any tissue in the body occurs in the retina. The retina's cells are therefore particularly susceptible to oxidative damage. Thus, animal models have found that zeaxanthin can prevent degeneration of retinal photoreceptors.

● **Acts as a light filter for the retina**   Furthermore, the long chain on the carotenoids gives these pigments their color, by absorbing light of various wavelengths. This absorption of light is biologically important since the yellow pigments lutein and zeaxanthin absorb blue light and ultraviolet light (forms of high-energy light). This absorption helps protect the macula from high-energy light exposure and oxidative damage. In fact, some studies show that lutein and zeaxanthin in the macula absorb anywhere from 40 to 90% of the high-energy blue light! In addition to being concentrated in the photoreceptor outer segments, lutein and zeaxanthin are concentrated in the nerve fiber layer that serves as the connection between the photoreceptors and the processing neurons of the retina. This nerve fiber layer sits on top of the photoreceptors in the macula and, because of the lutein and zeaxanthin, it acts to filter the light that passes through on its way to the photoreceptors.

There is also evidence to suggest that the absorption of blue light assists in improving the quality of the image we see. Lutein and zeaxanthin in the retina act by blocking excess light, improving the eye's contrast sensitivity, or the ability of the eye to distinguish different shades of contrast in dim light and in very bright light. Lutein and zeaxanthin pigments in the macula can absorb the shorter-wavelength blue light, reducing what is called "chromatic aberrations." This chromatic aberration would result in a blurred blue edge to the object that we see in the center of our vision. Alternative theories suggest that the macular pigments help prevent glare in bright daylight conditions.

● **Plays a role in a cell to cell communication protein**
In addition to their antioxidant and light-absorbing capabilities, carotenoids help upregulate expression of the gene to make connexin proteins and they stabilize connexin proteins as they are being made. These connexin proteins are important in cell to cell communication, and the loss of this communication is thought to play a role in the development of cancer.

● **Helps lower cholesterol**
Carotenoids share similar synthesis pathways as cholesterol and may help lower cholesterol levels by interfering in this pathway or by inhibiting cholesterol-forming enzymes such as HMGCoA in this pathway. Also, carotenoids are believed to

prevent the lipid oxidation in blood vessels that leads to atherosclerosis (blood vessel cholesterol clots and plaques that can result in heart disease and stroke, as well as artery or vein clots in the retina or optic nerve strokes).

● **Strengthens the immune defense system**   In addition, the carotenoids and notably vitamin A also play an essential role in immune protection. While vitamin A and the carotenoids assist in maintaining a healthy immune system, there is considerable controversy and unknown mechanism of how they function in this role. A deficiency in carotenoids and vitamin A can impair function of certain types of white blood cells, called neutrophils. The deficiency can also impair the ability of other types of white blood cells, known as macrophages, from ingesting and killing bacteria, while simultaneously causing an increased amount of inflammation, or the presence of excess white blood cells. It can also impair the response of other types of white blood cells, called T-cells.

Human Studies on Utility

Currently, there are numerous human studies on zeaxanthin use in eye disease reported in the scientifically-reviewed medical literature. These studies involve

the eye disease macular degeneration, cataract, and retinitis pigmentosa. These studies are described below.

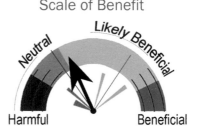

Looking at the mechanisms of action, there is good reason to use zeaxanthin in moderation for macular degeneration and cataract.

● Older studies suggested benefit of zeaxanthin for the retina and for retinitis pigmentosa

In the 1940's to 1960's, several German researchers looked at the benefits of commercially-available xanthophylls. Some studies of healthy people found that taking the xanthophylls for several months improved their night vision. Other researchers found that night vision improved in people with a night-blindness retinal disease, called retinitis pigmentosa. On the other hand, some of the researchers found no benefits. One study found that there was no change in the electrical activity of the retinal cells after use of the xanthophylls. These studies were mostly small studies, often without control groups, making them quite difficult to interpret; however, they did provide a suggestion of the benefits of xanthophylls.[64]

Summary of Studies for Macular Degeneration:

Over a dozen clinical trials have been performed looking at the role of zeaxanthin in both preventing and treating macular degeneration. These clinical trials are of many different types, some of which are very well-designed and well-performed studies.

As a whole, the clinical studies provide no definitive answer as to whether zeaxanthin is beneficial. Many of the studies found no benefit to zeaxanthin for macular degeneration. However, there is some suggestion that is may be beneficial, as 5 out of the 13 studies found a benefit. Looking

Zeaxanthin for
Macular Degeneration
Scale of Benefit

at the mechanisms of action, there is good reason to use zeaxanthin in moderation for macular degeneration.

The studies can be summarized as follows: one study found that those with macular degeneration had less zeaxanthin in their retinas. Two studies found a benefit in the past use of zeaxanthin in decreasing the risk of macular degeneration while another provided no benefit in the past use of zeaxanthin in decreasing the risk of macular degeneration. Interestingly, one study found that the past use of zeaxanthin actually increased the risk of macular degeneration, but this increased risk was in those who used zeaxanthin with high amounts of linoleic acid (see section on omega-6 oils). Thus, this finding supports the need for a well-balanced diet. Eating beneficial nutrients along with the bad may still cause harm. Several studies have shown no links (neither protective nor harmful) between levels of zeaxanthin in the blood and macular degeneration, though two studies found that higher levels of zeaxanthin in the blood are associated with a decrease in the risk of macular degeneration. In following people over time, three large, well-performed studies found that those who took zeaxanthin did not have any benefit in preventing macular degeneration compared to those who did not take zeaxanthin.

● **In one study: decreased zeaxanthin in the retina associated with macular degeneration** A study of over 100 autopsy cases found that those eyes with macular degeneration had lower levels of lutein and zeaxanthin in their retinas as compared to eyes without macular degeneration.[67]

● **In one study: no benefits in past use of zeaxanthin found on risk of macular degeneration** A study of over 3,500 people age 49 and over found no link (neither protective nor harmful) between the risk of developing macular degeneration over a 5 year period and people who took the following nutrients, alone or in combination, in the past: zeaxanthin and lutein,

lycopene, beta-carotene, vitamin A, or zinc. Surprisingly, however, the study found, that those who took vitamin C supplements combined with a diet high in vitamin C had a 2-fold increase in their risk of developing macular degeneration.[2] This finding is quite surprising, as one would expect vitamin C to protect against macular degeneration, as opposed to increasing the risk of macular degeneration. However, the finding highlights the problems associated with these types of studies: namely, that the findings may occur coincidentally and other true findings may be missed. It is sometimes difficult to explain the findings or apply them to real life.

● **One study found a harm: past use of zeaxanthin (with high amounts of linoleic acid) associated with *increased* risk of macular degeneration** A study of 2,000 people found that a diet high in lutein and zeaxanthin possibly decreased the risk of having dry or wet macular degeneration. However, when combined with a diet high in linoleic acid (a precursor of omega-6 fatty oils), the study found the risk of having dry or wet macular degeneration actually by increased by 2- to 5-fold![68] This finding of an increased risk with lutein and zeaxanthin is contrary to what one expects, but in the context of a diet high in linoleic acid, it supports the theory that a well-balanced diet is essential in protecting one's eyes. High amounts of linoleic acid by itself may be harmful (see section on omega-6 oils).

444

- **Though one study found harm, two studies found a benefit: past use of zeaxanthin associated with decreased risk of macular degeneration**   A large study of over 8,000 people age 40 and over found no link (neither protective nor harmful) between the risk of having macular degeneration (dry or wet) and a diet high in lutein and zeaxanthin. However, when the study population was divided, the study found that younger people age 40 to 59 who consumed diets high in lutein and zeaxanthin in the past had a 90% decrease in the risk of having *early* macular degeneration. Also, the study found that older people age 60 to 79 who consumed diets high in lutein and zeaxanthin in the past had a 90% decrease in the risk of having *advanced or severe* macular degeneration.[69]

A study of over 1,000 people age 55 to 80 found that those who consumed a diet high in lutein and zeaxanthin had a nearly 60% decrease in the risk of having wet macular degeneration compared to those who did not consume a diet high in lutein and zeaxanthin. Similarly, dietary beta-carotene decreased the risk by 40%, while dietary vitamin A and dietary carotenoids each decreased the risk by over 40%. The authors found no link (neither protective nor harmful) between macular degeneration and a diet high in vitamin C or E.[5]

- **In several studies: no link between blood levels of zeaxanthin and macular degeneration**   A study of over 900 people age 60 to 80 found that the blood levels of lutein and of zeaxanthin were no different among people divided into 3 groups: with early macular degeneration, with advanced or severe macular degeneration, and without any macular degeneration.[71]

A study of over 300 people from a group of nearly 5,000 people found no difference in the blood levels of zeaxanthin and lutein, beta-carotene, or lycopene between those with or without macular degeneration. They also found that those who had macular degeneration had lower blood levels of vitamin E compared to those without macular degeneration. Interestingly, they also found that fewer people with macular degeneration use vitamin C than people without macular degeneration.[7]

Another study of nearly 100 people found no difference in the blood levels of zeaxanthin and lutein, carotenoids, beta-carotene, lycopene, vitamin A, vitamin C, zinc, or selenium between those with or without macular degeneration (looking at both early and severe or advanced macular degeneration). However, the study found that those who had severe or advanced macular degeneration had lower blood levels of vitamin E compared to those without macular degeneration. They found no differences in the blood levels of vitamin E between those with or without early macular degeneration.[6]

● **Though the three studies above found no link, two studies found a benefit: decreased risk of macular degeneration in those with higher blood levels of zeaxanthin**   A study of nearly 400 people age 66 to 75 found that those with higher blood levels of zeaxanthin had a 50% decrease in the risk of having macular degeneration (dry or wet). The study found no link (neither protective nor harmful) between higher blood levels of lutein and macular degeneration. Interestingly, the study also found no link between macular degeneration and higher blood levels of zeaxanthin and lutein together.[72]

A study of over 1,000 people age 55 to 80 found that having higher blood levels of carotenoids decreased the risk of having wet macular degeneration by 60% compared to those who had lower blood levels of carotenoids.[11] Looking at specific carotenoids, the study found that having higher blood levels of zeaxanthin and lutein decreased the risk of having macular degeneration by 70%. Higher blood levels of beta-carotene also decreased the risk by 70% and higher blood levels of lycopene decreased the risk by 60%. Also, higher blood levels of a combination of three or more of four nutrients (carotenoids, vitamin C, vitamin E, and selenium) decreased the risk by 70%. The study found no link (neither protective nor harmful) between higher blood levels of vitamin C, vitamin E, or selenium by

themselves and macular degeneration.[12]

● **In large studies: no benefits from the use of zeaxanthin on the future risk of macular degeneration over time**   A study of over 75,000 people (nurses and health professionals) followed over time for up to 18 years found no link (neither protective nor harmful) between the risk of developing macular degeneration (wet or dry) and a diet high in any of the following nutrients: zeaxanthin and lutein, carotenoids, beta-carotene, lycopene, vitamin A, vitamin C, or vitamin E. The study did find that those who consumed more than 3 servings of fruit each day were 1/3 less likely to develop *wet* macular degeneration over time compared to those who consumed less than 1½ servings of fruit each day. No link (neither protective nor harmful) was found when looking at increased fruit consumption for dry macular degeneration, nor when looking at increased vegetable consumption for dry or wet macular degeneration.[15]

Looking over a 5-year period, a study of 2,000 people from a group of nearly 5,000, found no link (neither protective nor harmful) between macular degeneration and a diet high in zeaxanthin and lutein, beta-carotene, carotenoids, vitamin C, vitamin E, or zinc.[14]

A study of nearly 4,000 people, looking forward over an average of 8 years, found no link (neither protective nor harmful) between macular degeneration and a diet high in zeaxanthin and lutein, beta-carotene, lycopene, vitamin A, vitamin C, iron, or zinc. However, a diet high in vitamin E decreased the risk of having macular degeneration by 20%. A diet high in multiple nutrients (beta-carotene, vitamin C, vitamin E, and zinc together) decreased the risk of having macular degeneration by about ½![18]

 Summary of Studies for Cataract: Nearly a half dozen clinical trials have been performed looking at the role of zeaxanthin in preventing cataract. These clinical trials are of various types, some of which are very well-designed and well-performed studies.

As a whole, the studies provide no definitive answer that zeaxanthin is beneficial. However, 3 of the 5 studies found a benefit. Looking at the mechanisms of action, there may be good reason to use zeaxanthin in moderation for cataract.

Zeaxanthin for
Cataract
Scale of Benefit

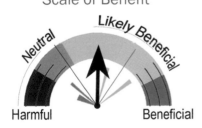

The studies can be summarized as follows: one study found no benefits from the past use of zeaxanthin on the risk of cataract, while three larger studies that did find a benefit in the past use of zeaxanthin in decreasing the risk of cataract.

One study found no link (neither protective nor harmful) between blood levels of zeaxanthin and the risk of cataract. There are no studies that have been reviewed by the scientific community that following over time people taking zeaxanthin.

● **In one study: no benefits in past use of zeaxanthin found on risk of cataract**
A study of nearly 500 people age 53 to 73 found no link (neither protective nor harmful) between the intake of zeaxanthin and lutein, beta-carotene, carotenoids, or lycopene and the risk of having cataracts. However, the study did show that the past intake of *higher* amounts of vitamin C decreased the risk of having cataracts by nearly 70%. It also found that long-term intake of vitamin C for over 10 years decreased the risk of having cataracts by nearly 65%. Similarly, past intake of *higher* amounts of vitamin B2 decreased the risk of having cataracts by over 60%, and past intake of *higher* amounts of folate decreased the risk by about 10%. It also found that long-term intake of vitamin E for over 10 years decreased the risk of having cataracts by over 50%, even though the study found no link (neither protective nor harmful) between the past intake of *higher* amounts of vitamin E and the risk of having cataracts. The finding of no beneficial link with higher doses of vitamin E may be related to increased risks associated with the higher doses. Furthermore, the use of a multivitamin for over 10 years reduced the risk of having cataract by over 40%.[20]

- **Though the one study above found no link, three large studies found a benefit: past use of zeaxanthin associated with decreased risk of cataract**   A 12-year study of over 75,000 nurses age 45 and over found that those who consumed the highest amounts of lutein and zeaxanthin in their diets had an over 20% reduction in the development of cataracts that required surgery.[75]

   A similar 8-year study of over 35,000 male health professionals age 45 and over found that those who consumed the highest amounts of lutein and zeaxanthin in their diets had a nearly 20% reduction in the development of cataracts that required surgery.[76]

   A study of over 1,300 people age 43 to 84 found that higher intake of lutein and zeaxanthin was associated with a decrease in the risk of having cataract by about a ½. No link (neither protective nor harmful) was found between cataract and the past use of vitamin C or of vitamin E over 10 years.[77]

- **In one study: no link between blood levels of zeaxanthin and cataract** A study of nearly 400 people age 66 to 75 found no link (neither protective nor harmful) between higher levels of zeaxanthin, vitamin C, or vitamin E and the risk of having any type of cataract. However, the study found that higher levels of beta-carotene and alpha-carotene in the blood decreased the risk of having one type of cataract but not another. Similarly, higher levels of lutein in the blood decreased risk of having one type of cataract, whereas higher levels of lycopene in the blood decreased risk of having another type of cataract.[28]

Body Absorption, Metabolism, & Excretion

   Digestion of fruits and vegetables occurs in the stomach with the assistance of stomach acids that help break down the fruits and vegetables to release the zeaxanthin. Zeaxanthin is insoluble in water, and therefore needs to be dissolved in fat micelles (spherical soap-bubble-like conglomerates of fat) that can carry zeaxanthin into the bloodstream from the intestines. Accordingly, eating a small quantity of fat with zeaxanthin assists in the absorption of zeaxanthin and greatly increases the amount that is delivered to the bloodstream. Zeaxanthin is then transported to specific tissues with the assistance of fatty-proteins.

   Excretion of zeaxanthin occurs mostly through the kidneys. Some excretion occurs through the digestive tract while excess zeaxanthin is often dumped back into the digestive tract through bile (a green fluid produced by the liver that is stored in the gallbladder to assist in digestion).

Deficiency

It has been shown that zeaxanthin and lutein levels are reduced in people with cystic fibrosis compared to healthy control people. Cystic fibrosis is an inherited lung disease and pancreas disease in which there is poor absorption of certain vitamin and nutrients, including zeaxanthin and lutein, vitamins A, D, and E. However, a study that found the decreased zeaxanthin and lutein levels did not show any difference in visual functioning in people with cystic fibrosis.

Toxicity & Side Effects

Excess zeaxanthin and lutein can result in a yellow-bronze discoloration of the skin, called carotenodermia or xanthosis cutis. It is harmless and can be reversed upon cessation of the supplementation.

Interactions with Other Nutrients

Fat in one's diet is an essential component of good carotenoid nutrition. Fat is required for absorption of zeaxanthin and lutein by the digestive system. However, in people with excess fat stores in their bodies, zeaxanthin and lutein can accumulate in body fat rather than be sent to the eyes when needed.

Furthermore, HDL (good type of cholesterol) is required for transportation of lutein and zeaxanthin to the retinas. In people with less of HDL, there is less lutein and zeaxanthin in their retinas. In fact, this finding may be one of the reasons why women undergoing menopause have a higher risk of macular degeneration since their HDl levels decrease during menopause.

Ideal Dosage

The recommended dose of zeaxanthin is 4 to 8 mg each day. Interestingly, zeaxanthin can be made from lutein within the cells of the retina.

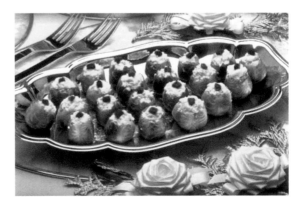

Sources (Where to Find It)

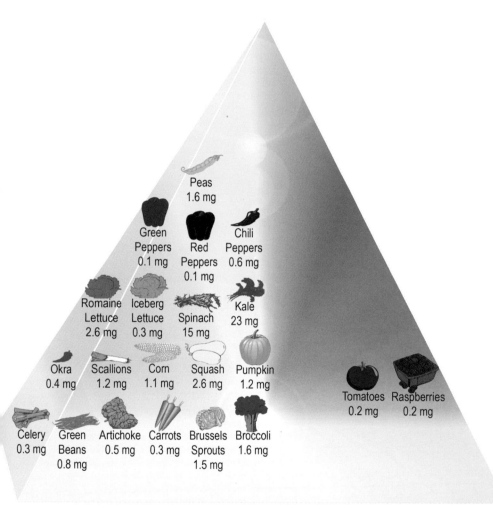

Peas
1.6 mg

Green
Peppers
0.1 mg

Red
Peppers
0.1 mg

Chili
Peppers
0.6 mg

Romaine
Lettuce
2.6 mg

Iceberg
Lettuce
0.3 mg

Spinach
15 mg

Kale
23 mg

Okra
0.4 mg

Scallions
1.2 mg

Corn
1.1 mg

Squash
2.6 mg

Pumpkin
1.2 mg

Tomatoes
0.2 mg

Raspberries
0.2 mg

Celery
0.3 mg

Green
Beans
0.8 mg

Artichoke
0.5 mg

Carrots
0.3 mg

Brussels
Sprouts
1.5 mg

Broccoli
1.6 mg

Pyramid Key:

Fats & Sweets

Dairy   Meats & Nuts

Vegetables   Fruits

Breads & Grains

Sources above are for lutein and zeaxanthin together. The top sources are spinach and kale. Other high sources include squash, romaine lettuce, peas, broccoli, and Brussels sprouts.

*See Guides on Pages 467-468.

ZINC

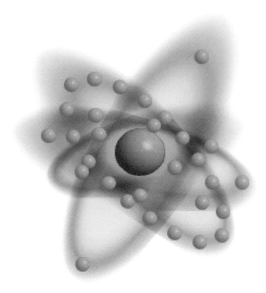

Category

Zinc is an essential metal.

Cellular Location

Zinc is the second-most abundant trace metal in the human body. Zinc is in high concentrations in the liver, muscles and bones, and skin and hair. The highest concentration of zinc in the body is in the eye, notably in the retina.

Structure

Zinc is found as an ionic metal. Its symbol on the periodic table of elements is Zn, and its atomic number is 30.

Mechanisms of Action

Zinc plays an essential role in hundreds of proteins and, in particular, enzymes. Zinc is essential in the making of DNA and RNA. It also can act both as an antioxidant and an oxidant.

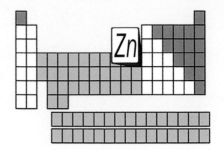

Biological & Ocular Importance

● **Essential in the process of making DNA & RNA** Zinc is essential in the functioning of DNA polymerase and RNA polymerase (enzymes that are involved in making DNA and RNA).

● **Activates genes in cells** Zinc plays an important role in the structure of proteins, by forming a finger-like stabilizing element called a zinc-finger. These zinc-finger proteins often function as transcription factors (proteins that turn specific genes on or off). Therefore, changes in zinc levels within cells can change the molecular makeup of these cells through the activation of genes.

● **Helps in healthy wound healing and preventing clouding of the cornea** The numerous enzymes that require zinc are essential for growth and development, healthy neurological function, and a healthy immune system. It also plays a role in wound healing, such as after eye injury or after surgery. Also, corneal swelling or clouding can be aggravated or even caused by low zinc levels.

● **Prevents loss of eyebrows & eyelashes** Zinc prevents loss of hair or alopecia. When zinc levels are low, this loss of hair can occur in the eyebrows or lashes.

● **Boosts the immune defense system** Zinc is important for the immune function of the body and eye. It may boost the immune system and protect against infections or help treat infections. It is frequently used to decrease the duration of the common cold. White blood cells, which are the body's circulating immune-defense cells, undergo a tremendous amount of DNA and RNA synthesis. Zinc acts in the enzymes involved in synthesizing DNA and RNA. Furthermore, zinc is required for the activity of numerous enzymes that are involved in immunity, such as the enzyme thymulin. Zinc also plays a role in the formation of cytokines (proteins that communicate between the body's immune-defense cells).

● Suggested for numerous diseases ranging from inflammatory diseases to diabetes

Zinc has been suggested as a treatment or preventative measure for numerous diseases. It has been used to treat diabetes and arthritis, though it may not be treating the actual disease, but rather some of the consequences of the disease, such as the impaired immune system in diabetes or inflammation in arthritis. However, there is some suggestion that zinc may improve the production of insulin in diabetes and decrease blood sugars in diabetics.

● Acts as an antioxidant though can also act as a toxic oxidant

Zinc in its elemental state can act as an antioxidant by losing electrons, though in its ionic form as Zn^{2+}, it can act as an oxidant by gaining electrons. However, zinc is not as chemically reactive because its valence (outer shell) electrons are held more closely to it, and its outer shell and subshell are full. Thus, unlike some other reactive metals, such as copper, iron, and magnesium, it does not have multiple oxidation states.

● Essential for antioxidant enzymes

Zinc, along with copper (see section on copper), plays a central role in the enzyme superoxide dismutase, a powerful antioxidant enzyme. One form of superoxide dismutase works within cells and requires both copper and zinc. As such, zinc is important for its role in the antioxidant enzyme. Typically, though, it is a deficiency of copper that affects the functioning of this enzyme.

● Stabilizes cell membranes

Zinc also works in cell membranes to stabilize them and to prevent oxidation of the lipids that form the membranes.

● Essential for melanin that protects against light damage

Zinc plays an essential role in the melanin (a pigment, which plays a major role in retinal pigment epithelium by absorbing excess light in order to protect against the light toxicity). Melanin plays an essential antioxidant role controlling ultraviolet light-produced oxidants and by binding iron. Retinal cells are particularly susceptible to oxidative damage. Zinc also plays this antioxidant role by helping in the formation of catalase and metallothionein, two potent antioxidant enzymes of the retina. Metallothionein can also function with other metals such as cadmium, copper, and mercury. In fact, the highest levels of zinc in the eye are found in the retina.

● Assists other enzymes in the retinal pigment epithelium

Zinc also plays a role in enzymes, in the retinal

pigment epithelium, which are involved in the mammoth task of digesting photoreceptor outer segment discs that are shed each day (see introduction).

● Regulates neurotransmitter signaling molecules

Zinc may also regulate the signaling of neurotransmitters in the synapses between the neurons of the retina, which is the process whereby signals are sent from the photoreceptors to other processing cells within the retina.

● Essential for the light-sensing pigments of the retina

Zinc deficiency has been associated with retinal degeneration, notably night-blindness and retinitis pigmentosa. In fact, serum zinc levels are sometimes found to be decreased in people with retinitis pigmentosa, and serum copper levels are sometimes found to be elevated in these people (see section on copper). When zinc levels are extremely low, there is an association with decreased vitamin A metabolism, particularly in photoreceptors. Zinc is involved in a dehydrogenase enzyme, retinol dehydrogenase (also known as retinene reductase), which is essential for vitamin A metabolism in photoreceptors. Vitamin A is required for production of light-sensing pigments of the retina (the rhodopsin in rod photoreceptors and the iodopsins in the cone photoreceptors).

Vitamin A is a retinol that is converted in the retina to retinoic acid or retinal, which is then linked to the opsin proteins to form the iodopsins and rhodopsin (see section on vitamin A). Zinc also facilitates vitamin A's "mobilization" out of the liver via vitamin A binding proteins. In fact, zinc deficiency has been associated with decreased formation of these vitamin A binding proteins by the liver. Furthermore, and very importantly, zinc has been recently found to play a structural role in the shape and folding of the rhodopsin protein. Zinc also assists in activating the light-sensing rhodopsin protein; thus, zinc deficiency is associated with decreased ability to see in the dark.

● Causes injury to neurons & oxidative damage

On a cellular level, high levels of zinc can be damaging to cells by enhancing the production of oxidants that abnormally alter the function of mitochondria (the energy-producing organelles in the body's cells). This disruption in the mitochondrial function affects other ionic balances within cells, while also blocking the function of other large compounds within cells, such as "neurotrophic" growth factors.

There is a growing body of evidence that zinc is involved in the death of neuronal cells in the retina, especially during events like retinal ischemia (a process in which blood flow to the retina is reduced). However, it is uncertain whether the higher levels of zinc observed are a cause or a result of the neuronal injury. In fact, perhaps the elevated zinc levels could be a result of the neuronal injury, which then causes even more neuronal injury. In addition, other evidence shows that zinc may be a neuroprotectant (a protective compound that prevents neuronal cells from being injured during events like retinal ischemia).

● **Plays a role in vitamin A's protective effects on the surface of the eye** Zinc's role in vitamin A metabolism is not only important for the retina, but also for other ocular tissues, such as the surface of the eye, where vitamin A plays an essential role (see section on vitamin A). In addition, through its assistance in the synthesis (body's formation) of the protein that carries vitamin A in the bloodstream, zinc helps maintain appropriate vitamin A levels in the blood. Similarly, vitamin A deficiency has been associated with decreases in the zinc-binding protein, which results in decreased zinc absorption and decreased zinc levels in the bloodstream (see section on vitamin A).

● **Prevents cataract** Zinc also prevents formation of cataract. Low zinc levels are associated with cataract formation. However, several studies have shown that some people with cataracts were found to have high zinc levels in their cataracts. It is uncertain whether that high level of zinc is the instigator of the cataract, or represents a secondary effect of the cataract, or is effectively an attempt by the body to prevent the cataract progression.

Human Studies on Utility

Currently, there are numerous human studies on zinc use in eye disease reported in the scientifically-reviewed medical literature. These studies involve the eye disease macular degeneration, cataract, and retinitis pigmentosa. These studies are described below.

● **In some studies: decreased risk of retinitis pigmentosa in those with higher blood levels of zinc**

In a study of 26 people with retinitis pigmentosa, zinc levels in the blood were found to be lower on average in the people with retinitis pigmentosa compared to healthy controls. Copper levels in the blood were found to be higher on average in the people with retinitis pigmentosa.[174] Other studies, mostly smaller ones, have confirmed these results as well; yet, others have shown no difference in zinc or copper levels.[175, 176, 177, & 178] These findings are difficult to interpret,

> Looking at the mechanisms of action, there may be good reason to use zinc in moderation for macular degeneration and cataract.

as it is not known whether the finding of a decrease in the zinc or copper is related to the retinitis pigmentosa, aggravates or causes the retinitis pigmentosa, or is caused by the retinitis pigmentosa.

Summary of Studies for Macular Degeneration:

Over a dozen clinical trials have been performed looking at the role of zinc in both preventing and treating macular degeneration. These clinical trials are of various types, some of which are very well-designed and well-performed studies.

As a whole, the clinical studies provide no definitive answer as to whether zinc is beneficial, and, in fact, the majority of studies found no benefit to zinc for macular degeneration. However, there is some evidence from 6 of the 15 studies that it may be beneficial, particularly in combination with other antioxidant nutrients. Looking at the mechanisms of action, there is good reason to use beta-carotene in moderation for macular degeneration.

The studies can be summarized as follows: four large studies found no benefits from the past use of zinc on the risk of macular degeneration, while another large study did find a benefit in the past use of zinc in decreasing the risk of macular degeneration.

One study has found no link (neither protective nor harmful) between levels of zinc in the blood and macular degeneration, while two studies have found a decreased risk of macular degeneration in those with higher blood levels of zinc. In following people over time, four studies found that those who took zinc did not have any benefit in preventing macular degeneration compared to those who did not take zinc. However, one poorly controlled study found that the use of zinc slowed the loss of vision in macular degeneration,

Zinc for
Macular Degeneration
Scale of Benefit

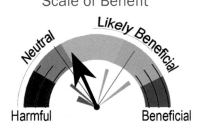

and another study found that the use of a multi-vitamin with zinc decreases the future risk of macular degeneration over time. More importantly, another study found that zinc by itself did not have any benefit in preventing macular degeneration, but in combination with other nutrients, it decreased the risk of macular degeneration by one-half! Finally, one study has noted that people with macular degeneration have "four-fold" reductions in zinc levels in their retinas.

● **In several studies: no benefits in past use of zinc found on risk of macular degeneration** A study of over 3,500 people age 49 and over found no link (neither protective nor harmful) between the risk of developing macular degeneration over a 5 year period and people who took the following nutrients, alone or in combination, in the past: zinc, lycopene, lutein and zeaxanthin, beta-carotene, or vitamin A. Surprisingly, however, the study found, that those who took vitamin C supplements combined with a diet high in vitamin C had a 2-fold increase in their risk of developing macular degeneration.[2] This finding is quite surprising, as one would expect vitamin C to protect against macular degeneration, as opposed to increasing the risk of macular degeneration. However, the finding highlights the problems associated with these types of studies: namely, that the findings may occur coincidentally and other true findings may be missed. It is sometimes difficult to explain the findings or apply them to real life.

Looking forward over time, a study of nearly 3,000 people age 49 and over found no link (neither protective nor harmful) between the risk of having macular degeneration and taking any of the following nutrients (alone or in combination) in the past: zinc, beta-carotene, vitamin A, vitamin B1, vitamin B2, vitamin B3, vitamin B6, vitamin B12, vitamin C, vitamin E, or folate.[13]

Also, a study of nearly 3,000 people age 49 and over found no link (neither protective nor harmful) between the risk of having macular degeneration a diet with higher amounts of zinc, vitamin A, vitamin C, or beta-carotene in the past.[4]

A study of nearly 2,000 people found that those with the early stages of macular degeneration had a tendency (that was not statistically significant) to consume less zinc than those without macular degeneration.[179]

● **Though the several studies above found no link, one large study found a benefit: past use of zinc associated with decreased risk of macular degeneration**
Looking at a group of nearly 2,000 people from a study population of nearly 5,000 people, researchers found a decreased risk of early-stage macular degeneration for those who consumed diets high in zinc. However, the study found no link (neither protective nor harmful) between the risk of developing macular degeneration and a diet high in vitamin C, vitamin E, or carotenoids.[3]

● **In one study: no link between blood levels of zinc and macular degeneration**
Another study of nearly 100 people found no difference in the blood levels of zinc, carotenoids, beta-carotene, lutein and zeaxanthin, lycopene, vitamin A, vitamin C, or selenium between those with or without macular degeneration

(looking at both early and severe or advanced macular degeneration). However, the study found that those who had severe or advanced macular degeneration had lower blood levels of vitamin E compared to those without macular degeneration. They found no differences in the blood levels of vitamin E between those with or without early macular degeneration.[6]

● **Two studies found a benefit: decreased risk of macular degeneration in those with higher blood levels of zinc**   A study of over 100 people, found that those who had macular degeneration had lower blood levels of zinc compared to those without macular degeneration. However, the study found no difference in the blood levels of carotenoids, vitamin A, vitamin C, vitamin E, or selenium between those with or without macular degeneration. [39]

Another study of 40 people found that those who had macular degeneration had lower blood levels of zinc and lower levels vitamin E of compared to those without macular degeneration.[167]

● **In four studies: no benefits from the use of zinc on the future risk of macular degeneration over time**
Looking over a 5-year period, a study of 2,000 people from a group of nearly 5,000, found no link (neither protective nor harmful) between macular degeneration and a diet high in zinc, beta-carotene,

carotenoids, lutein and zeaxanthin, vitamin C, or vitamin E.[14]

A larger and more recent well-performed study divided over 104,000 people into several groups, ranging from zinc in doses of about 25 to 40 mg per day from supplements and food sources, down to the lowest dose group taking about 8 to 10 mg per day. The study, however, failed to show any link between higher doses of zinc and preventing or minimizing macular degeneration.[180] The bioavailability of the zinc, or the true zinc dosage, was unclear in this study because different zinc preparations resulted in different zinc amounts that were actually delivered to the body.

A study of over 100 people found no link (neither protective nor harmful) between zinc (80 mg per day of bioavailable zinc over 2 years) and the risk of macular degeneration.[181]

A small study of 71 people with macular degeneration found no benefit to the macular degeneration or to vision in those who took a daily antioxidant combination, for over 1½ years, that consisted of zinc (12.5 mg), beta-carotene (20,000 IU), vitamin B2 (25 mg), vitamin C (750 mg), vitamin E (200 IU), chromium (100 µg), selenium (50 µg), taurine (100 mg), N-acetyl cysteine (100 mg), glutathione (5 mg), and selected bioflavonoids, compared to placebo.[17] It is impossible, however, to ascertain the individual effect of zinc from this type of study.

● **In a fifth study: no benefits from the use of zinc**

by itself on the future risk of macular degeneration over time, but use of zinc with multiple nutrients decreases future risk of macular degeneration   A study of nearly 4,000 people, looking forward over an average of 8 years, found no link (neither protective nor harmful) between macular degeneration and a diet high in zinc, iron, beta-carotene, lutein and zeaxanthin, lycopene, vitamin A, or vitamin C. However, a diet high in vitamin E decreased the risk of having macular degeneration by 20%. A diet high in multiple nutrients (beta-carotene, vitamin C, vitamin E, and zinc together) decreased the risk of having macular degeneration by about ½![18]

● **Though four studies above found no link, two studies found a benefit: use of zinc decreases the future risk of macular degeneration over time**   A study in 1988 of over 150 people found that zinc (80 mg daily of bioavailable zinc over 1 to 2 years) slowed the loss of vision in macular degeneration.[182] Unfortunately, though, this study did not have the appropriate controls to truly verify this finding.

A recent 10-year study of over 3,000 people age 55 and over found that taking a daily antioxidant combination of vitamin C (500 mg), vitamin E (400 IU), and beta-carotene (15 mg), with or without zinc (80 mg) and copper (2 mg) reduced the risk of developing severe or wet macular degeneration, in people with certain features of dry macular

degeneration within their retinas. The risk of developing severe or advanced macular degeneration decreased by 34% in people taking the antioxidant combination with zinc and copper, by 24% in people taking the antioxidant combination alone without zinc and copper, and by 30% in people taking the zinc and copper without the antioxidant combination. Looking at vision, the antioxidant combination with zinc and copper decreased the risk of losing vision from macular degeneration by 25% in these people with certain features of dry macular degeneration. There was no benefit to vision for people who took the antioxidant combination alone, without the zinc and copper, or the zinc and copper alone. This study has been used widely to recommend the multivitamin combination for macular degeneration, though the results are only applicable to people with certain features of macular degeneration in their retinas. Moreover, what confounds the interpretation of the data is the use of multivitamins in two-thirds of the people.[19]

Summary of Studies for Cataract: Four clinical trials have been performed looking at the role of zinc in preventing cataract. These clinical trials are of many different types, some of which are very well-designed and well-performed studies.

As a whole, the clinical studies provide no definitive answer as to whether zinc is beneficial, and, in fact, the majority of the studies found no

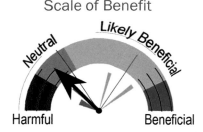

Zinc for
Cataract
Scale of Benefit

Neutral   Likely Beneficial

Harmful   Beneficial

benefit to zinc for cataract. Overall, studies provide little evidence to use zinc for cataract. Looking at the mechanisms of action, there is good reason to use zinc in moderation for cataract.

The studies can be summarized as follows: one found a benefit in the past use of zinc in decreasing the risk of cataract. Another study found no link (neither protective nor harmful) between higher levels of zinc in the blood and the risk of cataract.

In following people over time, two large studies found that those who took zinc did not have any benefit in preventing cataract compared to those who did not take zinc.

● In one study: past use of zinc associated with decreased risk of cataract

A study of nearly 3,000 people found that the past intake of zinc, iron, vitamin A, vitamin B1, vitamin B2, and vitamin B3 decreased the risk of having certain types of cataract by 30 to 50%.[62] It is interesting to note that in this study, iron was associated with a decrease in risk of having cataract,

and not an increased risk, as some physicians have predicted. Furthermore, it is surprising that no link (neither protective nor harmful) was found between vitamin C use and cataract, despite other studies showing a benefit.

● In one study: no link between blood levels of zinc and cataract

A study of 165 people found no link (neither beneficial nor harmful) between cataracts and zinc, copper, magnesium, vitamin A, and vitamin E levels in the blood. However, the study found that those who had cataracts had lower levels of carotenoids and vitamin D in their blood compared to those who did not have cataracts. On the other hand, the study found that those who had cataracts had higher levels of selenium in their blood.[41]

● In two studies: no benefits from the use of zinc on the future risk of cataract over time

A recent 10-year study of over 3,000 people found that taking an antioxidant combination of beta-carotene (15 mg), vitamin C (500 mg), and vitamin E (400 IU), with or without zinc and copper each day reduced the risk of macular degeneration over time, but found no link (neither protective nor harmful) to the risk of cataracts over time.[29]

A study of over 2,000 people given a multivitamin or a placebo for 5 years found a 36% decrease in the risk of developing cataracts in those people who were age 65 to 74. Of note, there was no difference in risk in the younger group age 45 to 64. These results exemplify the positive benefit of multivitamins; however, it is difficult to apply these results to a healthy population, as the study was performed on somewhat nutritionally-deprived people in rural China.[33]

The researchers also looked at specific nutrients in a group of over 3,000 people from the same population. They found no link (neither beneficial nor harmful) over the 5-year period between the risk of cataract and those who took vitamin A and zinc, or those who took selenium with beta-carotene and vitamin E, or those who took vitamin C and molybdenum. In contrast, in those who took vitamin B2 (5.2 mg) and vitamin B3 (40 mg) daily for 5 years had a 41% decrease in the risk of developing cataracts, compared to those who took placebo.[33]

Body Absorption, Metabolism, & Excretion

Zinc is rapidly absorbed in the intestines. Anywhere from 40 to 90% of the zinc ingested is absorbed, though the absorption decreases on a full stomach.

Much of the excretion of zinc comes from its secretion by the intestines out of the bloodstream and into the gastrointestinal tract and then the stool. A small amount is excreted by being filtered by the kidneys and a small amount is excreted with bile (a green fluid produced by the liver that is stored in the gallbladder to assist in digestion).

Deficiency

Deficiency is often caused by severe burns, diarrhea, pancreatic disease, liver disease including alcoholic hepatitis, or digestive absorption disease such as celiac sprue.

A genetic disorder of zinc impairment and transport, known as acrodermatitis enteropathica, results in zinc deficiency and causes scaly skin rashes as well as hair loss, including loss of eyelashes and eyebrows. There are also reports of increased eye infections associated with this disorder, as well as cataract formation, corneal abnormalities, retinal degeneration, and optic nerve degeneration.

Dietary zinc deficiency can cause some the same problems as above. Mild zinc deficiency is associated with growth retardation in children, mild neurological and psychological impairments in children, as well as increased susceptibility to infections.

Very mild zinc deficiency can abnormally alter one's ability to taste and smell.

In the eye, zinc deficiency can cause cataracts, corneal ulcers, optic nerve degeneration, and retinal degeneration. In some people with retinitis pigmentosa, a retinal disease characterized by night-blindness, zinc deficiency has been shown to be an associated factor. Mild zinc deficiency has been associated with difficulties with night vision as well as tearing and dryness of the eye's surface. Fortunately though, the night-blindness associated with zinc deficiency is often easily reversed with appropriate dietary levels of zinc.

During pregnancy, zinc deficiency is associated with early delivery and low birth weight.

Deficiency of zinc is also associated with cancer of the esophagus.

Toxicity & Side Effects

In moderation, zinc is essential in maintaining the appropriate amount of vitamin A that is required for proper retinal function. However, excess zinc can cause toxicity by excess oxidation, either through the stimulation of the metabolism of vitamin A into excess toxic forms in the retina, or by lowering copper levels.

Excess zinc consumption can lead to an imbalance of the proper ratio of zinc-to-copper, which can result in higher cholesterol levels. Actually, excess zinc can lead to low copper levels since zinc produces an enzyme, known as metallothionein, which binds copper in the intestines and prevents copper absorption. One of the main problems that occurs with copper deficiency is anemia (insufficiency of the red blood cells that carry oxygen) (see section on copper).

As with copper, acute excess zinc can result in stomach pains, nausea, vomiting, and diarrhea. These effects are believed to be mediated by the sulfate that often comes with zinc supplements. Other reported side effects include a metal taste in the mouth, headaches, dizziness, tiredness, and weakness.

While high doses of zinc have been associated with longer life spans, high doses of zinc also have been associated with increased risk of prostate cancer, Alzheimer's disease, and diabetes.

Although zinc may improve blood sugar levels in diabetics, there is some suggestion that, at high doses, zinc can be harmful in diabetics. It increases the amount of glucose-attacked proteins. When glucose levels are high, glucose attacks proteins, resulting in advanced glycation end products, or AGEs, that then damage various structures in the body and eye (see introduction).

Furthermore, while zinc is believed to be beneficial in boosting the immune defense system, at very high doses of over 300 mg, it may actually impair the immune system.

Interactions with Other Nutrients

There are numerous interactions between zinc and other nutrients. The important concept is that a balance should be achieved between the intake of zinc and other nutrients.

As stated above, zinc and vitamin A work together in the retina as well as other ocular tissues, such as the surface of the eye, where vitamin A plays an essential role (see section on vitamin A). Zinc facilitates vitamin A's "mobilization" out of the liver. A study of over 200 women with night-blindness from vitamin A deficiency who also had zinc deficiency demonstrated that both vitamin A and zinc were required to treat the night-blindness. Neither vitamin A nor zinc alone could effectively treat the night-blindness.[140]

Copper works with zinc to balance cholesterol levels. An imbalance in the ratio between copper and zinc can result in higher cholesterol levels because of improper absorption of either the zinc or the copper. This ratio should be 1-fold copper to 10-fold zinc. Deficiency of zinc can lead to excess copper as zinc and copper compete with each other for absorption in the digestive system; whereas, excess zinc can lead to low copper levels since zinc produces an enzyme, known as metallothionein, which binds copper in the intestines and prevents copper absorption.

Thus, zinc deficiency is unwanted because excess copper can be detrimental to the retina. Low serum zinc levels have been associated with high serum copper levels in some cases of retinitis pigmentosa (see section on copper).

It has been shown that over-the-counter and prescription supplements of iron can lead to decreased absorption of zinc, and thus decreased zinc levels. However, this decrease is not known to occur when supplementing iron levels through natural dietary sources.

Similarly, high levels of calcium can cause decreased zinc absorption in the intestines, but this finding has been shown to be the case in postmenopausal women and not necessarily in younger people. When calcium is combined with phytic acid levels, zinc absorption is further decreased. Since phytic acid chelates (binds and removes) metals, including zinc, within the intestines, preventing the bound metals from being absorbed into the bloodstream, which results in zinc deficiency with supplementation of high levels of phytic acid (see section on phytic acid). Other nutrients, such as alpha-lipoic acid and bioflavonoids that chelate can also cause zinc deficiency.

There is controversial data that suggests that folate absorption interacts with zinc absorption, such that low zinc levels cause low folate absorption, while high folate levels cause low zinc absorption.

However, the studies are not consistent on these findings. Nevertheless, a zinc-dependent enzyme is involved in folate absorption, and, as such, the need to balance zinc and folate supplementation is important.

In addition, high doses of zinc can result in blocked magnesium absorption.

Furthermore, zinc, copper, iron, and magnesium may inhibit the absorption of vitamin B2 as well.

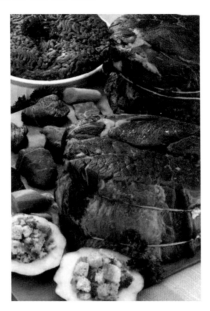

Ideal Dosage

Dietary zinc consumption is approximately 8 to 10 mg per day. The recommended dose of zinc in boys age 11 to 18 and men is 15 mg per day, and in girls age 11 to 18 and women is 12 mg per day. In pregnancy, the recommended dose increases to 15 mg per day.

It may be best to obtain a dose of about 20 to 30 mg per day. Care must be taken to avoid excess zinc. Furthermore, it is essential to consume zinc in a proper ratio with copper in order to maintain proper cholesterol levels. This ratio should be 10-fold zinc to 1-fold copper. Thus, it may be best to match with a dose of copper of about 2 to 3 mg per day.

In order to ensure that zinc is used efficiently, it should be taken in conjunction with vitamin A, and, if there is pancreatic disease, it should be taken along with pancreatic enzymes as well.

The formulation of the zinc is essential in determining the true dosage of the zinc that is bioavailable. For example, an anhydrous formulation of zinc sulfate that provides 25 mg actually provides about 10 mg of bioavailable zinc to the body.

Sources (Where to Find It)

Fruits, Vegetables, & Sweets:

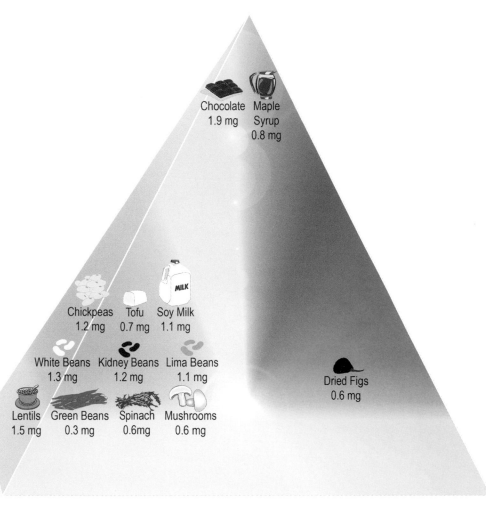

Chocolate
1.9 mg

Maple
Syrup
0.8 mg

Chickpeas
1.2 mg

Tofu
0.7 mg

Soy Milk
1.1 mg

White Beans
1.3 mg

Kidney Beans
1.2 mg

Lima Beans
1.1 mg

Lentils
1.5 mg

Green Beans
0.3 mg

Spinach
0.6mg

Mushrooms
0.6 mg

Dried Figs
0.6 mg

Pyramid Key:

Fats & Sweets

Dairy   *Meats & Nuts*

Vegetables   *Fruits*

Breads & Grains

*See Guides on Pages 467-468.

465

Dairy, Meats, & Grains:

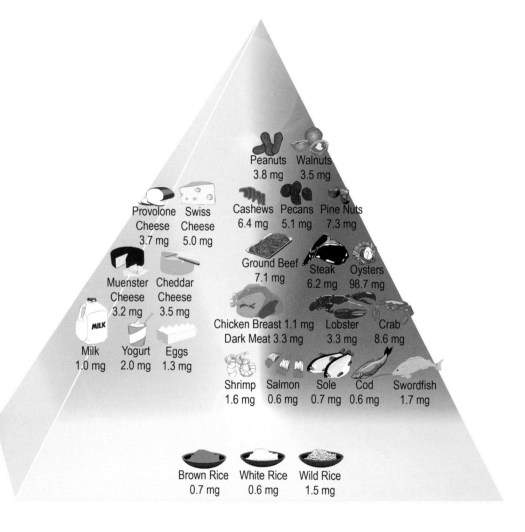

The top source of zinc is oysters. Other top sources are nuts (particularly pine nuts, pecans, and cashews), meats (such as ground beef and steak), and cheeses (including Swiss cheese and provolone cheese).

Food Portion Size Guide

Approximate portion sizes for selected foods in the pyramids:

alfalfa sprouts	4 cups		lemon	2/3 cup (2 lemons)
apricots	1 cup (4 apricots)		lentils	1/2 cup
artichoke	2/3 cup		lettuce	2 cups
asparagus	2/3 cup (8 spears)		mango	2/3 cup (1/2 mango)
bananas	3/4 cup (1 banana)		mangoes	2/3 cup
beans, green	1 cup		melon, honeydew	2/3 cup
beans, kidney	2/3 cup		mushrooms	1 & 1/2 cup
beans, lima	2/3 cup		nuts	3/4 cup
beans, pinto	2/3 cup		okra	3/4 cup
beans, white	1/2 cup		onions	3/4 cup
beets	3/4 cup		orange	2/3 cup (1 orange)
blackberries	3/4 cup		papaya	3/4 cup
blackeyed peas	2/3 cup		parsley	4 cups
blueberries	3/4 cup		pasta sauce	1/2 cup
broccoli, cooked	3/4 cup		peach	2/3 cup (1 peach)
broccoli, raw	1 & 1/3 cup		peas	3/4 cup
Brussels sprouts	3/4 cup		peppers, hot chili	1/2 cup (2 & 1/2 peppers)
cabbage, red	1 & 2/3 cup		peppers, sweet	3/4 cup (1 pepper)
cantaloupe	3/4 cup		pineapple	3/4 cup
carrots, cooked	3/4 cup		plums	1/2 cup (2 plums)
carrots, raw	1 cup		potato	1/2 cup (1/2 potato)
cauliflower	2/3 cup		potato, sweet	1/2 cup (1/2 potato)
celery	1 cup		prunes	1/2 cup
cheese, cottage	1/2 cup		pumpkin	1/2 cup
cheese, ricotta	1/2 cup		raisins	3/4 cup
chestnuts	3/4 cup		raspberries	1 cup
chickpeas	1/2 cup		rice, brown	1/2 cup
chocolate	2/3 cup		rice, white	3/4 cup
coconut	1 & 1/4 cup		scallions	1 & 1/4 cup
collards	2/3 cup		soybeans	2/3 cup
collards	2/3 cup		spinach, cooked	2/3 cup
corn	2/3 cup (2 ears)		spinach, raw	4 cups
couscous	3/4 cup		squash	2/3 cup
cucumber	1/3 cup		starfruit	1 cup
dates	2/3 cup		strawberries	2/3 cup
egg	1/2 cup (2 extra large eggs)		sunflower seeds	1 cup
grapefruit	2/3 cup (1/2 grapefruit)		tofu	2/3 cup
grapes	3/4 cup		tomato	1/2 cup (1 tomato)
green peas	3/4 cup		watermelon	3/4 cup
kale	1 cup		yogurt	1/2 cup
kiwi	1/3 cup (1 & 1/2 kiwis)			

Key: 1 cup 3/4 cup 2/3 cup 1/2 cup 1/3 cup 1/4 cup

Pyramid Guide:

- All foods listed are in 4 oz portions (approximately 115 grams).

- Drinks and soups are in 8 fl oz portions (1 cup).

- Note that the nutritional contents of the foods listed are approximate. Actual values will vary from sample to sample.

- Some foods are processed and fortified with extra nutrients, and so their nutrient content may vary from the listings in the pyramids.

Bibliography

1. Paker L, Kraemer K, Rimbach G. Molecular aspects of lipoic acid in the prevention of diabetes complications. Nutrition 2001;17:888-895.
2. Flood V, Smith W, Wang JJ, et al. Dietary antioxidant intake and incidence of early age-related maculopathy: the Blue Mountain Eye Study. Ophthalmology 2002;109:2272-8.
3. Mares-Perlman JA, Klein R, Klein BE, et al. Association of zinc and antioxidant nutrients with age-related maculopathy. Arch Ophthalmol 1996;114:9917.
4. Smith W, Mitchell P, Webb K, Leeder SR. Dietary antioxidants and age-related maculopathy. Ophthalmology 1999;106:761-7.
5. Seddon JM, Ajani, UA, Sperduto RD, et al. Dietary carotenoids, vitamins A, C, and E, and advanced age-related macular degeneration. JAMA 1994;272:1413-20.
6. Simonelli F, Zarrilli F, Mazzeo S, et al. Serum oxidative and antioxidant parameters in a group of Italian patients with age-related maculopathy. Clin Chim Acta 2002;320:111-5.
7. Mares-Perlman JA, Brady WE, Klein R, et al. Serum antioxidants and age-related macular degeneration in a population-based case-control study. Arch Ophthalmol 1995;113:1518-23.
8. Smith W, Mitchell P, Rochester C. Serum beta carotene, alpha tocopherol and age-related maculopathy: the Blue Mountains Eye Study. Am J Ophthalmol 1997;124:838-40.
9. Sanders TA, Haines AP, Wormald R, et al. Essential fatty acids, plasma cholesterol, and fat-soluble vitamins in subjects with age-related maculopathy and matched control subjects. Am J Clin Nutr 1993;57:428-33.
10. West S, Vitale S, Hallfrisch J, et al. Are antioxidants or supplements protective for age-related macular degeneration? Arch Ophthalmol 1994;112:222-7.
11. The Eye Disease Case-Control Study Group. Risk factors for neovascular age-related macular degeneration. Arch Ophthalmol 1992;110:1701-8.
12. The Eye Disease Case-Control Study Group. Antioxidant status and neovascular age-related macular degeneration. Arch Ophthalmol 1993;111:104-9.

13. Kuzniarz M, Mitchell P, Flood VM, Wang JJ. Use of vitamin and zinc supplements and age-related maculopathy: the Blue Mountains Eye Study. Ophthalmic Epidemiol 2002;9:283-95.
14. VandenLangenberg GM, Mares-Perlman JA, Klein R, et al. Associations between antioxidant and zinc intake and the 5year incidence of early age-related maculopathy in the Beaver Dam Eye Study. Am J Epidemiol 1998;148:204-14.
15. Cho E, Seddon JM, Rosner B, et al. Prospective study of intake of fruits, vegetables, vitamins, and carotenoids and risk of age-related maculopathy. Arch Ophthalmol 2004;122:883-892.
16. Teikari JM, Laatikainen L, Virtamo J, et al. Six-year supplementation with alpha-tocopherol and beta-carotene and age-related maculopathy. Acta Ophthalmol Scand 1998;76:224-9.
17. Age-Related Macular Degeneration Study Group. Multicenter ophthalmic and nutritional age-related macular degeneration study—part 2: antioxidant intervention and conclusions. J Am Optom Assoc 1996;67:30-49.
18. Van Leeuwen R, Boekhoorn S, Vingerling JR, et al. Dietary intake of antioxidants and risk of age-related macular degeneration. JAMA 2005 294:3101-7.
19. Age-Related Eye Disease Study Research Group. A randomized, placebo-controlled clinical trial of high-dose supplementation with vitamins C and E, beta carotene, and zinc for age-related macular degeneration and vision loss: AREDS report no. 8. Arch Ophthalmol 2001;119:1417-36.
20. Jacques PF, Chylack LT Jr, Hankinson SE, et al. Long-term nutrient intake and early age-related nuclear lens opacities. Arch Ophthalmol 2001;119:1009-19.
21. Mares-Perlman JA, Brady WE, Klein BE, et al. Serum carotenoids and tocopherols and severity of nuclear and cortical opacities. Invest Ophthalmol Vis Sci 1995;36:276-88.
22. Tavani A, Negri E, La Vecchia C. Food and nutrient intake and risk of cataract. Ann Epidemiol 1996;6:41-6.
23. Jacques PF, Taylor A, Hankinson SE, et al. Long-term vitamin C supplement use and prevalence of early age-related lens opacities. Am J Clin Nutr 1997;66:911-6. Companion study: Taylor A, Jacques PF, Chylack LT Jr, et al. Long-term intake of vitamins and carotenoids and odds of early age-related cortical and posterior subcapsular lens opacities. Am J Clin Nutr 2002;75:540-9.
24. McCarty CA, Mukesh BN, Fu CL, Taylor HR. The epidemiology of cataract in Australia. Am J Ophthalmol 1999;128:446.
25. Ferrigno L, Aldigeri R, Rosmini F, et al. Associations between plasma levels of vitamins and cataract in the Italian-American Clinical Trial of Nutritional Supplements and Age-Related Cataract (CTNS): CTNS Report #2. Ophthalmic Epidemiol 2005;12:71-80.
26. Lyle BJ, Mares-Perlman J, Klein BE, et al. Serum carotenoids and tocopherols and incidence of age-related nuclear cataract. Am J Clin Nutr 1999;69:272.
27. Mares-Perlman JA, Brady WE, Klein BE, et al. Diet and nuclear lens opacities. Am J Epidemiol 1995;141:322-34.
28. Gale CR, Hall NF, Phillips DI, Martyn CN. Plasma antioxidant vitamins and carotenoids and age-related cataract. Ophthalmology 2001;108:1992-8.

29. Age-Related Eye Disease Study Research Group. A randomized, placebo-controlled, clinical trial of high-dose supplementation with vitamins C and E and beta carotene for age-related cataract and vision loss: AREDS report no. 9. Arch Ophthalmol 2001;119:1439-52.
30. Teikari JM, Virtamo J, Rautalahti M, et al. Long-term supplementation with alpha-tocopherol and beta-carotene and age-related cataract. Acta Ophthalmol Scand 1997;75:634-40.
31. Christen WG, Manson JE, Glynn RJ, et al. A randomized trial of beta carotene and age-related cataract in US physicians. Arch Ophthalmol 2003;121:372-8.
32. Christen WG, Glynn RJ, Sperduto RD, et al. Age-related cataract in a randomized trial of beta-carotene in women. Ophthalmic Epidemiol 2004;11:401-12
33. Sperduto RD, Hu TS, Milton RC, et al. The Linxian cataract studies. Two nutrition intervention trials. Arch Ophthalmol 1993;111:1246-53.
34. Chylack LT Jr, Brown NP, Bron A, et al. The Roche European American Cataract Trial (REACT): a randomized clinical trial to investigate the efficacy of an oral antioxidant micronutrient mixture to slow progression of age-related cataract. Ophthalmic Epidemiol 2002;9;49-80.
35. Glacet-Bernard A, Coscas G, Chabanel A, et al. A randomized, double-masked study on the treatment of retinal vein occlusion with troxerutin. Am J Ophthalmol 1994;118:421-9.
36. Robertson JM, Donner AP, Trevithick JR. A possible role for vitamins C and E in cataract prevention. Am J Clin Nutr 1991;53:346S-51S.
37. Feher J, Kovacs B, Kovacs I, et al. Improvement of visual functions and fundus alterations in early age-related macular degeneration treated with a combination of acetyl-L-carnitine, n-3 fatty acids, and coenzyme Q10.
Ophthalmologica 2005;219:154-66.
38. Feher J, Papale A, Mannino G, et al. Mitotropic compounds for the treatment of age-related macular degeneration. The metabolic approach and a pilot study. Ophthalmologica 2003;217:351-7.
39. Ishihara N, Yuzawa M, Tamakoshi A. Antioxidants and angiogenetic factor associated with age-related macular degeneration (exudative type). Nippon Ganka Gakkai Zasshi 1997;101:248-51.
40. Jacques PF, Chylack LT Jr. Epidemiologic evidence of a role for the antioxidant vitamins and carotenoids in cataract prevention. Am J Clin Nutr 1991;53:352S-5S.
41. Jacques PF, Hartz SC, Chylack LT Jr, et al. Nutritional status in persons with and without senile cataract: blood vitamin and mineral levels. Am J Clin Nutr 1988;48:152-8.
42. Hankinson SE, Stampfer MJ, Seddon JM, et al. Nutrient intake and cataract extraction in women: a prospective study. BMJ 1992f;305:335-9.
43. Rejdak R, Toczolowski J, Krukowski J. Oral citicoline treatment improves visual pathway function in glaucoma. Med Sci Monit 2003;9:PI24-8.
44. Parisi V, Manni G, Colacino G, Bucci MG. Cytidine-5'-diphosphocholin (citicoline) improves retinal and cortical responses in patients with glaucoma. Ophthalmology 1999;106:1126-34.
45. Giraldi JP, Virno M, Covelli G, et al. Therapeutic value of citicoline in the treatment of glaucoma (computerized and automated perimetric investigation). Int Ophthalmol 1989 Jan;13:109-12.

46. Virno M, Pecori-Giraldi J, Liguori A, De Gregorio F. The protective effect of citicoline on the progression of the perimetric defects in glaucomatous patients (perimetric study with a 10-year follow-up). Acta Ophthalmol Scand Suppl 2000;(232):56-7.
47. Lodi R, Iotti S, Scorolli L, et al. The use of phosphorus magnetic resonance spectroscopy to study in vivo the effect of coenzyme Q10 treatment in retinitis pigmentosa. Mol Spects Med 1994;15(suppl):s221-30.
48. Mohan M, Sperduto R, Angra SK, et al. India-US case-control study of age-related cataracts. Arch Ophthalmol 1989;107:670-6.
49. Akyol N, Orhan D, Keha EE, Kilic S. Aqueous humour and serum zinc and copper concentrations of patients with glaucoma and cataract. Br J Ophthalmol 1990;74:661-2.
50. Cahill MT, Stinnett SS, Fekrat S. Meta-analysis of plasma homocysteine, serum folate, serum vitamin B(12), and thermolabile MTHFR genotype as risk factors for retinal vascular occlusive disease. Am J Ophthalmol 2003;136:1136-50.
51. Kuzniarz M, Mitchell P, Cumming RG, Flood VM. Use of vitamin supplements and cataract: the Blue Mountains Eye Study. Am J Ophthalmol 2001;132:19-26.
52. Knox DL, Chen MF, Guilarte TR, et al. Nutritional amblyopia. Folic acid, vitamin B-12, and other vitamins. Retina 1982;2:288-93.
53. Mares-Perlman JA, Klein BE, Klein R, Ritter LL. Relation between lens opacities and vitamin and mineral supplement use. Ophthalmology 1994;101:315-25.
54. Fies P, Dienel A. Ginkgo extract in impaired vision--treatment with special extract EGb 761 of impaired vision due to dry senile macular degeneration. Wien Med Wochenschr. 2002;152:423-6.
55. Lebuisson DA, Leroy L, Rigal G. Treatment of senile macular degeneration with Ginkgo biloba extract. A preliminary double-blind drug vs. placebo study. Presse Med 1986;15:1556-8.
56. Raabe A, Raabe M, Ihm P. Therapeutic follow-up using automatic perimetry in chronic cerebroretinal ischemia in elderly patients. Prospective double-blind study with graduated dose ginkgo biloba treatment. Klin Monatsbl Augenheilkd 1991;199:432-438.
57. Huang SY, Jeng C, Kao SC, et al. Improved haemorrheological properties by Ginkgo biloba extract (Egb 761) in type 2 diabetes mellitus complicated with retinopathy. Clin Nutr 2004;23:615-21.
58. Lanthony P, Cosson JP. The course of color vision in early diabetic retinopathy treated with Ginkgo biloba extract. A preliminary double-blind versus placebo study. J Fr Ophthalmol 1988;11:671-2.
59. Chung HS, Harris A, Kristinsson JK, et al. Ginkgo biloba extract increases ocular blood flow velocity. J Ocul Pharmacol Ther 1999;15:233-40.
60. Quranta L, Bettelli S, Uva MG, et al. Effect of Ginkgo biloba extract on preexisting visual field damage in normal tension glaucoma. Ophthalmology 2003;110-359-62.
61. Leske MC, Chylack LT Jr, Wu SY. The lens opacities case-control study. Risk Factors for Cataract. Arch Ophthalmol 1991;109:244-51.
62. Cumming RG, Mitchell P, Smith W. Diet and Cataract: the Blue Mountains Eye Study. Ophthalmology 2000;107:450-6.
63. Leske MC, Wu SY, Hyman L, et al. Biochemical factors in the lens opacities case-control study. Arch Ophthalmol 1995;113:1113-1119.

64. Nussbaum JJ, Pruett RC, Delori FC. Historic perspectives. Macular yellow pigment. The first 200 years. Retina 1981;1:296-310.
65. Aleman TS, Duncan JL, Bieber ML, et al. Macular pigment and lutein supplementation in retinitis pigmentosa and usher syndrome. Invest Ophthalmol Vis Sci 2001;42:1873-81.
66. Dagnelie G, Zorge IS, McDonald TM. Lutein improves visual function in some patients with retinal degeneration: a pilot study via the Internet. Optometry 2000;71:147-64.
67. Bone RA, Landrum JT, Mayne ST, et al. Macular pigment in donor eyes with and without AMDL a case-control study. Invest Ophthalmol Vis Sci 2001;42:235-40.
68. Vu HT, Robman L, McCarty CA, et al. Does dietary lutein and zeaxanthin increase the risk of age related macular degeneration? The Melbourne Visual Impairment Project. Br J Ophthalmol 2006;90:389-90
69. Mares-Perlman JA, Fisher AI, Klein R, et al. Lutein and zeaxanthin in the diet and serum and their relation to age related maculopathy in the third national health and nutrition examination survey. Am J Epidemiol 2001;153:424-32.
70. Snellen E, Verbeek A, Van Den Hoogen G, et al. Neovascular age-related macular degeneration and its relationship to antioxidant intake. Acta Ophthalmol Scand 2002;80:368-71.
71. Dasch B, Fuhs A, Schmidt J, et al. Serum levels of macular carotenoids in relation to age-related maculopathy. The Muenster Aging and Retina Study (MARS). Graefes Arch Clin Exp Ophthalmol 2005;243:1028-35.
72. Gale CR, Hall NF, Phillips DI, Martyn CN. Lutein and zeaxanthin status and risk of age-related macular degeneration. Invest Ophthalmol Vis Sci 2003;44:2461-5.
73. Richer S. ARMD—pilot (case series) environmental intervention data. J Am Optom Assoc 1999;70:24-36.
74. Richer S, Stiles W, Statkute L, et al. Double-masked, placebo-controlled, randomized trial of lutein and antioxidant supplementation in the intervention of atrophic age-related macular degeneration: the Veterans LAST study (Lutein Antioxidant Supplementation Trial). Optometry. 2004;75:216-30.
75. Chasan-Taber L, Willett WC, Seddon JM, et al. A prospective study of carotenoid and vitamin A intakes and risk of cataract extraction in US women. Am J Clin Nutr 1999;70:509-16.
76. Brown L, Rimm EB, Seddon JM, et al. A prospective study of carotenoid intake and risk of cataract extraction in US men. Am J Clin Nutr 1999;70:517-24.
77. Lyle BJ, Mares-Perlman JA, Klein BE, e al. Antioxidant intake and risk of incident age-related nuclear cataracts in the Beaver Dam Eye Study. Am J Epidemiol 1999;149:801.
78. Olmedilla B, Granado F, Blanco I, Vaquero M. Lutein, but not alpha-tocopherol, supplementation improves visual function in patients with age-related cataracts: a 2-y double-blind placebo-controlled pilot study. Nutrition 2003;19:21-4.
79. Cardinault N, Abalain JH, Sairafi, B, et al. Lycopene but not lutein nor zeaxanthin decreases in serum and lipoproteins in age-related macular degeneration patients. Clin Chim Acta 2005;357:34-42.
80. Gaspar AZ, Gasser P, Flammer J. The influence of magnesium on visual

field and peripheral vasospasm in glaucoma. Ophthalmologica 1995;209:11-13.

81. Miljanovic B, Trivedi KA, Dana MR, et al. Relation between dietary n-3 and n-6 fatty acids and clinically diagnosed dry eye syndrome in women. Am J Clin Nutr 2005;82:887-93.

82. Aragona P, Bucolo C, Spinella R, et al. Systemic omega-6 essential fatty acid treatment and pge1 tear content in Sjogren's syndrome patients. Invest Ophthalmol Vis Sci 2005;46:4474-9.

83. Cumming RG, Mitchell P, Smith W. Diet and cataract: the Blue Mountains Eye Study. Ophthalmology 2000;107:450-6.

84. Arnarsson A, Jonasson F, Sasaki H, et al. Risk factors for nuclear lens opacification: The Reykjavik Eye Study. Dev Opthalmol 2002;35:12-20.

85. Suzuki H, Morikawa Y, Takahashi H. Effect of DHA oil supplementation on intelligence and visual acuity in the elderly. World Rev Nutr Diet 2001;88:68-71.

86. Ren H, Magulike N, Ghebremeskel K, Crawford M. Primary open-angle glaucoma patients have reduced levels of blood docosahexaenoic and eicosapentaenoic acids. Prostaglandins Leukot Essent Fatty Acids 2006;74:157-63.

87. Sorokin EL, SMoliakova GP, Bachaldin IL. Clinical efficacy of eiconol in patients with diabetic retinopathy. Vestn Oftalmol 1997;113: 37-9.

88. Cho E, Hung S, Willett WC, et al. Prospective study of dietary fat and the risk of age-related macular degeneration. Am J Clin Nutr 2001;73:209-18.

89. Smith W, Mitchell P, Leeder SR. Dietary fat and fish intake and age-related macullopathy. Arch Ophthalmol 2000;118:401-4.

90. Chua B, Flood V, Rochtchina E, et al. Dietary fatty acids and the 5-year incidence of age-related maculopathy. Arch Ophthalmol 2006;124:981-986.

91. Seddon JM, Rosner B, Speduto RD, et al. Dietary fat and risk for advanced age-related macular degeneration. Arch Ophthalmol. 2001;119:1191-9.

92. Seddon JM, Cote J Rosner B. Progression of age-related macular degeneration: association with dietary fat, transunsaturated fat, nuts, and fish intake. Arch Ophthalmol 2003;121:1728-37.

93. Ouchi M, Ikeda T, Nakamura K, et al. A novel relation of fatty acid with age-related macular degeneration. Ophthalmologica 2002;216:363-7.

94. Pagliarini S, Moramarco A, Wormald RP, et al. Age-related macular disease in rural southern Italy. Arch Ophthalmol 1997;115:616-22.

95. Seddon JM, George S, Rosner B. Cigarette smoking, fish consumption, omega-3 fatty acid intake, and associations with age-related macular degeneration. The US twin study of age-related macular degeneration. Arch Ophthalmol 2006;124:995-1001.

96. Heuberger RA, Mares-Perlman JA, Klein R, et al. Relationship of dietary fat to age-related maculopathy in the Third National Health and Nutrition Examination Survey. Arch Ophthalmol 2001;119:1833-8.

97. Mares-Perlman JA, Brady WE, Klein R, et al. Dietary fat and age-related maculopathy. Arch Ophthalmol 1995;113:743-8.

98. Scorolli L, Scalinci SZ, Limoli PG, etr al. Photodynamic therapy for age related macular degeneration with and without antioxidants. Can J Opthalmol 2002;37:399-404.

99. Hoffman DR, Uauy R, Birch DG. Metabolism of omega-3 fatty acids in patients with autosomal dominant retinitis pigmentosa. Exp Eye Res 1995;60:279-89.

100. Hoffman DR, Locke KG, Wheaton DH, et al. A randomized, placebo-controlled clinical trial of docosahexaenoic acid supplementation for x-linked retinitis pigmentosa. Am J Ophthalmol 2004;137:704-18.

101. Berson EL, Rosner B, Sandberg MA, et al. Clinical trial of docosahexaenoic acid in patients with retinitis pigmentosa receiving vitamin A treatment. Arch Ophthalmol 2004;122:1297-1305.

102. Berson EL, Rosner B, Sandberg MA, et al. Further evaluation of docosahexaenoic acid in patients with retinitis pigmentosa receiving vitamin A treatment. Arch Ophthalmol 2004;122:1306-14.

103. Dagnelie G, Zorge IS, McDonald TM. Lutein improves visual function in some patients with retinal degeneration: a pilot study via the Internet. Optometry 2000;71:147-64.

104. Birch EE, Hoffman, DR, Uauy R, et al. Visual acuity and the essentiality of docosahexaenoic acid and arachidonic acid in the diet of term infants. Pediatr Res 1998;44:201-209.

105. Birch, EE, Castañeda YS, Wheaton DH, et al. Visual maturation of term infants fed long-chain polyunsaturated fatty acid-supplemented or control formula for 12 mo. Am J Clin Nutr 2005;81:871-9.

106. Hoffman DR, Birch EE, Castañeda YS, et al. Visual function in breast-fed term infants weaned to formula with or without long-chain polyunsaturates at 4 to 6 months: a randomized clinical trial. J Pediatr 2003;142:669-77.

107. Innis SM, Gilley J, Werker J. Are human milk long-chain polyunsaturated fatty acids related to visual and neural development in breast-fed term infants? J Pediatr 2001;139:532-8.

108. Jenson CL, Voigt RG, Prager TC, et al. Effects of maternal docosahexaenoic acid intake on visual function and neurodevelopment in breastfed term infants. Am J Clin Nutr 2005;82:125-32.

109. Austad N, Scott DT, Janowsky JS, et al. Visual, cognitive, and language assessments at 39 months: a follow-up study of children red formulas containing long-chain polyunsaturated fatty acids to 1 year of age. Pediatrics 2003;112:177-83.

110. Auestad N, Halter R, Hall RT, et al. Growth and development in term infants fed long-chain polyunsaturated fatty acids: a double-masked, randomized, parallel, prospective, multivariate study. Pediatrics 2001;108:372-81.

111. Auestad N, Montalto MB, Hall RT, et al. Visual acuity, erythrocyte fatty acid composition, and growth in term infants fed formulas with long chain polyunsaturated fatty acids for one year. Pediatr Res 1997;41:1-10.

112. Jensen CL, Prager TC, Fraley JK, et al. Effect of dietary linoleic/alpha-linolenic acid ratio on growth and visual function of term infants. J Pediatr 1997;131:173-5.

113. Makrides M, Neumann MA, Jeffrey B, et al. A randomized trial of different ratios of linoleic to alpha-linolenic acid in the diet of term infants: effects on visual function and growth. Am J Clin Nutr 2000;71:120-9.

114. O'Connor DL, Hall R, Adamkin D, et al. Growth and development in preterm infants fed long-chain polyunsaturated fatty acids: a

prospective, randomized controlled trial. Pediatrics 2001;108:359-71.

115. Carlson SE, Werkman SH, Rhodes PG, Tolley EA. Visual-acuity development in healthy preterm infants: effect of marine-oil supplementation. Am J Clin Nutr 1993;58:35-42.

116. Birch DG, Birch EE, Hoffman DR, Uauy RD. Retinal development in very-low-birth-weight infants fed diets differing in omega-3 fatty acids. Invest Ophthalmol Vis Sci 1992;33:2365-76.

117. Birch EE, Birch DG, Hoffman DR, Uauy. Dietary essential fatty acid supply and visual acuity development. Invest Ophthalmol Vis Sci 1992;33:3242-3253.

118. SanGiovanni JP, Parra-Cabrera S, Colditz GA, et al. Meta-analysis of dietary essential fatty acids and long-chain polyunsaturated fatty acids as they relate to visual resolution acuity in healthy preterm infants. Pediatrics 2000;105:1292-8.

119. Malcolm CA, Hamilton R, McCulloch DL, et al. Scotopic electroretinogram in term infants born of mothers supplemented with docosahexaenoic acid during pregnancy. Invest Ophthalmol Vis Sci 2003;44:3685-91.

120. Malcolm CA, McCulloch DL, Montgomery C, et al. Maternal docosahexaenoic acid supplementation during pregnancy and visual evoked potential development in term infants: a double blind, prospective, randomised trial. Arch Dis Child Fetal Neonatal Ed 2003;88:383-90.

121. Hayasaka S, Saito T, Nakajima H, et al. Clinical trials of vitamin B6 and proline supplementation for gyrate atrophy of the choroid and retina. Br J Ophthalmol. 1985;69:283-90

122. Tsang NC, Penfold PL, Snitch PJ, Billson F. Serum levels of antioxidants and age-related macular degeneration. Doc Ophthalmol 1992;81:387-400.

123. Knekt P, Heliovaara M, Rissanen A, et al. Serum antioxidant vitamins and risk of cataract. BMJ 1992;305:1392.

124. Lillico A, Jacobs B, Reid M, et al. Selenium supplementation and risk of glaucoma in the NPC trial selenium and cancer projects group. Rucson, AZ: Arizona Cancer Center, University of Arizona;2002.

125. Zhang M, Bi LF, Ai YD, et al. Effects of taurine supplementation on VDT work induced visual stress. Amino Acids 2004;26:59-63.

126. Morales-Pasantes H, Quiroz H, Quesada O. Treatment with taurine, diltiazem, and vitamin E retards the progressive visual field reduction in retinitis pigmentosa: a 3-year follow-up study. Metab Brain Dis 2002;17:183-97

127. Reccia R, Pignalosa B, Grasso A, Campanella G. Taurine treatment in retinitis pigmentosa. Acta Neurol 1980;2:132-6.

128. Patel S, Ferrier C, Plaskow J. Effect of systemic ingestion of vitamin and trace element dietary supplements on the stability of the pre-corneal tear film in normal subjects. Adv Exp Med Biol 1994;350:285-7.

129. Vetrugno M, Maino A, Cardia G, et al. A randomized, double masked, clinical trial of high dose vitamin A and vitamin E supplementation after photorefractive keratectomy. Br J Ophthalmol 2001;85:537-9.

130. Abboud IA, Hussman HG, Massoud WH. Vitamin A and chalazia. Exp Eye Res 1968;7:383-7.

131. Chatzinioff A, Nelson E, Stahl N, Clahane A. Eleven-CIS vitamin A in the treatment of retinitis pigmentosa. A negative study. Arch Ophthalmol

1968;80:417-9.
132. Berson EL, Rosner B, Sandberg M, et al. A randomized trial of vitamin A and vitamin E supplementation for retinitis pigmentosa. Arch Ophthalmol 1993;111:761-72.
133. Jacobson SG, Cideciyan Av, Regunath G, et al. Night blindness in Sorsby's fundus dystrophy reversed by vitamin A. Nat Genet 1995;11:27-32.
134. Goldberg J, Flowerdew G, Smith E, et al. Factors associated with age-related macular degeneration. An analysis of data from the first national health and nutrition examination survey. Am J Epidemiol 1988;128:700-10.
135. Delcourt C, Cristol JP, Tessier F, et al. Age-related macular degeneration and antioxidant status in the POLA study. POLA Study Group. Pathologies Oculaires Liees a l'Age. Arch Ophthalmol 1999;117:1384-90.
136. Blumenkranz MS, Russell SR, Robey MG, et al. Risk factors in age-related maculopathy complicated by choroidal neovascularization. Ophthalmology 1986;96:552-8.
137. Simon JA, Hudes ES. Serum ascorbic acid and other correlates of self-reported cataract among older Americans. Clin Epidemiol 1999;52:1207.
138. Chasan-Taber L, Willett WC, Seddon JM, et al. A prospective study of vitamin supplement intake and cataract extraction among US women. Epidemiology 1999;10:679.
139. Krepler K, Schmid R. Alpha-tocopherol in plasma, red blood cells and lenses with and without cataract. Am J Ophthalmol 2005;139:266-70.
140. Christian P, Khatry SK, Yamini S, et al. Zinc supplementation might potentiate the effect of vitamin A in restoring night vision in pregnant Nepalese women. Am J Clin Nutr 2001;73: 1045-51.
141. Asregadoo ER. Blood levels of thiamine and ascorbic acid in chronic open-angle glaucoma. Ann Ophthalmol 1979;11:1095-1100.
142. Williamson J. Lipotriad therapy in senile macular degeneration. Trans Ophthalmol Soc U K 1964;84:713-24.
143. Brown CA. Lipotriad. A double-blind clinical trial. Trans Ophthalmol Soc U K 1974;94:578-82.
144. Ellis JM, Folkers K, Minadeo M, et al. A deficiency of vitamin B6 is a plausible molecular basis of the retinopathy of patients with diabetes mellitus. Biochem Biophys Res Commun 1991;179:615-9.
145. Azumi I, Kosaki H, Nakatani H. Effects of metcobolamin (Methycobal) on the visual field of chronic glaucoma—a multicenter open study. Folia Ophthalmol Jpn 1983;34:873-8.
146. Saki T, Murata M, Amemiya T. Effect of long-term treatment of glaucoma with vitamin B-12. Glaucoma 1992;14:167-70.
147. Patel S, Plaskow J, Ferrier C. The influence of vitamins and trace element supplements on the stability of the pre-corneal tear film. Acta Ophthalmol 1993;71:825-9.
148. Peponis V, Bonovas, S, Kapranou A, et al. Conjunctival and tear film changes after vitamin C and E administration in non-insulin dependent diabetes mellitus. Med Sci Monit 2004;10:CR213-7
149. Millen AE, Gruber M, Klein R, et al. Relations of serum ascorbic acid and alpha-tocopherol to diabetic retinopathy in the third national health and nutrition examination survey. Am J Epidemiol 2003;158:225-33.

150. Christen WG, Ajani UA, Glynn RJ, et al. Prospective cohort study of antioxidant vitamin supplement use and the risk of age-related maculopathy. Am J Epidemiol 1999;149:476-84.
151. Vitale S, West S, Hallfrisch J, et al. Plasma antioxidants and risk of cortical and nuclear cataract. Epidemiology 1993;4:195-203.
152. The Italian-American Cataract Study Group. Risk factors for age-related cortical, nuclear and posterior subcapsular cataracts. Am J Epidemiol 1991;133:541-53.
153. Robertson JM, Donner AP, Trevithick JR. Vitamin E intake and risk of cataracts in humans. Ann N Y Acad Sci 1989;570:372-82.
154. Jacques PF, Chylack LT Jr, Taylor A. Relationships between natural antioxidants and cataract formation. In: Frei B, ed. Natural antioxidants human health and disease. Orlando, FL: Academic Press, 1994:513.
155. Maresa-Perlman JA, Lyle BJ, Klein R, et al. Vitamin supplement use and incident cataracts in a population-based study. Arch Ophthalmol 2000;118:1556-1563.
156. Mares-Perlman JA, Lyle BJ, Klein R, et al. Vitamin supplement use and incident cataracts in a population-based study (in process citation). Arch Ophthalmol 2000;118:1556-63.
157. Seddon JM, Christen WG, Manson JE, et al. The use of vitamin supplements and the risk of cataract among US male physicians. Am J Public Health 1994;84:788-92.
158. Birich TV, Birich TA, Marchenko LN. Vitamin E in multiple-modality treatment of primary glaucoma patients. Vestn Oftalmol 1984;102:10-3.
159. Johnson L, Schaffer D, Quinn G, et al. Vitamin E supplementation and the retinopathy of prematurity. Ann N Y Acad Sci 1982;393:473-95.
160. Schaffer DB, Johnson L, Quinn GE, et al. Vitamin E and retinopathy of prematurity. Follow-up at one year. Ophthalmology 1985;92:1005-11.
161. Finer NN, Schindler RF, Peters KL, Grant GD. Vitamin E and retrolental fibroplasia. Improved visual outcome with early vitamin E. Ophthalmology 1983;90:428-35.
162. Schaffer DB, Johnson L, Quinn GE, et al. Vitamin E and retinopathy of prematurity: the ophthalmologist's perspective. Birth Defects Orig Artic Ser 1988;24:219-35.
163. Quinn GE, Johnson L, Otis C, et al. Incidence, severity and time course of ROP in a randomized clinical trial of vitamin E prophylaxis. Doc Ophthalmol 1990;74:223-8.
164. Phelps DL, Rosenbaum AL, Isenberg SJ, et al. Tocopherol efficacy and safety for preventing retinopathy of prematurity: a randomized controlled, double-masked trial. Pediatrics 1987;79: 489-500.
165. Bursell SE, Clermont AC, Aiello LP, et al. High-dose vitamin E supplementation normalizes retinal blood flow and creatinine clearance in patients with type 1 diabetes. Diabetes Care 1999;22:1245-51.
166. Nussenblatt RB, Kim J, Thompson DJ, et al. Vitamin E in the treatment of uveitis-associated macular edema. Am J Ophthalmol 2006;141:193-4.
167. Belda JI, Romá J, Vilela C, et al. Serum vitamin E levels negatively correlate with severity of age-related macular degeneration. Mech Ageing Dev 1999;107:159-64.

168. Belda JI, Romá J, Vilela C, et al. Serum vitamin E levels negatively correlate with severity of age-related macular degeneration. Mech Ageing Dev 1999;107:159-64.
169. Taylor HR, Tikellis G, Robman LD, et al. Vitamin E supplementation and macular degeneration: randomized controlled trial. BMJ 2002;325:11.
170. Leske MC, Chylack LT Jr, He Q, et al. Antioxidant vitamins and nuclear opacities the longitudinal study of cataract. Ophthalmology 1998;105:831.
171. Nadalin G, Robman LD, McCarty CA, et al. The role of past intake of vitamin E in early cataract changes. Ophthalmic Epidemiol 1999;6:105-12.
172. Rouhiainen P, Rouhiainen H, Salonen JT. Association between low plasma vitamin E concentration and progression of early cortical lens opacities. Am J Epidemiol 1996;144:496.
173. McNeil JJ, Robman L, Tikellis G, et al. Vitamin E supplementation and cataract ran: randomized controlled trial. Ophthalmology 2004;111:75-84.
174. Karcioglu ZA, Stout R, Hahn HJ. Serum zinc levels in retinitis pigmentosa. Curr Eye Res 1984;3:1043-8.
175. Gahlot DK, Khosla PK, Makashir PD, et al. Copper metabolism in retinitis pigmentosa. Br J Ophthalmol 1976;60:770-4.
176. Ehlers N, Bulow N. Clinical copper metabolism parameters in patients with retinitis pigmentosa and other tapeto-retinal degenerations. Br J Ophthalmol 1977;61:595-6.
177. Marmor MF, Nelson JW, Levin AS. Copper metabolism in American retinitis pigmentosa patients. Br J Ophthalmol 1978;62:168-71.
178. Rao SS, Satapathy M, Sitaramayya A. Copper metabolism in retinitis pigmentosa patients. Br J Ophthalmol 1981;65:127-30.
179. Mares-Perlman A, Klein R, Klein BE, et al. Association of zinc and antioxidant nutrients with age-related maculopathy. Arch Ophthalmol 1996;114:991-7.
180. Cho E, Stampfer MJ, Seddon JM, et al. Prospective study of zinc intake and the risk of age-related macular degeneration. Ann Epidemiol 2001;11:328-36.
181. Stur M, Tittl M, Reitner A, Meisinger V. Oral zinc and the second eye in age-related macular degeneration. Invest Opthalmol Vis Sci 1996;37:1225-35.
182. Newsome DA, Swartz M, Leone NC, et al. Oral zinc in macular degeneration. Arch Ophthalmol 1988;106:192-8.